Neuroendocrine Correlates of Stress

BIOCHEMICAL ENDOCRINOLOGY

Series Editor: Kenneth W. McKerns

STRUCTURE AND FUNCTION OF THE GONADOTROPINS
Edited by Kenneth W. McKerns

SYNTHESIS AND RELEASE OF ADENOHYPOPHYSEAL HORMONES
Edited by Marian Jutisz and Kenneth W. McKerns

REPRODUCTIVE PROCESSES AND CONTRACEPTION
Edited by KennethW. McKerns

HORMONALLY ACTIVE BRAIN PEPTIDES: Structure and Function
Edited by Kenneth W. McKerns and Vladimir Pantić

REGULATION OF GENE EXPRESSION BY HORMONES
Edited by Kenneth W. McKerns

REGULATION OF TARGET CELL RESPONSIVENESS, Volumes 1 and 2
Edited by Kenneth W. McKerns, Asbjørn Aakvaag, and Vidar Hansson

HORMONAL CONTROL OF THE HYPOTHALAMO-PITUITARY-GONADAL AXIS
Edited by Kenneth W. McKerns and Zvi Naor

NEUROENDOCRINE CORRELATES OF STRESS
Edited by Kenneth W. McKerns and Vladimir Pantić

Neuroendocrine Correlates of Stress

Edited by

Kenneth W. McKerns

The International Foundation for Biochemical Endocrinology
Blue Hill Falls, Maine

and

Vladimir Pantić

Institute for Biological Research
Belgrade, Yugoslavia

PLENUM PRESS • NEW YORK AND LONDON

Library of Congress Cataloging in Publication Data

Neuroendocrine Aspects of Stress (1984: Cavtat, Croatia)
Neuroendocrine correlates of stress.

(Biochemical endocrinology)
"Proceedings of an international symposium entitled Neuroendocrine Aspects of Stress, held Sept. 9-15, 1984, in Cavtat, Yugoslavia"—T.p. verso.
Bibliography: p.
Includes index.
1. Stress (Physiology)—Congresses. 2. Neuroendocrinology—Congresses. 3. Hypothalamo-hypophyseal system—Congresses. I. McKerns, Kenneth W. II. Pantić, Vladimir. III. Title. IV. Series.
QP82.2.S8N48 1984 612′.4 85-12162
ISBN 0-306-42072-4

Proceedings of an international symposium entitled Neuroendocrine Aspects of Stress, held September 9–15, 1984, in Cavtat, Yugoslavia

A Division of Plenum Publishing Corporation
233 Spring Street, New York, N.Y. 10013

Printed in the United States of America

PREFACE

The beautiful town of Cavtat near Dubvronic, Yugoslavia was the site of the twelfth meeting of the International Foundation for Biochemical Endocrinology. It was sponsored by the Serbian Academy for Sciences and Arts and by the Foundation.

The Croatia Hotel in Cavtat was a splendid place for a meeting. The presentation of the subject matter relating to "Neuroendocrine Correlates of Stress" was interesting and informative. The topics included many forms of stress, their mediators and responses. They included: releasing factors; neurotransmitters in the hypothalamus; role of noradrenaline; the reaction of the hypothalamo-pituitary-adrenocortical axis to stress; immunological stress; thermal stress; immobilization stress; peptides in shock; stress-induced prolactin; stress and acupuncture; stress and behavior; spinal cord transection and stress; electroconvulsive stress; neuroendocrine cells and stress; protein kinase as a signal transducer; the effects of constant light and darkness on the pineal; sleep, stress and ovarian function; and finally, hormonal response to exercise.

Subsequently, the papers presented were rewritten for inclusion in this monograph.

The Chairmen for the sessions at Cavtat were K. McKerns and Stefan Manolov, V. Chong-Li and L. Rakič, S. Feldman and R. Milin, M. Lee and V. Liposits.

The next meeting of the Foundation will be held in Edinburgh near the end of September, 1985. The topic will be "Neuroendocrine Molecular Biology" with Professor George Fink as Honorary Chairman of the local organizing committee.

Kenneth W. McKerns
Vladimir Pantić

ACKNOWLEDGMENTS

The editors thank the organizing committee of the meeting at Cavtat, consisting of: Vladimir Pantić as Chairman; with Radoslav K. Anđus, Borislav Božović, Radivoj Milin, Vojislav Petrović, Ljubisav Racić and Dušan Gledić.

The Foundation is grateful for the financial support provided by the Serbian Academy. The American Cyanimid Company provided travel support for one participant.

The Foundation is indebted to Prof. Dr. Dušan Kanazir, the President of the Serbian Academy for continued interest and help.

CONTENTS

THE PARAVENTRICULO-INFUNDIBULAR CORTICOTROPIN RELEASING FACTOR (CRF)-IMMUNOREACTIVE SYSTEM OF THE RAT - I. MORPHOLOGICAL ASPECTS

Zsolt Liposits, István Lengvári, Sándor Vigh, Tamás Görcs, György Sétáló, and Béla Flerkó

Department of Anatomy, University Medical School Pécs, Hungary

INTRODUCTION

The hormone production of the anterior pituitary is influenced by neurosecretory materials produced in neurons of the prosencephalon (Szentágothai et al., 1962). The bioactive substances released from nerve endings of the median eminence and the pituitary stalk are taken up by hypophyseal portal vessels, which distribute them to the pars distalis of the pituitary gland (Harris, 1955). The stimulatory effect of diencephalic extracts upon the hormone secretion of adrenocorticotroph cells (Guillemin and Rosenberg, 1955; Saffran and Schally, 1955) proved the existence of corticotropin releasing factor (CRF). In the last three decades, several substances were proposed to be CRF's or at least modulators of the adrenocorticotroph hormone (ACTH) releasing substance (for review see Saffran and Schally, 1977; Yasuda et al., 1982). Vale et al. (1981) have rencently reported the isolation of a 41-amino acid peptide from ovine hypothalamic tissue, with potent activity to stimulate the secretion of ACTH and beta-endorphin. The synthetic CRF has also been demonstrated to cause a dose related release of pituitary ACTH and beta-endorphin both in vitro and in vivo (Rivier et al., 1982; Spiess et al., 1981; Turkelson et al., 1981). The availability of synthetic CRF has allowed the generation of antibodies for radioimmunoassay (RIA) quantitation and immunomorphological analysis of CRF-containing structures (Moldow and Fischman, 1982a; Vigh et al., 1982b).

The present study was focused on the morphology of

the paraventriculo-infundibular CRF-system of the rat, as the main neuronal circuit transporting CRF to the hypophyseal portal vessels.

For the detection of hormone containing structures the peroxidase-anti-peroxidase complex (PAP) method (Sternberger, 1979) and its modified silver-gold-post-intensified form (Liposits et al., 1983b) were used, both at light and electron microscopic levels. The generation and characterization of the primary antibody (SV-22, raised against synthetic ovine CRF coupled to bovine serum albumin) has already been published (Merchenthaler et al., 1982; Vigh et al., 1982a).

DISTRIBUTION OF CRF-IMMUNOREACTIVE STRUCTURES IN EXTRA-HYPOTHALAMIC BRAIN REGIONS

Fischman and Moldow (1982) measured the CRF-immunoreactivity of extrahypothalamic brain areas in normal adult rats - by RIA - and found a very wide distribution throughout the neuroaxis.

Immunohistological studies - carried out on colchicine pretreated rat brains - also revealed the presence of CRF-immunoreactive neurons and fibers in many regions of the brain (Merchenthaler et al., 1982, 1984a, b; Olschowka et al., 1982; Swanson et al., 1983). In the telencephalon, most of the CRF-neurons are located in the nucleus accumbens (Fig. 1b), the bed nucleus of the stria terminalis and the central amygdaloid nucleus. The olfactory bulb (Fig. 1a), cortical mantle and hippocampal formation also contain a moderate number of CRF-cells. The central tegmental area, the periaqueductal central gray (Fig. 1e) and the dorsal raphe region are the CRF-immunopositive parts of the mesencephalon. In the metencephalon the locus coeruleus, the dorsal and ventral parabrachial nuclei and the laterodorsal tegmental nucleus are involved in CRF production. In the myelencephalon, the medial vestibular nucleus (Fig. 1f), the nucleus of the solitary tract and the reticular nucleus showed immunoreaction. CRF-containing perikarya were observed in laminae V-VII, X and sympathetic intermediolateral column of the spinal cord after colchicine administration (Merchenthaler et al., 1983b). Many of the above mentioned areas belong to the limbic system and take part in the mediation of autonomic responses. The presence of CRF in these structures suggests that the neurohormone beyond the regulation of the hypophyseal adrenal axis may also act as a neuromodulator. The finding that exogenously administrated CRF acts directly on hippocampal, hypothalamic (Vale et al., 1983)

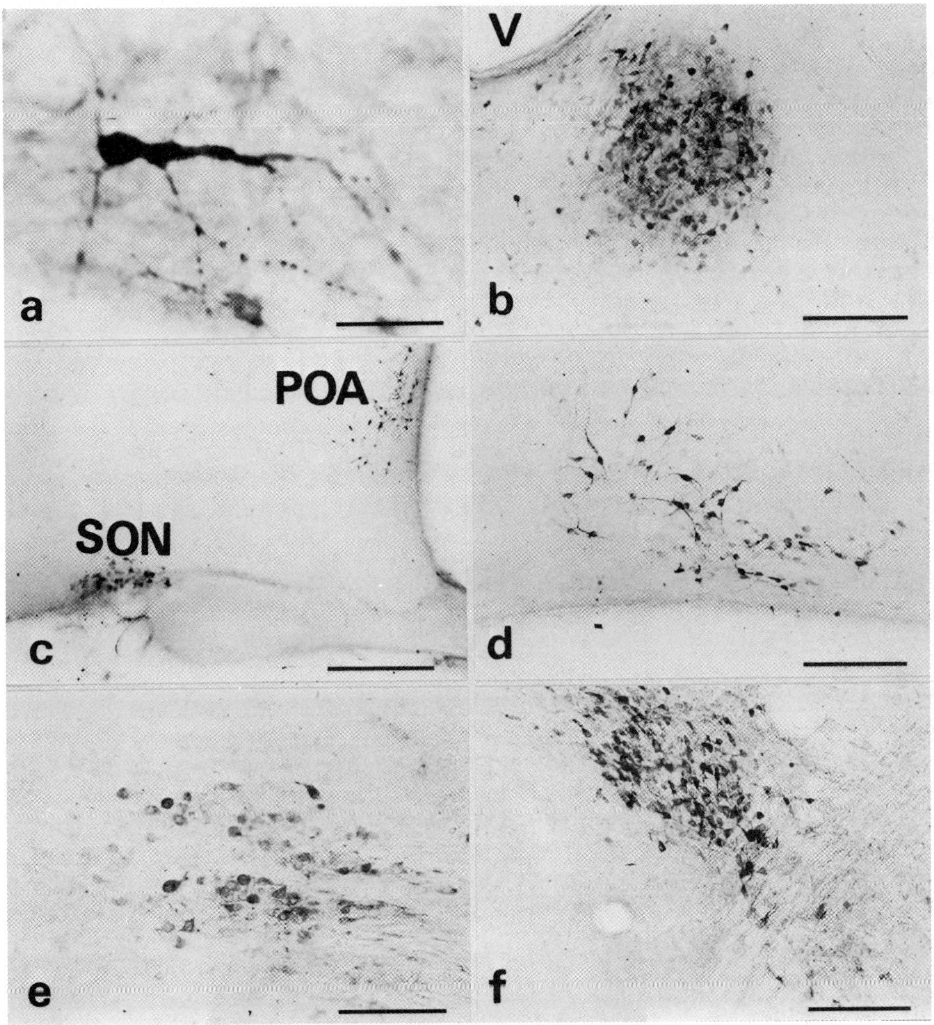

Fig. 1. Different brain regions of cholchicin treated male rats, exhibiting CRF-immunoreactivity. (a) Multipolar CRF-neuron in the olfactory bulb. Bar: 50 µm. (b) Immunolabeled cells in the nucleus accumbens. V: pars centralis ventriculi lateralis. Bar: 200 µm. (c) CRF-containing neurons in the supraoptic nucleus (SON) and medial pre-optic area (POA). Bar: 500 µm. (d) CRF-neurons of the preoptic area, shown in Fig.c, with higher power. Bar: 200 µm. (e) CRF-perikarya in the central gray of the mesencephalon. Bar: 200 µm. (f) Immunolabeled cells population in the medial vestibular nucleus. Bar: 200 µm.

and mesencephalic neurons (Sirinathsinghji et al., 1983) further supports the extrahypophysiotrophic, neuroregulatory function of CRF. The different CRF-cell groups of the brain are interconnected by immunoreactive fibers (Swanson et al., 1983), indicating that the local CRF-immunoreactive neuronal circuits might function in an integrated manner. The elevated catecholamine levels (Brown et al., 1982) and increased discharge rates of locus coeruleus neurons (Valentino et al., 1983) observed after intraventricular administration of CRF are indicative of the relationship between CRF and the sympathetic nervous system.

DISTRIBUTION OF CRF NEURONS IN THE DIENCEPHALON

The majority of the diencephalic CRF-neurons are located in the parvocellular subnuclei of the paraventricular nucleus (PVN; Fig. 2a). A small number of CRF-neurons are also present in the magnocellular division of the nucleus, which part is primarily involved in the synthesis of oxytocin, vasopressin and neurophysins. The medial preoptic area (Figs. 1c, d) and the supraoptic nuclei (Fig. 1c) are also sites of CRF production. Scattered cells were observed in the periventricular, dorsomedial, mammillary nuclei, the anterior hypothalamic area and the lateral basal hypothalamic region.

Before the immunohistological labelling of CRF-immunoreactive structures became possible Makara and colleagues proved - by the use of CRF bioassay - that fibers transporting CRF to the portal vessels originate in, or pass through, the paraventricular nucleus (PVN) and enter the basal hypothalamus via the retrochiasmatic area (Makara et al., 1981, 1982). The first immunohistological observations (Bloom et al., 1982; Bugnon et al., 1982; Kawata et al., 1982; Merchenthaler et al., 1982; Olschowka et al., 1982; Vigh et al., 1982b) confirmed this concept. Thus, from neuroendocrinological viewpoint the hypothalamic CRF-system became the focus of interest.

LIGHT MICROSCOPIC MORPHOLOGY OF THE PARAVENTRICULO-INFUNDIBULAR CRF-SYSTEM

In the paraventricular nuclei CRF is manufactured in multipolar and fusiform neurons. In the latter group, the CRF perikarya exhibit either smooth, or rough surface contour (Liposits et al., 1983b). Similar types of fusiform neurons, with luteinizing hormone-releasing

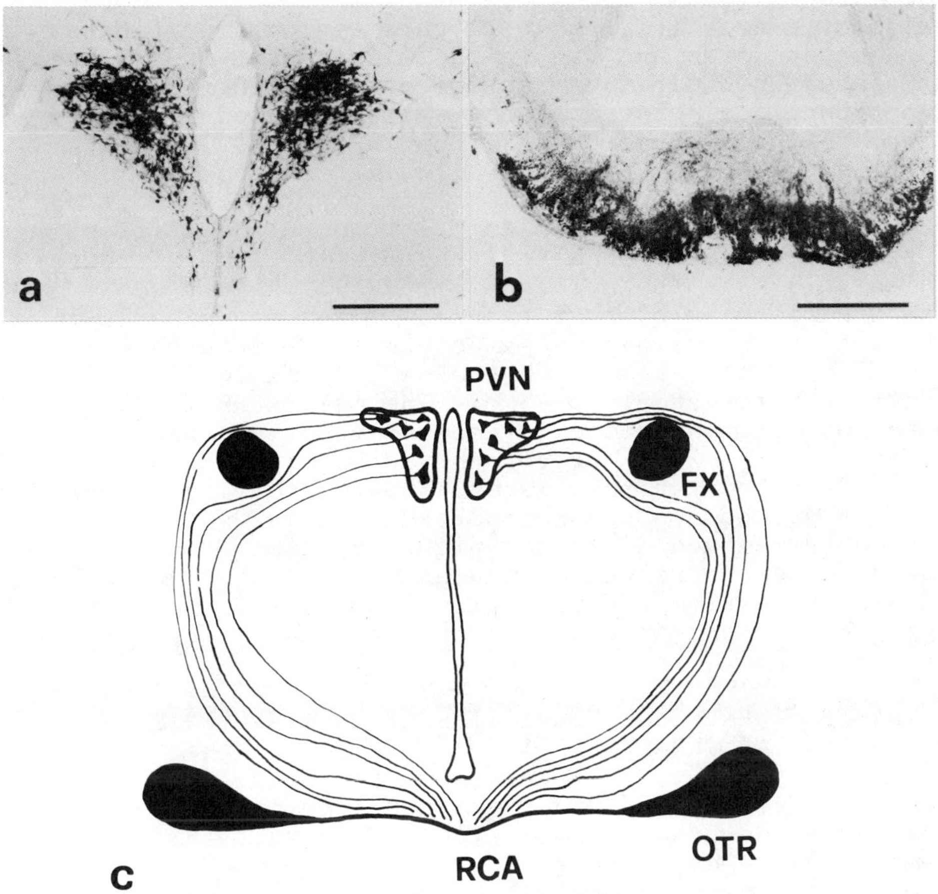

Fig. 2. The paraventriculo-infundibular CRF-system. (a) CRF-neurons located in the medial, parvocellular part of the paraventricular nucleus. Bar: 200 µm. (b) CRF-immunoreactive fibers in the median eminence. The majority of the immunolabeled axons occupy the external zone. Bar: 200 µm. Schematic drawing of the paraventriculo infundibular CRF-fiber projection. Fx: fornix, OTR: optic tract, PVN: paraventricular nucleus, RCA: retrochiasmatic area. (Figs. 2a, b are by courtesy of Dr. Merchenthaler.)

hormone (LH-RH)-content were observed in the preoptic region of the rat brain (Liposits et al., 1984). The axons of the paraventricular CRF-neurons flow out at the lateral side of the nucleus and forming an arc in the coronal plane reach the basal part of the retrochiasmatic area (Fig. 2c). In this region, the fibers turn caudalwards and run in the middle part of the median eminence. This fiber projection can be visualized in hyperfunctional states of the system, caused by adrenalectomy or hypophysectomy (Merchenthaler et al., 1983a; Paull and Gibbs, 1983) and following surgical lesion of the retrochiasmatic area (Liposits et al., 1983b). The majority of the paraventriculo-infundibular CRF-fibers enter the basal hypothalamus through the lateral retrochiasmatic gate (Antoni et al., 1983), while a substantial portion of them traverse first caudalwards in the lateral basal hypothalamus, thereafter turn to medial direction and reach the median eminence (Merchenthaler et al., 1984b). The CRF-fibers occupy both the internal and external layers of the median eminence (Fig. 2b), however the majority of them are located in the external layer. The terminals draw the contour of the hypophyseal portal vessels, which penetrate the median eminence. In the pituitary stalk the immunoreaction is restricted to the external zone. The number of CRF fibers in the posterior pituitary is low. The intermediate and anterior lobes are free of CRF-terminals.

ULTRASTRUCTURAL CHARACTERISTICS OF THE PARAVENTRICULO-INFUNDIBULAR CRF-SYSTEM

We have studied the fine structure of CRF neurons in colchicine treated rat (Liposits et al., 1983a, b) in order to elucidate the morphological signs of the hormone production and the termination of CRF-axons in the median eminence.

The centrally located nuclei of the cells are frequently indented. The immunolabel is bound to free ribosomes and rough endoplasmic reticulum, indicating the participation of these organelles in the synthesis of CRF (Fig. 3). The Golgi-apparatus, in which packaging of the hormone takes place did not show immunoreactivity (Fig. 3). The neurosecretory granules, budding from the Golgi rings are in 80-120 nm in diameter. Unlabeled axon terminals established synaptic connections with CRF-perikarya (Figs. 4a, d) and dendrites (Fig. 4b). The majority of the observed synapses belonged to the asymmetric type. In special form of the axo-somatic connection, the preterminal axon is deeply indented into the cytoplasm of the CRF-neuron, where it forms asymmetric type of synapse (Figs. 4c, d). According to the hypothesis of Léránth et al. (1983) CRF-neurons receive neuronal input from the magnocellular division

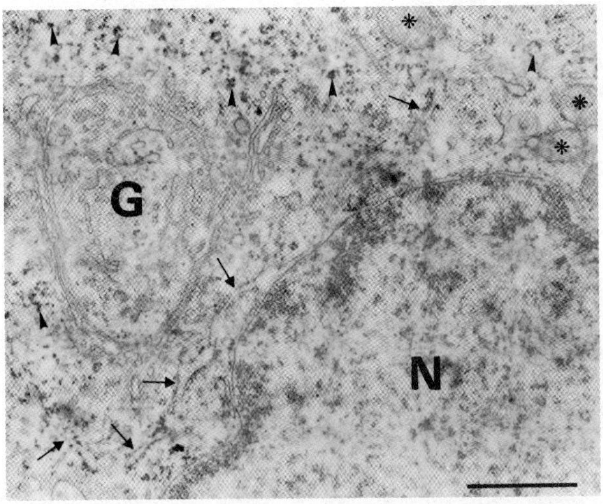

Fig. 3. Detail from a CRF-producing neuron of the paraventricular nucleus. The diaminobenzidine chromogen is bound to free ribosomes (arrowheads) and rough endoplasmic reticulum (arrows). The Golgi ring (G), nucleus (N) and mitochondria (asterisks) are non-reactive. Bar: 1 µm.

of the paraventricular nucleus via such synaptic connections.

We have observed synaptic bouton on the surface of infolding preterminal axon (Fig. 4c). This finding suggests, that the presynaptic element of the encompassed synapse is regulated - at least partly - via axo-axonic synapses, which presumably mediate inhibitory influence.

In CRF-axons reaching the median eminence the immunolabel is attached to neurosecretory granules and small electron lucent vesicles. The CRF terminals appear in the vicinity of the pericapillary space. Ependymal endings may separate the CRF-endings from the external limiting membrane (Fig. 5a), but most of the terminals lie directly on the membrane (Fig. 5b). Thus, the released neurohormone can rapidly be taken up by the capillary vessels.

The structure of CRF-fibers observed in the neurohypophysis was similar to those of the median eminence. The CRF-terminals, filled with neurosecretory granules (80-120 nm in diameter) and clear vesicles, located either directly on the external limiting membrane of

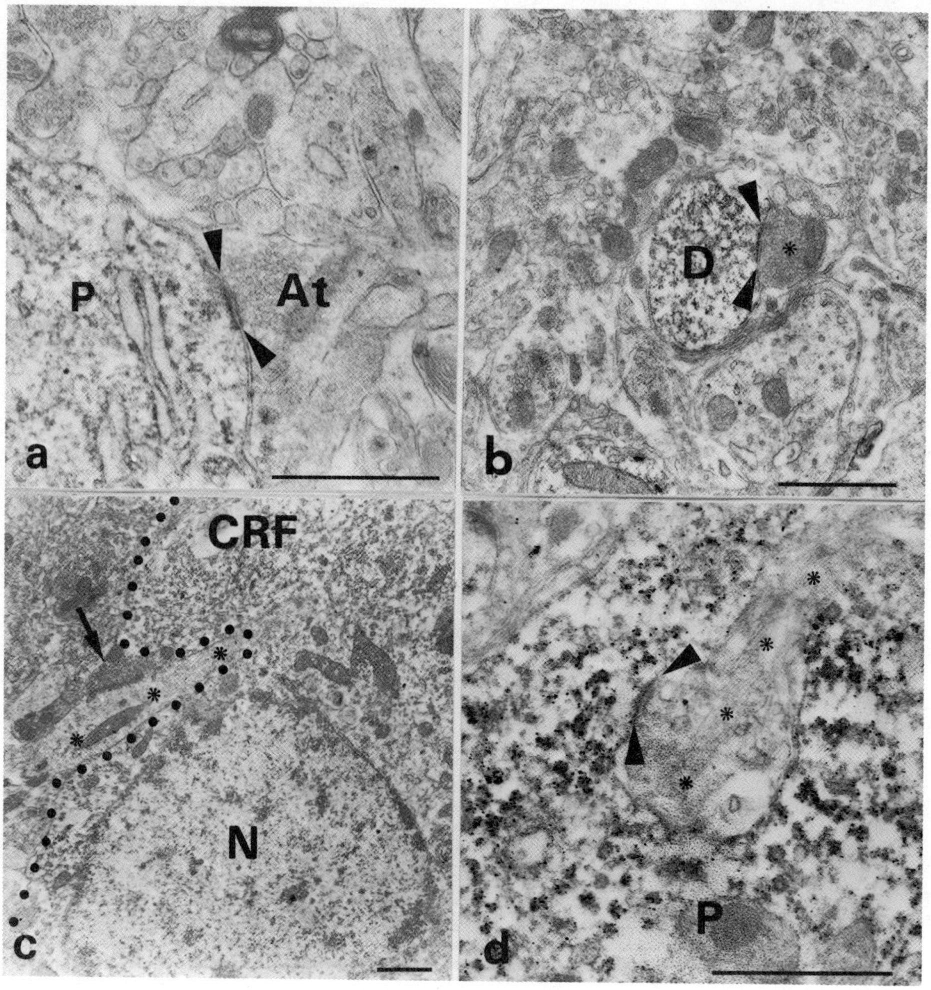

Fig. 4. Synaptic connections of CRF-neurons located in the paraventricular nucleus. (a) Axo-somatic synapse of asymmetric type. Arrowheads indicate the synaptic specialization. P: CRF-perikaryon, At: axon terminal. Bar: 1 µm. (b) Small bouton (asterisk) synapses on CRF dendrite (D). Arrowheads point to synaptic specialization. Bar: 1 µm (c) Axon (asterisks) being deeply indented into the cytoplasm of a CRF neuron (CRF). Note the axon terminal (arrow) on the surface of the preterminal axon. The cell border is labeled by dotted-line. N: nucleus. Bar: 1 µm. (d) Similar morphological arrangement, as shown in Fig. c. The synapse(arrowheads) is encompassed by the CRF perikaryon. Asterisks indicate the terminal. Bar: 1 µm.

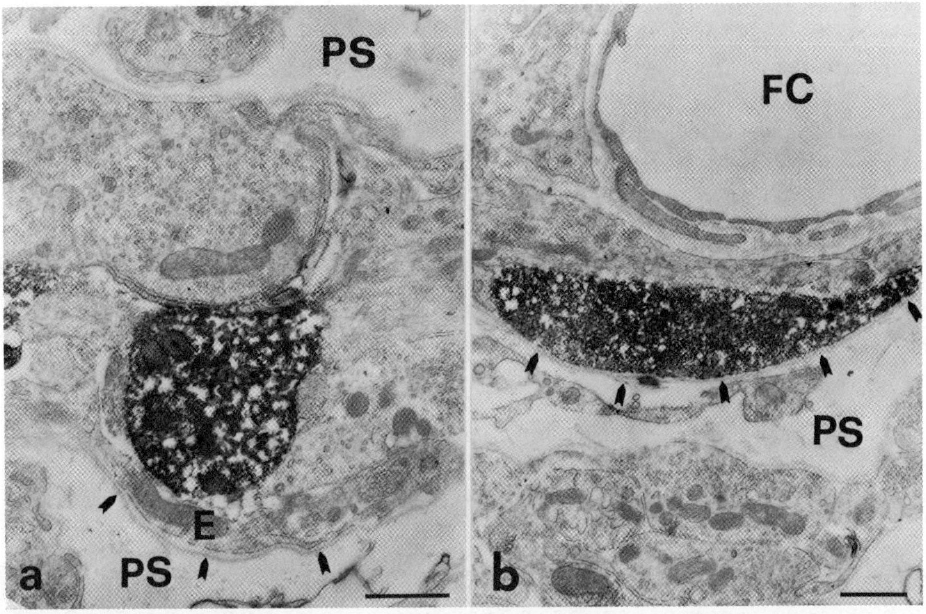

Fig. 5. CRF-immunoreactive axons terminating in the external layer of the median eminence. PS: pericapillary space, FC: fenestrated portal capillary. (a) Ependymal ending (E) separates the CRF terminal from the external limiting membrane (arrowheads). Bar: 1 μm. (b) Neuro-hemal junction established by a CRF terminal on the external limiting membrane (arrowheads). Bar: 1 μm.

the blood vessels or were separated from it by thin processes of pituicytes (Lengvári et al., 1984). In the above mentioned terminal fields, we have not observed any morphological signs referring to synaptoid contacts of CRF-fibers and other neural elements.

In order to see whether the paraventricular region is the only source of the hypophysiotrophic CRF, or other diencephalic CRF-cell populations also project to the median eminence, we detected the changes of CRF-immunoreactivity in the median eminence-pituitary stalk-posterior pituitary unit after the ablation of the paraventricular nuclei (Liposits et al., 1983b;

Lengvári et al., 1984). Since CRF-neurons located in the dorso-lateral part of PVN expand the border of the nucleus and reach the fornices, it seemed necessary to increase the lateral extension of the lesion up to 1,5 mm from the midline. In such cases the lesion destroyed, beside the PVN, also the periventricular nucleus, the perifornical region and partly the dorsomedial nuclei. The bilateral surgical destruction of the extended paraventricular region, resulted in a gradual decrease of CRF-immunoreactivity from the median eminence-pituitary stalk-posterior pituitary unit. Following the second postoperative week, the CRF-immunoreactivity practically disappeared from this area. The degenerating CRF fibers were also traced at ultrastructural level (Liposits et al., 1983b). From these studies we concluded that the CRF-innervation of the infundibular region originates from neurons of the paraventricular nucleus and scattered CRF-cells located in the periventricular, perifornical region and the dorsomedial nucleus. The paraventriculo-infundibular projection is mainly ipsilateral, only a narrow zone in the middle part of the median eminence receives fibers from the contralateral nucleus. After bilateral lesion of the paraventricular nuclei, Bruhn and colleagues observed, that the CRF-immunoreactivity of the stalk-median eminence unit (SME) was reduced by 87-90 % (from 2 ng/SME to 0,27 ng/SME), and the ACTH response to ether stress was greatly attenuated (Bruhn et al., 1984). Concerning the other CRF cell groups of the diencephalon, the immunolabeled cells of the mammillary body project to the thalamus via the mammillo-thalamic tract (Kovács et al., 1984), while the role of the supraoptic CRF remains to be determined.

EFFECT OF ADRENALECTOMY ON THE ULTRASTRUCTURE OF THE PARAVENTRICULO-INFUNDIBULAR CRF-SYSTEM

After elimination of the negative corticosteroid feedback upon the brain and the hypophysis (Russel et al., 1969; Yates et al., 1971) - by either hypophysectomy or adrenalectomy, the paraventriculo-infundibular CRF-system became detectable without colchicine pretreatment (Merchenthaler et al., 1983a; Paull and Gibbs, 1983). Moldow and Fischman (1982b) observed a slight decrease in the hypothalamic CRF-content one week after adrenalectomy or hypophysectomy, followed by an enormous increase during the second postoperative week.

In our material, we found intensely labeled CRF-neurons at the end of the first postoperative week. The most conspicuous phenomenon of these cells was the

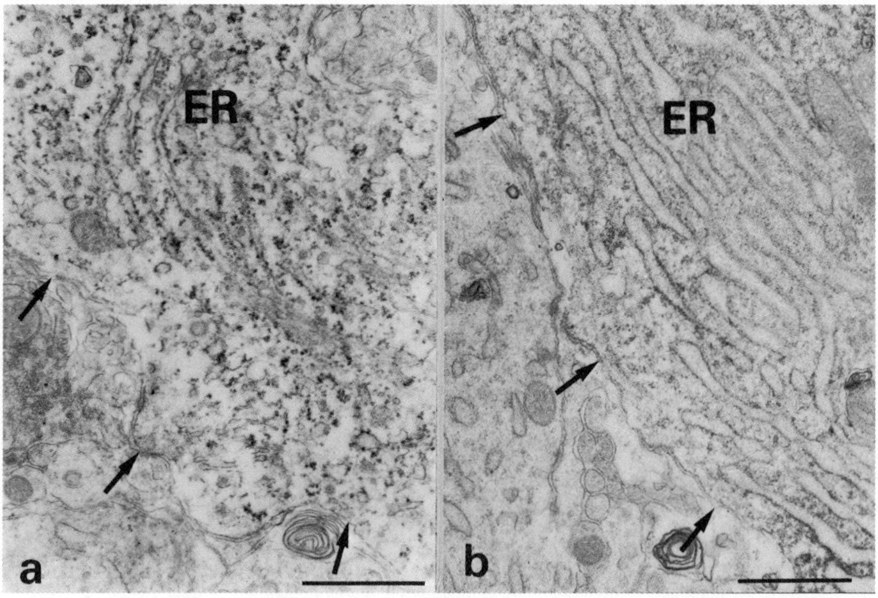

Fig. 6. Details from the cytoplasm of CRF-perikarya (arrows). ER: rough endoplasmic reticulum. (a) Colchicin pretreated animal. Bar: 1 µm. (b) Adrenalectomized rat, survived one week. Note the hypertrophy of the endoplasmic reticulum and the marked dilatation of its cisternae. Bar: 1 µm.

hypertrophy of the rough endoplasmic reticulum (Fig. 6b). The cisternae of the ergastoplasm showed dilatation compared to similar organelles of CRF-cells obtained from colchicine treated rats (Fig. 6a). This means, that the paraventricular CRF-neurons - liberated from the suppression of corticosteroids - are going to synthesize the hormone at an increased rate. As a consequence of the elevated hormone content of the CRF-axons, the paraventriculo-infundibular CRF-fiber loop became detectable. More CRF fibers were observed in the median eminence, especially in its internal zone. The presence of small CRF-fiber bundles traversing perpendicularly the median eminence is characteristic for the hyper-functional system. These fibers run paralelly with the processes of tanycyte cells (Fig. 7a). The tanycyte processes were not immunoreactive, indicating that the ventriculo-portal transport mechanism - in case of CRF - can be excluded. The CRF-terminals contact directly the

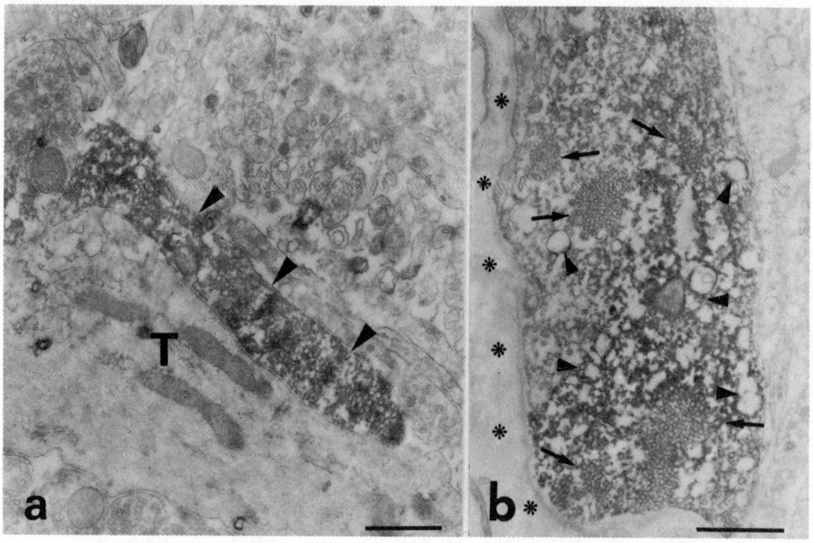

Fig. 7. CRF-containing axons in the median eminence of adrenalectomized rats. One week of survival. (a) Longitudinally sectioned CRF-fiber (arrowheads) in the neighbourhood of a tanycyte process (T). Bar: 1 µm. (b) Dilated CRF-terminal lying directly on the external limiting membrane. The profile contains many small electron-lucent vesicles, showing cluster formation (arrows) and vacuoles of different size (arrowheads). Asterisks label the pericapillary space. Bar: 1 µm.

external limiting membmrane in the palisadic layer of the median eminence of adrenalectomized rats. The axoplasm is filled with clusters of synaptic vesicles and vacuoles (Fig. 7b). The number of neurosecretory granules decreased. Between the vesicular elements, tubular structures resembling to constituents of the smooth endoplasmic reticulum were recognized. It may be hypothesized, that under hyperfunctional conditions, extragranular hormone transport mechanism exists also in CRF-neurons, similar to magnocellular neurohypophyseal axons of water deprivated animals (Alonso and Assenmacher, 1979). In this case the small vesicles might bud off the free ends of smooth endoplasmic reticulum and convey CRF to the axolemma for discharge.

Adrenalectomy was reported to induce vasopressin synthesis in CRF-producing neurons (Tramu et al., 1983), indicating that the withdrawl of adrenal steroid causes not only morphological but also biochemical alterations of the paraventriculo-infundibular CRF-tract.

ACTH-IMMUNREACTIVE INNERVATION OF PARAVENTRICULAR CRF NEURONS

Adrenocorticotroph hormone, as a member of the opiomelanocortin family (Mains et al., 1977) is synthesized beside the distal and intermediate lobes of the pituitary gland also in neurons of the medial basal hypothalamus (Krieger et al., 1977; Watson et al., 1978). The hypothalamic arcuate nucleus is the source of the central opiomelanocortin system (Joseph, 1980). The ACTH-immunoreactive fibers arise from the arcuate region and show a widespread distribution in the brain (Romagnano and joseph, 1983). Sawchenko et al. (1982) detected ACTH-immunoreactive fibers in the paraventricular nucleus, mostly in its parvocellular subdivision. The similarity in distribution of CRF and ACTH-immunoreactive structures in the paraventricular nucleus raised the possibility of a neuronal interaction between the two peptidergic systems. For simultaneous localization of the two peptides, we used the immunohistological double labelling method, which has been elaborated in our Department (Liposits et al., 1983c). The method provides possibility for simultaneous tracing of two different antigens at <u>ultrastructural level</u>. This advantage of the method may be utilized for the elucidation of peptid or transmitter specific afferentations of a given immunolabeled system.

Many varicose ACTH-(1-39)-immunoreactive fibers were detected in the parvocellular region of the paraventricular nucleus (Fig. 8a). At ultrastructural level, immunolabeled neurosecretory granules (80-120 nm in diameter) were observed in the axons (Fig. 8b). In the double labelling procedure, the ACTH-fibers were detected first by the silver gold intensified PAP-3,3'-diaminobenzidine (DAB) method, resulting black colour appearance of the profiles. In the second step, the CRF-immunoreactive elements were visualized by the brown coloured DAB endproduct.A substantial number of the beaded ACTH-fibers showed terminal type varicosities on the cell bodies and the proximal dendrites of CRF-neurons (Fig. 8c). The axo-somatic juxtaposition of ACTH-fibers and CRF-neurons was verified at ultrastructural level (Fig. 8d). This morphological arrangement indicates that the hypothalamic opiomelanocortin system regulates the function of the paraventriculo-infundibular

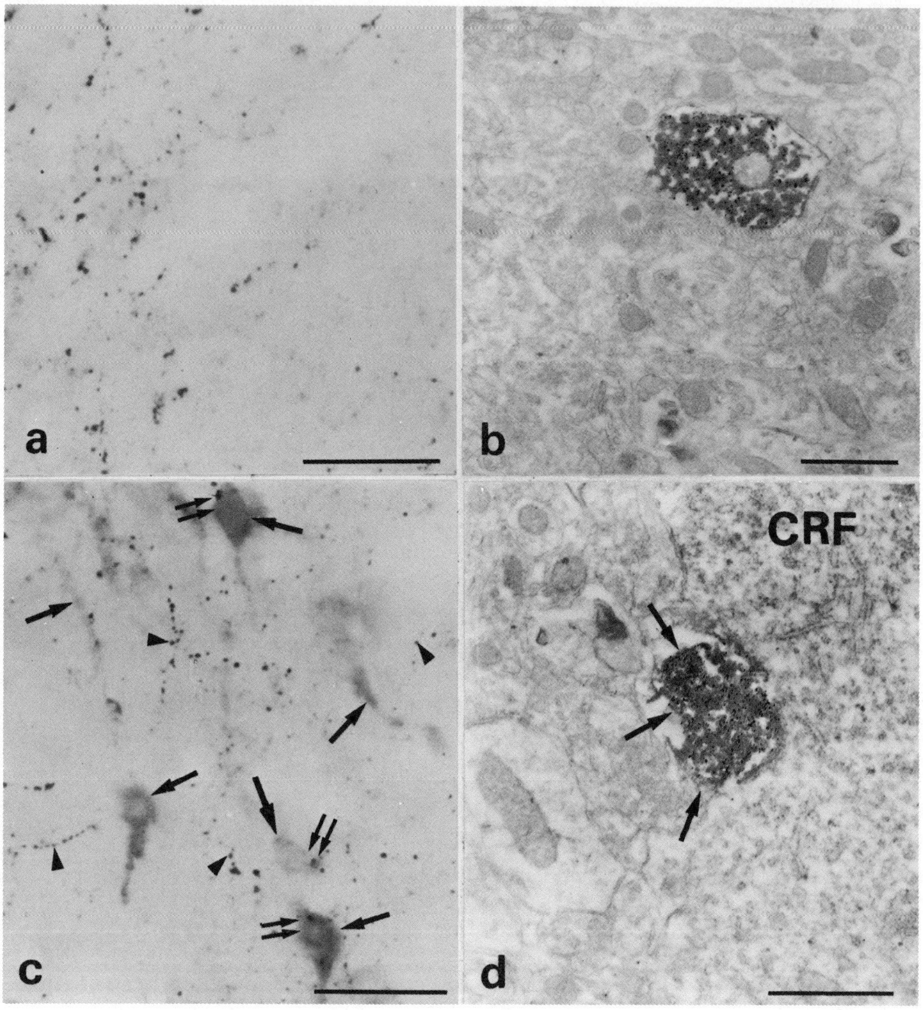

Fig. 8. ACTH-immunoreactive innervation of CRF-synthesizing neurons located in the paraventricular nucleus. Colchicin treated rat. (a) ACTH-containing fibers in the parvocellular part of the nucleus detected by the silver-gold intensified PAP-DAB method. Bar: 50 µm. (b) ACTH axon, filled with neurosecretory granules. Note the metallic grains over the labeled organelles. Bar: 1 µm. (c) Immunohistological double labelling for demonstration of the connection of the two different peptidergic systems. The black colored ACTH-fibers can easily be distinguished from the brown colored CRF-neurons (arrows). Double arrows point to CRF-cells receiving ACTH-afferentation.

Bar: 50 μm. (d) Double labelling at ultrastructural level. The picture corresponds to an axo-somatic juxtaposition, similar to those shown in Fig. c. The ACTH terminal (arrows) is labeled by intensified DAB chromogen, while the CRF-perikaryon (CRF) by the less electron-dense DAB-endproduct. Note the marked difference in electron-density between the original and intensified forms of DAB chromogen. Bar: 1 μm.

CRF-system. Recently Pilcher and Joseph (1984) have reported similar co-localization of CRF immunoreactive perikarya and ACTH-immunopositive fibers in the forebrain and the brainstem of the rat.

CONCLUDING REMARKS

Our present data indicate that the paraventriculo-infundibular CRF-system is the main source of CRF discharged into the portal circulation. The morphological changes of the paraventriculo-infundibular CRF-system, observed after adrenalectomy, prove the steroid hormone dependent function of the system. The different kind of axon terminals synapsing on CRF-neurons suggests the participation of different peptide and transmitter systems in the regulation of the hypothalamo-hypophyseal-adrenal axis. The hypothalamic ACTH-1-39-immunoreactive fibers were found to establish morphological connections with paraventricular CRF-cell groups, indicating the regulatory role of the central opiomelanocortin system upon the paraventriculo-infundibular CRF-system.

REFERENCES

Alonso, G., and Assenmacher, I., 1979, The smooth endoplasmic reticulum in neurohypophyseal axons of the rat: Possible involvement in transport, storage and release of neurosecretory material, Cell Tissue Res. 199:415.

Antoni, F.A., Palkovits, M., Makara, G. B., Linton, E. A., Lowry, P. J., and Kiss, L. Z., 1983, Immunoreactive corticotropin releasing hormone in the hypothalamoinfundibular tract, Neuroendocrinology, 36:415.

Bloom, F. E., Battenberg, E. L. F., Rivier, J., and Vale, W., 1982, Corticotropin releasing factor (CRF): immunoreactive neurons and fibers in the

rat hypothalamus. Regul. Peptides,4:43.
Brown, M. R., Fischer, L. A., Spiess, J., Rivier, C., Rivier, J., and Vale, W., 1982, Corticotropin--releasing factor: actions on the sympathetic nervous system and metabolism. Endocrinology, 111:928.
Bruhn, T. O., Plotsky, P. M., and Vale, W. W., 1984, Effect of paraventricular lesions on corticotropin releasing factor (CRF)-like immunoreactivity in the stalk-median eminence: studies on the adrenocorticotropin response to ether stress and exogenous CRF, Endocrinology, 114:57.
Bugnon, C., Fellmann, D., Gouget, A., and Cardot, J., 1982, Corticoliberin in the rat brain: immunocytochemical localization of a novel neuroglandular system, Neurosci. Lett., 30:25.
Fischman, A. J., and Moldow, R. L., Extrahypothalamic distribution of CRF-like immunoreactivity in the rat brain, Peptides, 1:149.
Guillemin, R., and Rosenberg, B., 1955, Humoral hypothalamic control of anterior pituitary: Study with combined tissue cultures, Endocrinology, 57:599.
Harris, G. W., 1955, Neural control of the pituitary gland. Monographs of the Physiological society, Number 3. London Edward Arnold (Publishers) Ltd.
Joseph, S. A., 1980, Immunoreactive adrenocorticotropin in rat brain: a neuroanatomical study using antiserum generated against synthetic ACTH(1-39), Amer. J. Anat., 158:533.
Kawata, M., Hashimoto, K., Takahara, J., and Sano, Y., 1982, Immunohistochemical demonstration of the localization of corticotropin releasing factor--containing neurons in the hypothalamus of mammals including primates. Anat. Embriol.. 165: 303.
Kovács, M., Lengvári, I., Liposits, Zs., Vigh, S., Schally, A. V., and Flerkó, B., 1984, CRF-immunoreactive neurons in the mammillary body of the rat, Cell Tissue Res. (submitted).
Krieger, D. T., Liotta, A., and Brownstein, M. J., 1977, Presence of corticotropin in brain of normal and hypophysectomized rats. Proc. nat. Acad. Sci. USA 74:648.
Lengvári, I., Liposits, Zs., Vigh, S., Schally, A. V., and Flerkó, B., 1984, The origin and ultrastructural characteristics of CRF-immunoreactive nerve fibers in the posterior pituitary of the rat, Cell Tissue Res., (submitted).

Léránth, Cs., Antoni, F. A., and Palkovits, M., 1983, Ultrastructural demonstration of ovine CRF-like immunoreactivity (oCRF-LI) in the rat hypothalamus: processes of magnocellular neurons establish membrane specializations with parvocellular neurons containing oCRF-LI, Reg. Peptides, 6:179.

Liposits, Zs., Görcs, T., Sétáló, Gy., Lengvári, I., Flerkó, B., Vigh, S., and Schally, A.V., 1983a, Ultrastructural characteristics of immunolabelled, corticotropin releasing factor (CRF)-synthesizing neurons in the rat brain. Cell Tiss. Res., 229: 191.

Liposits, Zs., Lengvári, I., Vigh, S., Schally, A. V., and Flerkó, B., 1983b, Immunohistological detection of degenerating CRF-immunoreactive nerve fibers in the median eminence after lesion of paraventricular nucleus of the rat. A light and electron microscopic study, Peptides, 4:941.

Liposits, Zs., Görcs, T., Török, A., Domány, S., and Sétáló, Gy., 1983c, Simultaneous localization of two different tissue antigens based on the silver intensified PAP-DAB and on the traditional PAP-DAB methods, Acta Morph. Acad. Sci. Hung., 31:365.

Liposits,Zs., Sétáló, G., Flerkó, B., 1984, Application of the silver-gold intensified 3,3'-diaminobenzidine chromogen to the light and electron microscopic detection of the LH-RH system of the rat brain, Neuroscience, (in press).

Mains, R.E., Eipper, B. A., and Ling, N., 1977, Common precursor to corticotropins and endorphins. Proc. Natl. Acad. Sci. USA, 74:3014.

Makara, G. B., Stark, E., Kárteszi, M., Palkovits, M., and Rappay, Gy., 1981, Effects of paraventricular lesions on stimulated ACTH release and CRF in stalk-median eminence of the rat, Am J. Physiol., 240:E441.

Makara, G. B., Kárteszi, M., Kiss, J. Z., Palkovits, M., Rappay, G., and Stark, E., 1982, Corticoliberin (CRF) activity in selected hypothalamic regions in rats with anterolateral hypothalamic cuts, Neuropeptides, 2:287.

Merchenthaler, I., Vigh, S., Petrusz, P., and Schally, A.V., 1982, Immunocytochemical localization of corticotropin releasing factor (CRF) in the rat brain., Am. J. Anat., 165:385.

Merchenthaler, I., Vigh, S., Petrusz, P., and Schally, A.V., 1983a, The paraventriculo-infundibular corticotropin releasing factor (CRF)-pathway as revealed by immunocytochemistry in long-term hypophysectomized or adrenalectomized rats. Reg. Peptides, 5:295.

Merchenthaler, I., Hynes, M. A., Vigh, S., Schally, A. V., and Petrusz, P., 1983b, Immunocytochemical localization of corticotropin releasing factor (CRF) in the rat spinal cord. Brain Res., 275: 373.

Merchenthaler, I., 1984a, Corticotropin releasing factor (CRF)-like immunoreactivity in the rat central nervous system. Extrahypothalamic distribution, 5:53, (Suppl. 1).

Merchenthaler, I., Hynes, M. A., Vigh, S., Schally, A. V., and Petrusz, P., 1984b, Corticotropin releasing factor (CRF): origin and course of afferent pathways to the median eminence (ME) of the rat hypothalamus. Neuroendocrinology, 39:296.

Moldow, R., and Fischman, A. J., 1982a, Radioimmunoassay of CRF-like material in rat hypothalamus, Peptides, 3:37.

Moldow, R. L., Fischman, A. J., 1982b, Hypothalamic CRF--like immunoreactivity in the rat after hypophysectomy or adrenalectomy, Peptides, 1:143.

Olschowka, J. A., O'Donohue, T. L., Mueller, G. P., and Jakobowitz, D. M., 1982, Hypothalamic and extrahypothalamic distribution of CRF-like immunoreactive neurons in the rat brain, Neuroendocrinology, 35:305.

Paull, W.K., Gibbs, F. P., 1983, The corticotropin releasing factor (CRF) neurosecretory system in intact, adrenalectomized, and adrenalectomized--dexamethasone treated rats, Histochemistry, 78:303.

Pilcher, W. H., and Joseph, S. A., 1984, Co-localization of CRF-ir perikarya and ACTH-ir fibers in rat brain, Brain Res., 299:91.

Rivier, C., Brownstein, M., Spiess, J., Rivier, J., and Vale, W., 1982, In vivo corticotropin-releasing factor-induced secretion of adrenocorticotropin, ß-endorphin, and corticosterone, Endocrinology, 110:272.

Romagnano, M., Jospeh, S. A., 1983, Immunocytochemical localization of $ACTH_{1-39}$ in the brainstem of the rat, Brain Res., 276:1.

Russel, S. M., Dhariwal, A. P. S., McCann, S. M., Yates, F. E., 1969, Inhibition by dexamethasone of the in vivo pituitary response to corticotropin releasing factor (CRF), Endocrinology, 85:512.

Saffran, M., and Schally, A. V., 1955, The release of corticotropin by anterior pituitary tissue in vitro, Can J. Biochem. Physiol., 33:408.

Saffran, M., and Schally, A. V., 1977, The status of the corticotropin releasing factor (CRF). Neuroendocrinology, 24:359.

Sawchenko, P. E., Swanson, L. W., and Joseph, S. A., 1982, The distribution and cells of origin of ACTH(1-39)-stained varicosities in the paraventricular and supraoptic nuclei. Brain Res., 232:365.

Sirinathsinghji, D. J. S., Rees, L. H., Rivier, J., and Vale, W., 1983, Corticotropin releasing factor is a potent inhibitor of sexual receptivitiy in the female rat, Nature, 305:232.

Spiess, J., Rivier, J., Rivier, C., and Vale, W., 1981, Primary structure of corticotropin-releasing factor from ovine hypothalamus, Proc. Natl. Acad. Sci. USA, 78:6517.

Sternberger, L. A., 1979, Immunocytochemistry, 2nd Edition, John Wiley and Sons, New York.

Swanson, L. W., Sawchenko, P. E., Rivier, J., and Vale, W. W., 1983, Organization of ovine corticotropin--releasing factor immunoreactive cells and fibers in the rat brain: An immunohistochemical study, Neuroendocrinology, 36:165.

Szentágothai, J., Flerkó, B., Mess, B., and Halász, B., 1962, Hypothalamic control of the anterior pituitary, Akadémiai Kiadó, Budapest.

Tramu, G., Croix, C., and Pillez, A., 1983, Ability of the CRF immunoreactive neurons of the paraventricular nucleus to produce a vasopressin-like material, Neuroendocrinology, 37:467.

Turkelson, C. M., Arimura, A., Culler, M. D., Fishback, J. B., Groot, K., Kanda, M., Luciano, M., Thomas, C. R., Chang, D., Chang, J. K., and Shimizu, M., 1981, In vivo and in vitro release of ACTH by synthetic CRF, Peptides; 2:425.

Vale, W., Spiess, J., Rivier, C., and Rivier, J., 1981, Characterization of a 41-residue ovine hypothalamic peptide that stimulates secretion of corticotropin and ß-endorphin, Science, 213:1394.

Vale, W., Rivier, C., Brown, M. R., Spiess, J., Koob, G., Swanson, L., Bilezikjian, L., Bloom, F., and Rivier, J., 1983, Chemical and biological characterization of corticotropin releasing factor, Recent Progress in Hormone Research, 39:245.

Valentino, R. J., Foote, S. L., and Aston-Jones, G., 1983, Corticotropin releasing factor activates noradrenergic neurons of the locus coeruleus, Brain Res., 270:363.

Vigh, S., Merchenthaler, I., Petrusz, P., Sueiras-Diaz, J., and Schally, A. V., 1982a, Specific antibodies against the corticotropin releasing factor (CRF): immunocytochemical localization of CRF in the rat brain. The End. Soc. 64th Annual Meeting, San Francisco, p. 84.

Vigh, S., Merchenthaler, I., Torres-Aleman, I., Sueiras--Diaz, J., Coy, D. H., Carter, W. H., Petrusz, P., and Schally, A. V., 1982b, Corticotropin releasing factor (CRF): immunocytochemical localization and radioimmunoassay (RIA), Life Sci., 31:2441.

Watson, S. J., Richer, C. W., Barchas, J. D., 1978, Adrenocorticotropin in rat brain: immunocytochemical localization in cells and axons, Science, 200:1180.

Yasuda, N., Greer, M. A., and Aizawa, T., 1982, Corticotropin releasing factor, Endocr. Rev., 3:123.

Yates, F. E., Russel, S. M., Dallman, M. F., Hedge, G. A., McCann, S. M., Dhariwal, A. P. S., 1971, Potentiation by vasopressin of corticotropin release induced by corticotropin-releasing factor, Endocrinology, 88:3.

THE PARAVENTRICULO-INFUNDIBULAR CORTICOTROPIN RELEASING FACTOR (CRF)-SYSTEM II. FUNCTIONAL ASPECTS

István Lengvári, Magdolna Kovács, Zsolt Liposits
Sándor Vigh, and Béla Flerkó

Department of Anatomy, University Medical School
Pécs, Hungary

INTRODUCTION

Recent isolation, characterisation and synthesis of CRF, a 41-residue polypeptide (Vale et al., 1981) made it possible to produce specific antibodies against it, which in turn resulted in immunohistochemical detection of CRF containing structures within the central nervous system (Merchenthaler et al., 1982: Swanson et al., 1983). One of the main characteristics of the central CRF system is that CRF containing cell bodies are found in diverse parts of the central nervous system. CRF containing cell bodies are demonstrated in several limbic areas, besides the hypothalamus (Liposits et al., 1983a: Merchenthaler et al., 1983), and even a few cells are scattered in the cerebral cortex (Merchenthaler, 1984: Fig. 1). It is evident that all of these cell groups are not directly responsible for the ACTH release of the anterior pituitary, as some of the areas containing CRF-immunopositive cells do not have classically demonstrated connection with the median eminence. In this presentation we try to answer two questions: (1) which CRF cell group is responsible for the pituitary ACTH release; and (2) what is the role of the other CRF cell groups.

THE PARAVENTRICULO-INFUNDIBULAR CRF SYSTEM

It is logical that our first attempt was to find those cells which innervate the median eminence. In our morphological study (Liposits et al., 1983b) we showed

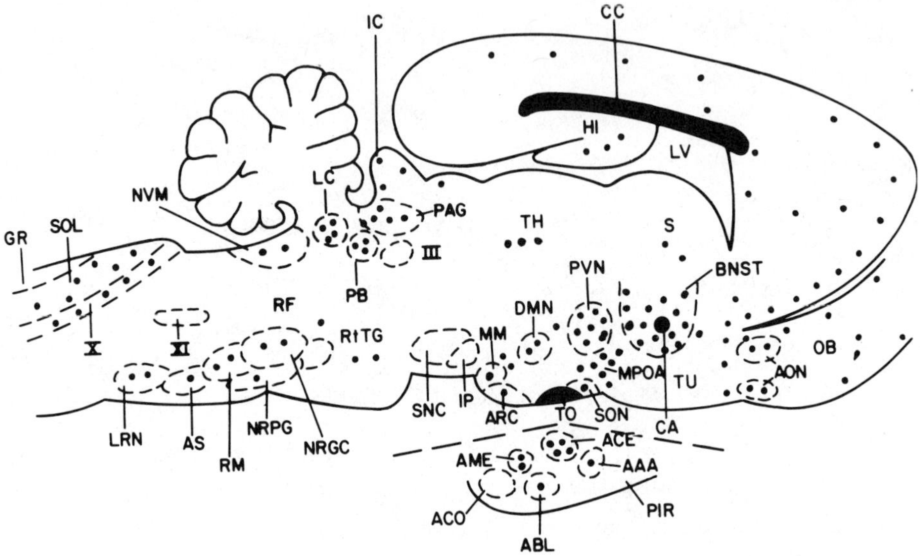

Fig. 1. An updated schematic drawing summarizing the distribution of CRF-immunopositive perikarya (solid circles) in a parasagittal segment of the rat brain. Abbreviations: AAA: anterior amygdaloid area, ABL: basolateral amygdaloid nucleus, ACE: central amygdaloid nucleus, ACO: anterior cortical nucleus, AME: medial amygdaloid nucleus, AON: anterior olfactory nucleus, ARC: arcuate nucleus, BNST: bed nucleus of the stria terminalis, CC: corpus callosum, DMN: dorsomedial nucleus, GR: nucleus gracilis, HI: hippocampus, IC: inferior colliculus, IP: interpeduncular nucleus, LC: locus ceruleus, LRN: lateral reticular nucleus, LV: lateral ventricle, MM: medial mammillary nucleus, MPOA: medial preoptic area, NRGC: nucleus reticularis gigantocellularis, NVM: nucleus vestibularis medialis, OB: olfactory bulb, PAG: periaqueductal gray, PB: parabrachial nucleus, PIR: piriform cortex, PVN: paraventricular nucleus, RF: reticular formation, RM: raphe magnus, RtTG: reticulotegmental nucleus of the pons, SCN: substancia nigra, SOL: solitary tract, SON: supraoptic nucleus, TH: thalamus, TO: tractus opticus, TU: tuberculum olfactorium. (By courtesy of Dr. I. Merchenthaler)

that complete removal of the hypothalamic paraventricular nuclei results in an almost complete disappearance of CRF immunopositive fibers from the median eminence two- or three weeks after the surgery. We tried to give direct evidence that the paraventricular nuclei indeed are the main sources of CRF, released into the pituitary

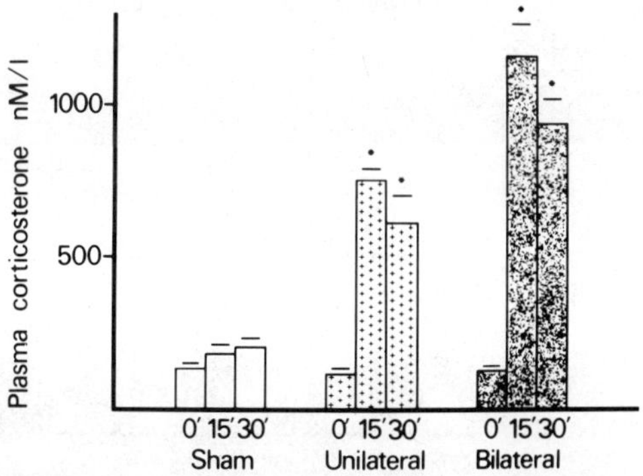

Fig. 2. Effect of sham stimulation and uni- and bilateral stimulation of the paraventricular nuclei on plasma corticosterone level. Each column represents the mean of 8-15 animals; horizontal bars indicate standard errors, asterisks denote significant difference from 0' values.

portal vessels (Lengvári et al., 1983). In dexamethasone--morphin-Nembutal blocked animals we electrochemically stimulated, unilaterally or bilaterally the paraventricular nuclei. As it is seen from Fig. 2., sham stimulation (e.g. only lowering the electrode to the level of the paraventricular nuclei) was ineffective. Unilateral stimulation of paraventricular nuclei resulted in a significant increase of plasma corticosterone, 15 minutes after the stimulation, which tended to lower after additional 15 minutes. Bilateral stimulation was more effective in term of corticosterone release, both 15 and 30 minutes after the stimulation. These clearly, but not exclusively show the role of paraventricular nuclei in ACTH release.

In a next set of experiments we tried to find that whether there is any part of the hypothalamus, electrochemical stimulation of which results in ACTH release after removal of the paraventricular nuclei (Lengvári

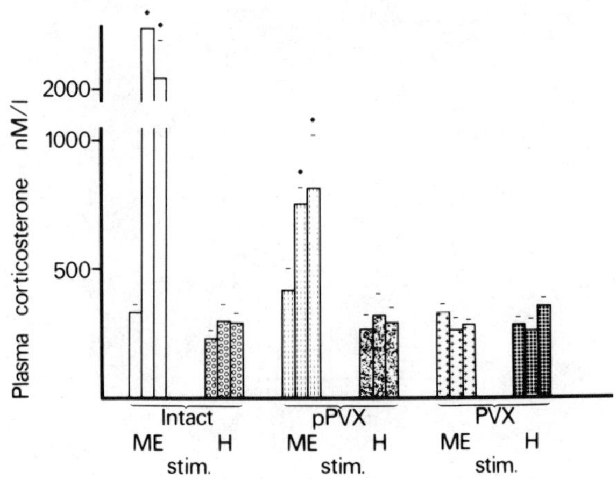

Fig. 3. Effect of stimulation of the median eminence (ME) and mediobasal hypothalamus (H) on plasma corticosterone in intact rats and after partial (pPVX) or complete (PVX) removal of the paraventricular nuclei. For further explanations see Fig. 2.

et al., 1985a). As it is seen in Fig. 3, in normal animals - as it is expected - stimulation of the median eminence causes a tremendous increase in plasma corticosterone, while stimulation of other parts of the hypothalamus (mainly the ventromedial and dorsomedial nuclei) is ineffective. Partial removal of the paraventricular nuclei reduces the effect of median eminence stimulation, while complete destruction of the mentioned nuclei prevents the effect of stimulation of the median eminence on plasma corticosterone.

These functional data, taken together with our morphological findings strongly suggest that practically all CRF terminals of the median eminence originates from the paraventricular nuclei. The possible role of paraventricular nuclei in regulating pituitary ACTH release was first suggested by Moll as early as 1960. Later

Dunn and Critchlow (1972) stimulated different parts of the hypothalamus, and stimulation of the paraventricular nuclei was the most effective in causing an increase in plasma corticosterone. Unfortunately, they reported only two cases of paraventriculat stimulation, which did not permit definitive conclusion, and this data became forgotten. It is very important to note that until the isolation of the "true" CRF, it was almost impossible to find an experimental set up, in which the possible effect of vasopressin could be excluded in experiments manipulating with the paraventricular nuclei. Vasopressin has been considered as one of the major candidate of CRF, and indeed it has an ACTH releasing potency (Vale et al., 1983). Moreover, there are several experimental data showing parallel changes in the content of neurosecretory material of the median eminence and the adrenal function.

If, on the basis of the presented evidences it is accepted that CRF fibers of the median eminence originate exclusively from the paraventricular nuclei, then it is difficult to explain some earlier results on the regulation of pituitary ACTH secretion. Halász et al. (1965) introduced a revolutionary new and simple method in the neuroendocrinology: with a very simple, bayonet shaped knife they were able to disrupt discrete brain pathways or isolate some brain regions without damaging the overlaying structures. This method has been widely used since 1965, and various conclusions have been drawn on the basis of partial or complete isolation of the medial basal hypothalamus. It was concluded that CRF was produced within the so-called hypophysiotrophic area (which is a well circumscribed part of the medial basal hypothalamus), because animals with isolated hypophysiotrophic area responded to a series of stresses with increased plasma corticosterone levels (Halász et al., 1967; Palka et al., 1969; Voloschin et al., 1968). The problem with these experiments is that the paraventricular nuclei were not considered as parts of the hypophysiotrophic area, and one would expect that during both complete and frontal isolation of the medial basal hypothalamus the majority of the fibers of the paraventriculo-infundibular CRF tract were severed. In an immunohistological study we attempted to explain this discrepancy (Lengvári et al., 1985b).

Frontal afferents to the hypophysiotrophic area were interrupted using a Halász-knife. Great care was taken to use exactly the same type of knife and similar stereotaxic coordinates which were used by Halász et al. (1967). Examination of the haematoxylin-eosin stained sections of operated brains showed that the knee of the knife rotated just in front of (Fig. 4) or through

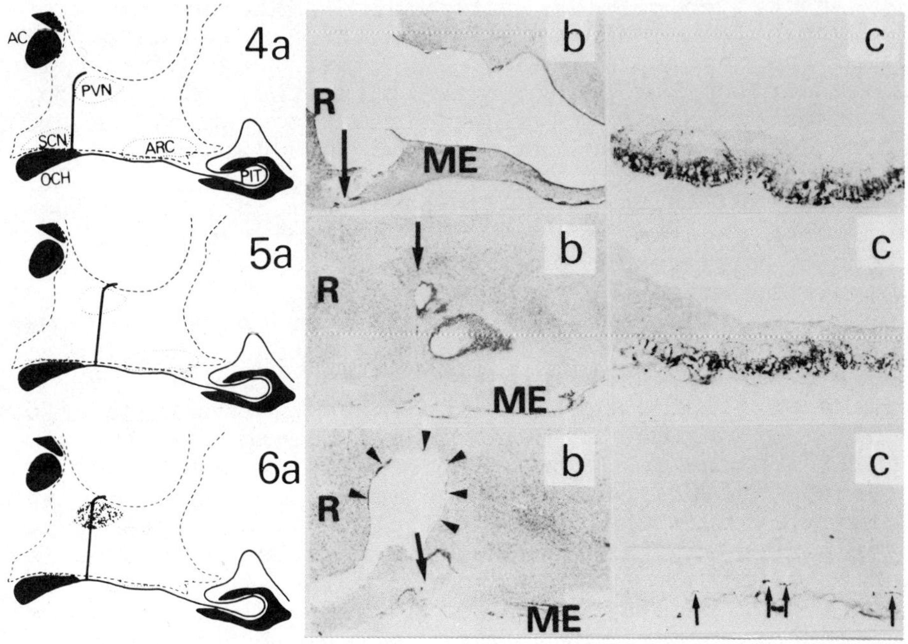

Figs. 4-6. The effect of frontal isolation of the mediobasal hypothalamus on the CRF innervation of median eminence. The different rostro-caudal locations of the cut lines are demonstrated on schematic drawings by solid lines (Figs. 4a, 5a, 6a) and on haematoxylin-eosin stained sections by arrows (Figs. 4b, 5b, 6b). Figs. 4c, 5c, 6c show the corresponding immunostained median eminences. All illustrations are in the sagittal plane. Abbreviations: AC: anterior commissure, ARC: arcuate nucleus, ME: median eminence, OCH: optic chiasma, PIT: pituitary gland, PVN: paraventricular nucleus, R: rostral, SCN: suprachiasmatic nucleus.

Figs. 5b and 6b) the paraventricular nuclei. It resulted in a cut either in front of the nuclei or through them. In the optimal case the tip of the knife reached the base of the brain in the middline just behind the optic chiasma and then the knive was rotated to both sides by 90°. Thus the cut extended up to the level of the supraoptic nuclei. Although we tried to reach the base of the skull during the surgery, it was not unusual for a 10-50 µm thick tissue gap to remain uncut in the arc of the cutline on the basal surface of the brain, presumably due to the characteristic configuration of the inner surface of the skull. If the knife cut the paraventricular nuclei into halves, they sometimes necrotized (Figs. 6a and b). In the immunostained material, the presence of CRF immunoreactive fibers of the median eminence was independent of the exact rostro-caudal localization of the cut line (Figs. 4c and 5c). The only cases in which the immunolabelled CRF fibers almost completely disappeared from the median eminence were those in which the paraventricular nuclei necrotized (Fig. 6c).

From this study it is clear that frontal isolation of the medial basal hypothalamus by the method of Halász et al. (1967) saves most of the fibers running from the paraventricular nuclei to the median eminence. The projection of CRF fibers from the paraventricular nuclei to the median eminence is similar to that of the magnocellular paraventriculo-hypophysial tract, i.e. they reach the retrochiasmatic area from the lateral direction as proposed by Makara et al. (1979), before immunostaining techniques of CRF-containing structures became available. Thus the number of CRF-fibers entering the medial basal hypothalamus depends on the medio-lateral extension of the cut in the retrochiasmatic area. The fact that in a few cases the paraventricular nuclei necrotize, probably because of damage of their blood supply from vessels coming from the basal surface of the brain (Ambach and Palkovits, 1974) was easily overlooked in earlier studies, because the importance of these nuclei in the production of CRF was not known. One of the main problems in judging deafferentation studies is that the exact histological localization of the intervention is infrequently given and most of the publications lack histological illustrations, probably because deafferentation was considered a very standard and uniform intervention. In general, the question whether the cut line reached the basal surface of the brain was neglected. It has to be pointed out that, when frozen or polyethylenglycol embedded materials are used, it is impossible to judge the completeness of the deafferentation, while fine gaps can be torn when the sections are floating. The importance of even small gaps in functional recovery of the medial basal hypothalamus was first mentioned by Sétáló et al. (1978) in case of LHRH fibers. Makara et al. (1979) reinvestigating the effect of complete deafferentation of the medial basal hypothalamus on ACTH secretion, again called attention to the importance of these tissue gaps, especially at the retrochiasmatic level.

The presented material gives some explanation for some controversial results of earlier deafferentation studies. It has been shown (Halász et al., 1967: Palka et al., 1969; Voloschin et al., 1968) that frontal deafferentation of the medial basal hypothalamus does not alter basal ACTH secretion or even increases it on the basis of plasma corticosterone level. It is evident from Figs. 4 and 5 that the paraventriculo-infundibular CRF-tract remains essentially intact after frontal deafferentation of the medial basal hypothalamus. The difference, seen in resting corticosterone levels of groups of operated animals, can be explained for instance by the fact that the surgery probably destroys, at least in part, the afferents to the CRF producing cells. It is probable that CRF immunoreactive cells receive both excitatory and inhibitory afferents, and different knives destroy different pathways during surgical interventions.

A general conclusion of the presented study is that without precise and detailed, and if possible, immunohistological control, no definitive conclusions should be drawn from studies based on deafferentation experiments. Deafferentation, even if done with great care, varies from animal to animal, and important individual differences could be overlooked.

If one wants to empty the median eminence of CRF immunopositive fibers then a Halász-knife with 2 mm of radius or a 4 mm wide piece of razor blade should be used, and the cut line should be behind the paraventricular nuclei (Fig. 7a). In these cases there are marked accumulations of CRF immunopositive material in perikarya of the paraventricular nuclei and in the cut line anteriorly, while the median eminence practically does not contain CRF positive fibers (Fig. 7b). An anterolateral cut on one side of the hypothalamus (Fig. 8a) results in an almost complete disappearance of CRF fibers in the ipsilateral side of the median eminence, however close to the middline a narrow zone remains well innervated of the operated side (Fig. 8b). With an additional cut in the middline (Fig. 9a), these CRF fibers disappear, while the contralateral side seems to be intact (Fig. 9b). A 4 mm long mediosagittal cut from the posterior edge of the optic chiasma to the pituitary stalk (Fig. 10a) results in the disappearance of CRF fibers from the median part of the median eminence (Fig. 10b). These data clearly show that a rather wide cut behind the paraventricular nuclei is necessary to disrupt all CRF fibers running to the median eminence. This again indicates that earlier deafferentation studies were ineffective in causing complete disappearance of CRF fibers from the median eminence. Another interesting point of these deafferentation studies is that the largest part of the median eminence receives CRF innervation from the ipsilateral paraventricular nucleus. There is, however a narrow strip in the middline to which CRF fibers run from both paraventricular nuclei.

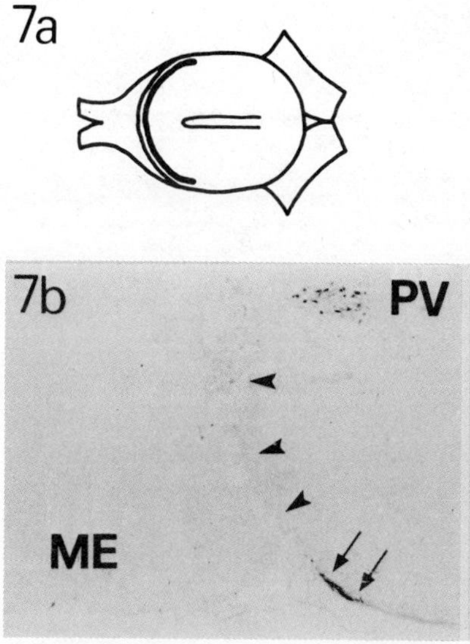

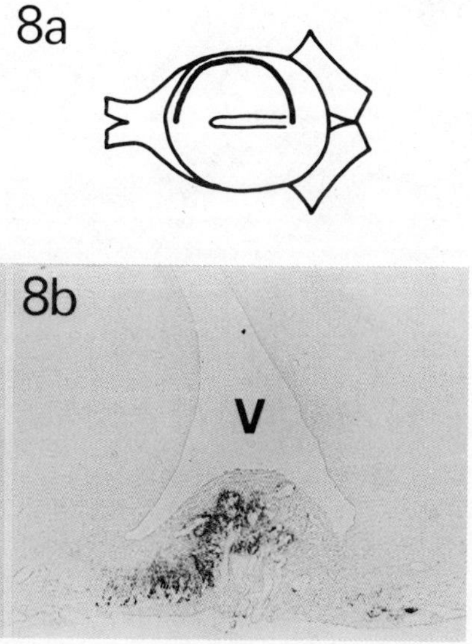

Fig. 7. (a) Schematic drawing of the basal surface of the hypothalamus showing a cut made with a Halász-knife (2mm radius; heavy line).
(b) CRF-immunostained middsagittal section; arrowheads indicating the cut-line. The median eminence (ME) does not contain CRF immunopositive fibers. Note the accumulation of immunopositive material in cell bodies of the paraventricular nucleus (PV) and in front of the cut-line (arrows).

Fig. 8. (a) Schematic drawing of unilateral anterolateral cut (heavy line).
(b) Coronal section of the immunostained median eminence. V: 3rd ventricle. (For further details see text.)

On the basis of our material the question cannot be answered, whether there is a definitive crossing of fibers somewhere in front of the median eminence, or the fibers cross the middline in the entire length of the median eminence.

EXTRAHYPOTHALAMIC CRF CELL GROUPS

The above data - in our opinion - clearly indicate that paraventricular nuclei are responsible for CRF release into the portal vessels and the subsequent ACTH release. Now we can turn to our second problem: what is the role of CRF cell groups other than the paraventricular

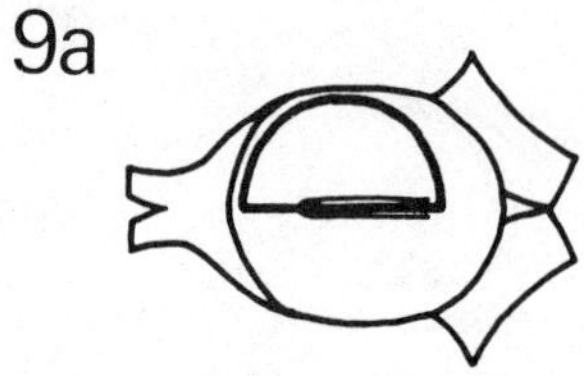

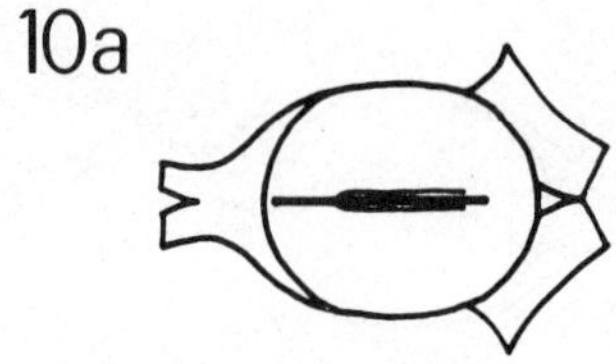

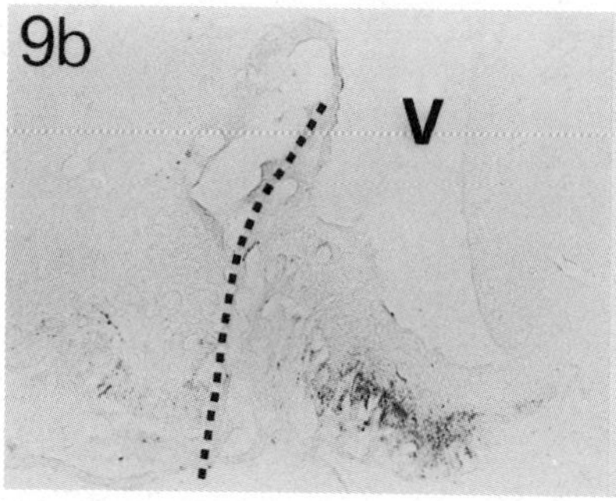

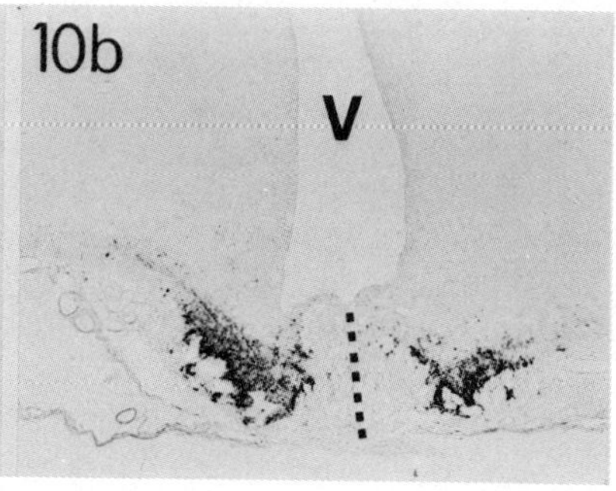

Fig. 9. (a) Schematic drawing of combined unilateral antero-lateral cut and middsagittal cut (heavy lines). (b) Coronal section of immunostained median eminence. Broken line indicates the sagittal cut. V: 3rd ventricle.

Fig. 10. (a) Schematic drawing of middsagittal cut (heavy line). (b) Coronal section of immunostained median eminence. Broken line indicates the cut. V: 3rd ventricle. (For further details see text.)

CRF. First we consider a very peculiar CRF-immunopositive cell population located in the mammillary region. These cells can be stained only after colchicine treatment. In our surprise, CRF positive cells were found in our material without colchicine pretreatment after removal of the paraventricular nuclei. This fact attempted us to further investigate these cells, both morphologically (Kovács et al., 1985) and functionally (Lengvári et al., 1984).

First we placed a wide cut behind the paraventricular nuclei either by lowering a 4 mm wide piece of razor blade or using a modified Halász knife. In these cases the median eminence was almost completely free of CRF--immunoreactive terminals, and again CRF-cells were easily stained in the mammillary region. These cells are round to oval, mainly bipolar, and the general characteristics of these cells resembled to the CRF-immunopositive cells in the paraventricular nuclei. A few morphometric parameters of the two cell populations were compared, and they were found similar. It is interesting to note that these cells do not respect the boundaries of any well definied mammillary nucleus.

In a next step we looked for the possible efferentation of the mammillary CRF cells (Kovács et al., 1985). The fact, that after making a wide frontal cut behind the paraventricular nuclei, the median eminence is free of CRF-immunoreactive terminals, excludes the possibility that these cells project directly to the median eminence. On the other hand, utilizing classical neuroanatomical tract tracing methods, no such connection has been detected (Cruce, 1975; 1976; Shen, 1983). To look for the efferentation of the mammillary CRF cells we used a very simple approach, which is widely accepted in mapping peptidergic pathways: if one cuts an axon, then there is an accumulation of neurosecretory material in the cutline on the side of the cell body. We made cuts (again either with a piece of razor blade or modified Halász-knife) in front of, through and behind the mammillary region. Accumulation of CRF immunopositive material was observed only in those cases in which the cut was in front of or went through the mammillary body, and there was no CRF accumulation if a cut was placed behind the mammillary body. In those cases in which accumulation of neurosecretory material was observed, it always happened behind the cutline. We have a few cases in which the accumulated material follows the mammillothalamic tract, suggesting that CRF positive neurons project into this tract. It was shown by tract-tracing methods (Cruce, 1975; 1976; Shen, 1983) that the main efferents of the mammillary complex are the mammillothalamic and mammillotegmental tracts. The latter probably does not contain efferent CRF fibers from the mammillary region, because there was no accumulation of neurosecretory material in cuts placed behind the mammillary complex. This means that the main - if not sole - efferent CRF pathway of the mammillary region is the mammillothalamic tract, axons of which terminate in the anterolateral, anteromedial and anterodorsal thalamic nuclei. The assumption that mammillary CRF-immunoreactive cells project to these part of the thalamus is well correlated to those studies, which demonstrated a relatively high CRF content of the thalamus by radioimmunoassay (Fishman and Holdow, 1982) and recent immunohistological data showing rich CRF innervation (Merchenthaler, 1984) and CRF perikarya (Merchenthaler et al., 1984) in the thalamus.

The question arises that what is the functional role of these CRF immunopositive cells in the mammillary region. To answer this question we stimulated the mammillary region of dexamethasone-morphine-Nembutal

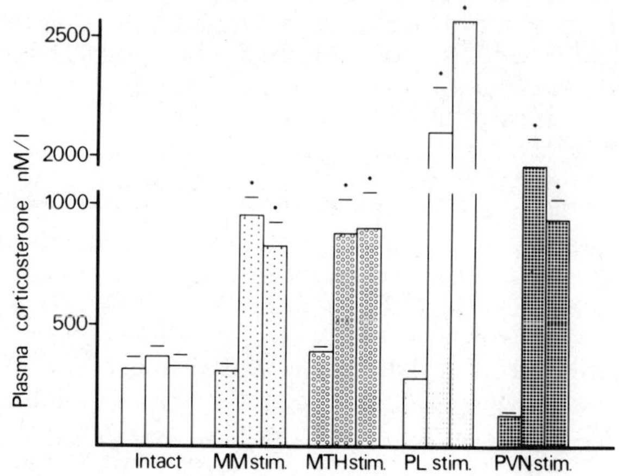

Fig. 11. The effect of sham stimulation (Intact) and stimulation of the mammillary body (MM), mammillothalamic tract (MTH) and posterior lobe (PL) on plasma corticosterone. For comparison the effect of paraventricular stimulation (PVN) is redrawn from Fig. 2. For further explanations see Fig. 2.

blocked rats (Lengvári et al., 1984). Bilateral stimulation of the mammillary body (which centered in the posterior mammillary nucleus and involved parts of the medial mammillary nucleus) was effective in causing a significant increase of plasma corticosterone levels both 15 and 30 minutes after stimulation, indicating previous ACTH release (Fig. 11). The increase of plasma corticosterone in these cases, however was smaller than after stimulation of the paraventricular nuclei, indicating that stimulation of the mammillary CRF cells is less effective in causing ACTH release than stimulation of the paraventricular nuclei. Similar changes in plasma corticosterone were observed when the stimulation involved the mammillothalamic tract. In a few cases the tip of the electrode reached the posterior lobe of the pituitary gland. As it is expected, such stimulation resulted in a tremendous increase of plasma corticosterone; this effect however is beyond the scope of our present subject.

It is evident from the presented material that stimulation of the mammillary region, in which CRF immunoreactive cells are detected leads to a significant increase of plasma corticosterone. This result is in accordance with results of the early fifties, which showed some stimulatory role of the mammillary region in stress response. Thus, it was demonstrated that electrical stimulation of the mammillary body of rabbits resulted in lymphopenia, which was similar to that following an emotional stress, while lesion of the mammillary body abolished or diminished the lymphopenic response following an emotional stress (de Groot and Harris, 1950). In cats and monkeys a marked increase of electrical activity, limited to the posterior hypothalamus was induced by stressful stimuli which resulted in eosinopenia (Porter, 1952), while stimulation of the same region led to eosinopenia (Porter, 1953). These studies, however have been forgotten and to our knowledge nobody has ever reinvestigated the role of the mammillary region in the regulation of ACTH secretion.

The above morphological and functional data strongly suggest that the mammillary CRF-immunoreactive cells are parts of a neural circuit which, under certain circumstances, can influence the activity of the paraventriculo--infundibular CRF-system. Without having more informations about the function of this system it would be mere speculation to tell more about the exact role of the mammillary CRF-system.

Finally we briefly mention some preliminary results concerning two other CRF cell groups. There is a well definied CRF cell population in the central and medial amygdaloid nucleus (Fellman et al., 1982; Merchenthaler, 1984). Stimulation of this area again resulted in an increase of plasma corticosterone (Fig. 12). Amygdala has long been known to have stimulatory effect on ACTH secretion, and our result is in accordance with this earlier results. Without having any information about the efferentation of amygdaloid CRF cell group it is not possible to tell anything about the mechanism by which amygdala affects ACTH secretion.

The other CRF cell group is situated around the anterior commissura: the cells belong to the nucleus proprius of anterior commissura, and in part to the nucleus accumbens septi. Stimulation of these cells causes a moderate but significant increase in plasma corticosterone (Fig. 12). This result is a little surprising as, in general, forebrain and rhinencephalic

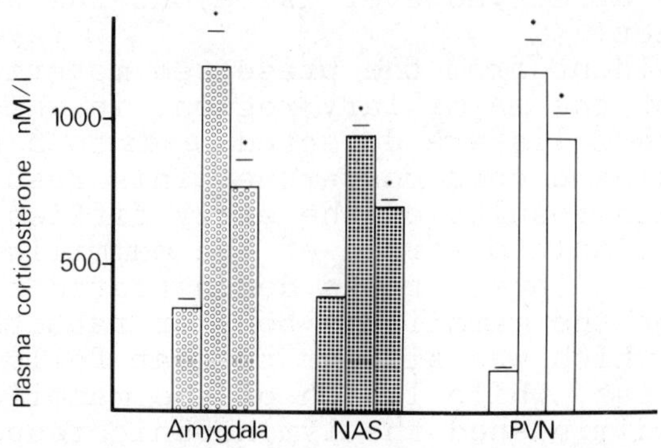

Fig. 12. The effect of stimulation of amygdala and a region around the commissure anterior (NAS) on the plasma corticosterone. For comparison the effect of paraventricular stimulation (PVN) is redrawn from Fig. 2. For further explanations see Fig. 2.

structures have been repeatedly reported to inhibit adreconocortical function, although this specific cell group can hardly identified in non-immunostained material. Further studies are in progress in our laboratory to elucidate the connections of the latter two CRF cell groups.

CONCLUDING REMARKS

The presented material permits to draw some conclusions which should be treated as working hypothesis only. In our opinion the pituitary ACTH secretion is under a two-level control. The first level is the paraventriculo-infundibular CRF (and probably paraventriculo-hypophyseal vasopressin) system. This system represents the final common pathway, i.e. every information which leads to stimulation or inhibition of pituitary ACTH secretion converges to the hypothalamic paraventricular nuclei. The second level is a sophisticated system of stimulatory and inhibitory areas. Most of these structures belong to the limbic system. Some of these limbic structures (such as mammillary complex, amygdala) contains CRF cells, too. It is interesting that those limbic structures which contain CRF cell bodies have long been considered as stimulatory areas of ACTH secretion.

It is to be said that immunohistology of the CRF system of the central nervous system opened new vistas in studying the regulation of ACTH secretion. It explained some earlier conflucting results, it solved some problems, but as it is usual, it gave several new questions.

REFERENCES

Ambach, G., and Palkovits, M., 1974, Blood supply of the rat hypothalamus. II. Nucleus paraventricularis, Acta Morph. Acad. Sci. hung., 22:311.

Cruce, A. F., 1975, An autoradiographic study of the projections of the mammillothalamic tract in the rat, Brain Res., 85:211.

Cruce, A. F., 1976, An autoradiographic study of the descending connections of the mammillary nuclei of the rat, J. Comp. neurol., 176: 631.

Dunn, J., and Critchlow, V., 1972, Electrically stimulated ACTH release in pharmacologically blocked rats, Endocrinology, 93:835.

De Groot, J., and Harris, G. W., 1950, Hypothalamic control of the anterior pituitary gland and blood lymphocytes, J. Physiol., 111:335.

Fellman, D., Bugnon, C., and Gouget, A., 1982, Immunocytochemical demonstration of corticoliberin-like immunoreactivity (CLI) in neurons of the rat amygdala central nucleus (ACN), Neurosci. Lett., 34:253.

Fishman, A. J., and Moldow, R. L., 1982, Distribution of CRF-like immunoreactivity in the rabbit. Peptides 3:842.

Halász, B., and Pupp, L., 1965, Hormone secretion of the anterior pituitary gland after physical interruption of all nervous pathways to the hypophyseotrophic area, Endocrinology 77:553.

Halász, B., Slusher, M., and Gorski, R. A., 1967, Adrenocorticotrophic hormone secretion in rats after partial or total deafferentation of the medial basal hypothalamus, Neuroendocrinology 2:43.

Kovács, M., Lengvári, I., Liposits, Zs., Vigh, S., Schally, A. V., and Flerkó, B., 1985, CRF-

-immunoreactive neurons in the mammillary body of the rat, in press.

Lengvári, I., Kovács, M., and Szelier, M., 1983, The effect of electrochemical stimulation of paraventricular nuclei on plasma corticosterone, Neuroendocrinol. Lett. 5:207.

Lengvári, I., Kovács, M., Liposits, Zs., and Szelier, M., 1984, The effect of stimulation of mammillary body on plasma corticosterone in rat, Neuroendocrinol. Lett. 6: 285.

Lengvári, I., Kovács, M., Liposits, Zs., and Szelier, M., 1985a, The lack of effect of electrochemical stimulation of the hypothalamus and median eminence on the plasma corticosterone level after lesion of the paraventricular nuclei, Exp. Clin. Endocrinol. in press.

Lengvári, I., Liposits, Zs., Vigh, S., Schally, A.V., and Flerkó, B., 1985b, Re-evaluation of "frontal deafferentation studies on the regulation of ACTH secretion in the light of CRF immunohistology, Endocrinol. experiment, in press.

Liposits, Zs., Görcs, T., Sétáló, Gy., Lengvári, I., Flerkó, B., Vigh, S., and Schally, A.V., 1983a, Ultrastructural characteristics of immunolabelled, corticotropin releasing factor (CRF)-synthesizing neurons in the rat brain. Cell Tiss. Res. 229:101.

Liposits, Zs., Lengvári; I., Vigh, S., Schally, A. V., and Flerkó, B., 1983b, Immunohistological detection of degenerating CRF-immunoreactive nerve fibers in the median eminence after lesion of paraventricular nucleus of the rat. A light and electronmicroscopic study, Peptides 4:941.

Makara, G. B., Stark, E., Rappay, Gy., Kárteszi, M., and Palkovits, M., 1979, Changes in corticotropin releasing factor of the stalk median eminence in rats with various cuts around the medial basal hypothalamus, J. Endocrinol. 83:165.

Merchenthaler, I., 1984, Corticotropin releasing factor (CRF)-like immunoreactivity in the rat central nervous system. Extrahypothalamic distribution. Peptides 5 (Suppl. 1):53.

Merchenthaler, I., Vigh, S., Petrusz, P., and Schally, A. V., 1982, Immunocytochemical localization of corticotropin releasing factor (CRF) in the rat brain, Am. J. Anat. 165:385.

Merchenthaler, I., Vigh, S., Petrusz, P., and Schally, A. V., 1983, The paraventriculo-infundibular corticotropin releasing factor (CRF)-pathway as revealed by immunochemistry in longterm hypophysectomized or adrenalectomized rats, Regul.

Pept. 5:295.
Merchenthaler, I., Vigh, S., Schally, A.V., Stumpf, W. E., and Arimura, A., 1984, Immunocytochemical localization of corticotropin releasing factor (CRF)-like immunoreactivity in the thalamus of the rat, Brain Res. in press.
Moll, J., 1960, Localization of hypothalamic lesions inhibiting adrenal weight maintenance in the rat, Acta Endocrinol. 34:19.
Palka, Y., Coyer, D., and Critchlow, V., 1969, Effects of isolation of medial basal hypothalamus on pituitary-adrenal and pituitary-ovarian functions, Neuroendocrinology 5:333.
Porter, R. W., 1952, Alterations in electrical activity of the hypothalamus induced by stress stimuli. Am. J. Physiol. 169:629.
Porter, R. W., 1953, Hypothalamic involvement in the pituitary-adrenocortical response to stress stimuli. Am. J. Physiol. 172:515.
Sétáló, G., Flerkó, B., Arimura, A., and Schally, A. V., 1978, Brain cells as producers of releasing and inhibiting hormones, Int. Rev. Cytol. Suppl. 7:1.
Shen, C. L., 1983, Efferent projections from the mammillary complex of the guinea pig: An autoradiographic study, Brain Res. Bull. 11:43.
Swanson, L. W., Sawchenko, P. E., Rivier, J., and Vale, W. W., 1983, Organization of ovine corticotropin--releasing immunoreactive cells and fibers in the rat brain: An immunohistochemical study. Neuroendocrinology 36:165.
Vale, W., Spiess, J., Rivier, C., and Rivier, J., 1981, Characterization of a 41-residue ovine hypothalamic peptide that stimulates secretion of corticotropin and ß-endorphin. Science 213:1394.
Vale, W., Rivier, C., Brown, M.R., Spiess, J., Koob, G., Swanson, L., Bilezikjian, L., Bloom, F., and Rivier, J., 1983, Chemical and biological characterization of corticotropin releasing factor, Recent Progr. Hormone Res. 39:245.
Voloshin, L., Joseph, S. A., and Knigge, K. M., 1968, Endocrine function in male rats following complete and partial isolation of the hypothalamo-pituitary unit. Neuroendocrinology 3:387.

ROLE OF NEUROTRANSMITTERS AND ELECTROPHYSIOLOGICAL CHANGES IN THE HYPOTHALAMUS RELATED TO CENTRAL ADRENOCORTICAL REGULATION

Shaul Feldman and David Saphier

Department of Neurology
Hadassah University Hospital and Hebrew University-Hadassah Medical School
Jerusalem, Israel

Because afferent neural inputs to the hypothalamus modify considerably the secretion of the adrenal cortex, this laboratory has been involved in the elucidation of the neural pathways which mediate the adrenocortical responses following the stimulation of a variety of afferent stimuli. More recently we have tried to determine the possible role of neurotransmitters involved in the mediation of these responses. In view of the fact that neural stimuli, which produce ACTH secretion, cause also changes in the electrical activity of hypothalamic neurons, we have recently studied in paraventricular nucleus (PVN), which plays a central role in this mechanism, possible electrophysiological correlates of neuroendocrine phenomena in acute and chronic preparations. The purpose of this article is to review briefly previous studies and to describe more recent experiments in the above mentioned areas.

1. Effect of Neural Stimuli on Adrenocortical Responses and the Pathways Involved

Numerous studies have demonstrated that extrahypothalamic structures are involved in the transmission or modulation of adrenocortical responses (Feldman, 1981). In our previous experiments in rats, it was found, that stimulation of afferent sensory modalities, i.e. photic, acoustic, sciatic nerve or olfactory stimulation, as well as the electrical stimulation of the frontal cortex, hippocampus, septum, midbrain reticular formation, or amygdala in the rat, will cause an initial rise in plasma corticosterone (CS). Partial

This research has been supported by the Lena P. Harvey Endowment Fund for Neurological Research.

hypothalamic deafferentations, and limbic extrahypothalamic lesions have a differential effect on the adrenocortical response following the stimulation of these various modalities. These studies have shown that the effects of photic and acoustic stimuli were mediated by the medial forebrain bundle (MFB) and by posterior inputs to the hypothalamus, while the responses following sciatic and olfactory stimuli involved forebrain limbic structures and an anterior hypothalamic input. The limbic pathways involved are the ventral hippocampus, fimbria and the medial septal nucleus for the somatosensory and amygdala and stria terminalis for the olfactory modalities (Feldman and Conforti, 1980a, 1980b). Direct measurements of ACTH secretion following sensory stimuli in intact and brain lesioned rats, have confirmed the data obtained with CS determinations indicating that the sensory modalities do not stimulate the adrenal cortex by a direct neural input, but through the hypothalamo-pituitary-adrenal axis (Feldman et al., 1981; Siegel et al., 1980, 1981). These experiments have thus demonstrated that the four sensory modalities studied, utilize different neural pathways for the activation of the ACTH response.

For the study of the pathways by which limbic structures project to the hypothalamus, chronically implanted electrodes were introduced into the dorsal or ventral hippocampus, medial septal nucleus, the basolateral amygdala, or the midbrain reticular formation. Both anterior and posterior hypothalamic deafferentations diminshed very significantly the rise in plasma CS levels following the stimulation of the above limbic structures, while the adrenocortical response to ether stress in these animals remained intact (Feldman et al., 1982).

In our previous studies, we have found that anterior hypothalamic deafferentation does not abolish the adrenocortical response to ether stress, while other investigators have reported that such a cut with a knife with a diameter of 1.9 mm will block this response (Makara et al., 1980). One of the reasons for this descrepency may be the fact that we have used a knife with a diameter of 1.4 mm only. Such deafferentation may spare the afferent corticotropin releasing factor (CRF) fibers which project from the PVN to the median eminence and enter the mediobasal hypothalamus (MBH) from the MFB more posterolaterally, beyond the extent of our deafferentation. Another factor maybe the time which elapsed between the deafferentation and the stress. We have found that while one week after anterior hypothalamic deafferentation with a wide knife the adrenocortical response was suppressed, it returned to normal after four weeks. This phenomenon has been described in deafferented rats in which a small gap in the cut has remained (Makara et al., 1980). The possibility, that there remained a few unsevered fibers at the base of the brain cannot be discounted also in our experiments. At any rate, we find that in our hands the preparation with partial hypothalamic deafferentations is very useful in differentiating the neural pathways involved in the mediation of adrenocortical responses to a variety of peripheral and central neural stimuli.

The significant finding in the above studies, that posterior hypothalamic deafferentation blocked the adrenocortical response to forebrain limbic stimulation would indicate the importance of neural afferents impinging upon the hypothalamus from the caudal direction. It is also possible, that in order to obtain a full adrenocortical response following stimulation, of forebrain limbic structures which innervate the hypothalamus from the rostral direction, a tonic caudal neural input is essential (Feldman et al., 1982).

In view of the fact that the MFB is a major fiber system which conducts impulses in both anterior and posterior directions, its possible role in the propagation of cortical and limbic influences on CS secretion was studied. It was found that bilateral MFB lesions had no effect on the adrenocortical responses following ventral hippocampal or septal stimulation, but they were very significantly depressed following the stimulation of the frontal cortex, dorsal hippocampus, basolateral amygdala, or the midbrain reticular formation. (Feldman et al., 1983; Feldman and Conforti, 1984). Thus, it is evident that the MFB has a major, thou a differential role, in the transmission of afferent impulses to the hypothalamus which cause an increase in CS secretion.

Recent studies have emphasized the role of CRF in the PVN in the regulation of ACTH secretion and the importance of the retrochiasmatic area as the major afferent input to the median eminence in the mediation of adrenocortical responses to stressful stimuli (Antoni et al., 1983). However, undoubtedly other factors are also involved in this mechanism. Among them, as evident from our studies, is the conduction of impulses along the MFB, as well as a posterior input to the hypothalamus. This pathway seems to be essential for the activation of the hypothalamo-pituitary-adrenal axis in response to some specific neural stimuli. Some of the described afferents in our experiments are related to MBH. However, recent studies (Sawchenko and Swanson, 1983) indicate that the MBH nuclei project to the PVN region in which are located CRF-containing cells, which send their axons to the median eminence. Thus, extrahypothalamic impulses which increase ACTH secretion may reach the PVN CRF-secreting neurons via the MBH.

2. Role of Neurotransmitters in Adrenocortical Secretion

There exists an extensive literature dealing with the role of neurotransmitters in adrenocortical secretion (Weiner and Ganong, 1978). However, there is considerable controversy in this area. Various discrepencies in the literature on the effects of a given neurotransmitter administered systemically or locally, maybe the result of different methodological approaches, such as the site and time of drug administration, age, sex, species and end point of pituitary-adrenal functions studied (Krieger, 1973).

Concerning the role of norepinephrine (NE) in the rat, the evidence in favour of inhibition of ACTH secretion includes the finding that alpha-methyltyrosine, which is a catecholamine synthesis inhibitor, phentolamine, the alpha-adrenergic blocking agent, as well as reserpine, which depletes brain NE, all increase ACTH secretion (Weiner and Ganong, 1978). In vitro studies have also demonstrated the inhibitory effect of NE, as it abolished the stimulatory effect of acetylcholine on CRF release (Jones et al., 1976). As most reported studies have used systemic or intraventricular administration, and in view of our interest to identify the neurotransmitter involved in specific neural pathways, we have used the topical injection of 6-hydroxydopamine (6-OHDA) into the brain. The rats which received bilateral 6-OHDA injections in the MFB two weeks previously, showed a reduction of about 60% in hypothalamic NE as compared to vehicle injected animals, However, there was no change in the concentration of hypothalamic dopamine (Feldman, et al., 1983). In preliminary studies it was found that in these animals the adrenocortical response to ether stress and to acoustic and sciatic nerve stimulation remained intact. However, this response to photic stimulation was decreased significantly when compared to intact rats (Feldman et al., 1984a).

Subsequently, we have studied plasma CS and serum ACTH levels in vehicle and 6-OHDA injected rats into the MFB at 0 time and 2,4,10 and 30 min following the onset of 4/sec photic stimulation.

As evident from Figs. 1 and 2 the basal CS and ACTH levels were very significantly ($p < 0.01$ and < 0.001, respectively) elevated in the rats which received 6-OHDA, when compared to the control vehicle injected animals. Fig 1 demonstrates the significant increase in the plasma CS levels at 2,4,10 and 30 min following the onset of photic stimulation in the vehicle injected rats, when compared with the basal level. On the other hand, in the 6-OHDA injected animals there was no significant change at 2 and 4 min as the result of photic stimulation and significant increase in the plasma CS occurred only at 10 and 30 min in relation to the basal level (Fig. 1). As evident from Fig. 2, there was a very significant increase in serum ACTH levels at 2 min following onset of photic stimulation in the vehicle injected rats and it remained significantly elevated approximately at the same level at 4, 10 and 30 min when compared to the basal value. Contrary to this finding in the 6-OHDA injected rats, at 2 min there was a significant decrease in serum ACTH level, and reduced levels in comparison to the basal value persisted at 10 and 30 min following the onset of photic stimulation (Feldman et al., 1984b).

The destruction of the NE fibers in the MFB produced two phenomena, namely a marked elevation of the basal ACTH and CS levels, and an inhibition in ACTH and CS responses to photic stimulation.

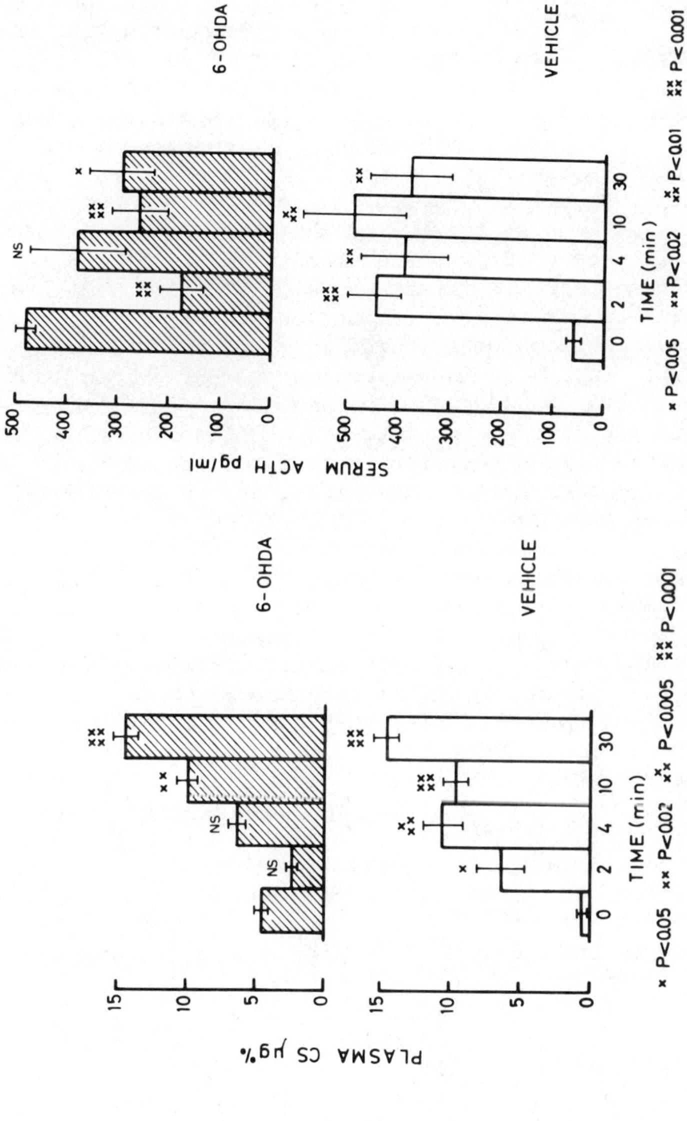

Fig. 1 & 2. Plasma CS and serum ACTH concentrations in rats with bilateral MFB injections of vehicle or 6-OHDA before and 2,4,10 and 30 min following the onset of photic stimulation.
Number of animals tested was 5-7 per point (Feldman et al., 1984b).

The first phenomenon is probably related to the reported tonic inhibitory effect of a central NE system on ACTH secretion (Weiner and Ganong, 1978). This is based on experiments in which it was found that the injection of 6-OHDA into the ventral NE bundle, or the third ventricle produced a transient increase in basal plasma CS levels (Cuello et al., 1974;Fuxe et al., 1973). The second finding is the delayed reponse of the plasma CS following photic stimulation in rats with 6-OHDA injection, when compared with the vehicle injected rats. This inhibitionin response was also observed in the serum ACTH levels. In fact, the post-stimulation levels in the 6-OHDA injected rats, were even reduced in comparison to the basal ACTH levels. We have no explanation, at the present time, for this phenomenon. A similar finding was observed in rats with hypothalamic deafferentation following photic stimulation (Siegal et al., 1980), and maybe also related to the reduced content of NE in the hypothalamic island (Brownstein et al., 1976). These results thus indicate that the intactness of the hypothalamic NE system in general and possible the conduction, in NE MFB fibers, play a role in the mediation of ACTH and CS responses following photic stimulation, Though, 6-OHDA inhibited markedly both ACTH and CS secretion, there was a delayed plasma CS response, which was not accompanied by a corresponding increase in ACTH secretion. This may suggest that in addition to the ACTH mediated effect on CS, there may also be a direct hypothalamic influence on the adrenal cortex (Holzwarth et al., 1980).

In view of our earlier studies on the role of the medial septal nucleus, in the transmission of somatosensory impulses to the hypothalamus we have injected 6-OHDA into this area and studied the effects of photic and sciatic nerve stimulation on adrenocortical responses. As evident from Fig. 3 the response to photic stimulation was not affected, while the rise in plasma CS following sciatic nerve stimulation was inhibited significantly when compared with the vehicle injected rats. This would indicate that NE has a role in the mediation of this adrenocortical response via the septum.

Recent studies attributed a central role to the dorsal medial parvocellular part of the PVN in the regulation of ACTH secretion as it is the major source of CRF containing neurons which send their axons to the median eminence. (Swanson et al., 1983). Electrolytic lesions of the PVN have been reported to block ACTH secretion following stressful stimuli (Bruhn et al., 1984). To investigate the possibility that NE plays a role in the neuroendocrine mechanisms related to ACTH secretion in the parvocellular PVN we have studied the effects of 6-OHDA injected into this region. The neurotoxin caused a depletion of NE of about 60% in the PVN, but only of 30% in the MBH. As evident from Fig. 4 the basal plasma CS was significantly elevated in the 6-OHDA injected rats. The adrenocortical responses following ether stress, photic, acoustic

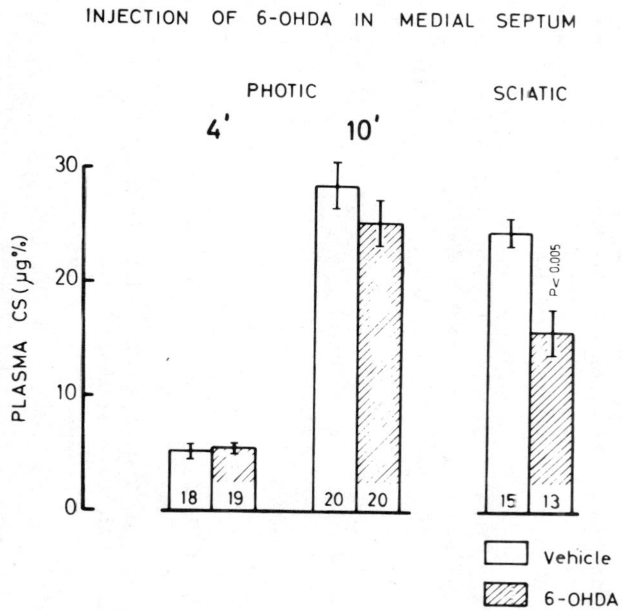

Fig. 3 Plasma CS concentration in rats with vehicle or 6-OHDA injection into the medial septal nucleus 4 and 10 min following onset of photic and sciatic nerve stimulation Number of animals indicated.

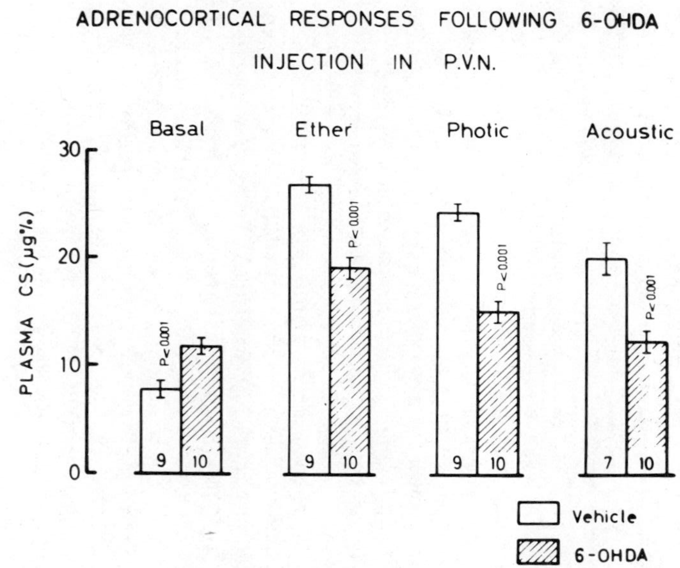

Fig. 4 Plasma CS concentration in rats with bilateral injection of vehicle or 6-OHDA into the PVN under basal conditions and following ether stress or photic and acoustic stimulation.

and sciatic nerve stimulation, were all significantly inhibited in these animals, when compared with the vehicle injected rats.

Though the inhibition of adrenocortical secretion was not as drastic as reported in rats with the destruction of the PVN the present preliminary data would suggest that NE participates, at least partially, in the release of CRF in the PVN, under basal conditions and following stressful stimuli.

Another aspect of NE involvement in adrenocortical regulation which we have studied is its modulation of glucocorticoid negative feedback effects. The site of the negative feedback have been the subject of numerous studies and it is now clear that the effect is exerted both at the level of the pituitary and the hypothalamus. Recent evidence also indicates that dexamethasone (dex) inhibites the secretion of CRF in the portal circulation of the rat following haemorrage (Plotsky and Vale, 1984). Previous experiments have suggested that extrahypothalamic structures are involved in the feedback effect of dex upon the adrenocortical response to ether stress (Feldman and Conforti, 1976; 1980). Thus, we have demonstrated that posterior hypothalamic deafferentation, dorsal hippocampectomy or dorsal fornix section, reduce the inhibitory effect of dex on the CS response to ether stress, while bilateral MFB lesions enhanced the suppressive effect of the glucocorticoid. These experiments suggested the existance of extrahypothalamic regions with tonically facilitatory or inhibitory effects which altered the sensitivity of the hypothalamus to feedback action of glucocorticoid hormones.

In view of the chemical heterogenicity of the MFB (Nieuwenhuys, 1982) we have attempted to determine which of the MFB fibers are involved. Therefore, we have studied the dex negative feedback effects on the adrenocortical response following ether stress in rats with 6-OHDA or vehicle injected into the MFB. As evident from Fig. 5, in animals in which the NE fibers were destroyed, the efficiency of the dex feedback action was enhanced, similar to the results obtained with MFB electrolytic lesions. Thus, these results indicate that the NE fibers are, at least partially, responsible for the MFB mediated modulation of hypothalamic sensitivity to glucocorticoid hormones.

Review of the literature concerning the role of serotonin (5-HT) in the rat, reports effects of stimulation, inhibition or no effect at all on ACTH secretion. (Weiner and Ganong, 1978; Karteszi et al., 1981). The evidence that central release of 5-HT stimulates CRF secretion, is based on the findings that its precursor 5-hydroxytryptophane increases ACTH secretion and intraventricular administration of 5-HT has the same effect. The addition of 5-HT to incubated hypothalamus, also causes an increase in CRF secretion (Jones et al., 1976). Other investigators have reported however, that 5-HT implants in the hypothalamus or intraventricular

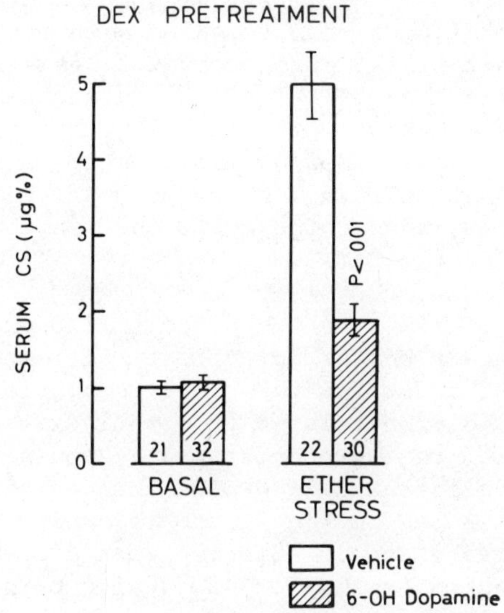

Fig. 5 Basal and ether stress induced serum CS levels in vehicle or 6-OHDA injected animals 4 h subsequent to administration of 10 µg i.p. of dex (Feldman et al., 1983).

administration of 5-HT inhibits ACTH secretion and p-chlorophenylalanine, a serotonin depleting drug, enhanced the increase in ACTH production by ether stress or electric shock. Also, stimulation of the raphe nuclei decreased stress responses while lesions of this region had an opposite effect. As mentioned above, there are probably different reasons for these discrepencies and these may also be related to the fact that different stressful stimuli were studied. To examine the possibility that 5-HT has a differential role in the mediation of impulses which produce ACTH secretion, we have studied the effects of ether stress and of photic, acoustic and sciatic nerve stimulation on adrenocortical responses in rats which were injected with either vehicle or with 5,7-dihydroxytryptamine (5,7-DHT) into the dorsal and median raphe nuclei two weeks previously. The injection of the neurotoxin resulted in a depletion of 72% of 5-HT in the hypothalamus when compared with controls. The 5-HT depletion did not affect the adrenocortical response to ether stress or to acoustic stimulation at 4 and 10 min after stimulus onset, as well as to the stimulation of the sciatic nerve. However, the rise in plasma CS levels following photic stimulation, both at 4 and 10 min after the onset of stimulus, was significantly reduced in the 5,7-DHT injected rats, when compared to the vehicle injected animals (Feldman et al., 1984c).

Thus, it is of interest that hypothalamic depletion of NE or 5-HT had only an effect on the adrenocortical response to photic stimulation, without affecting the other modalities studies. This phenomenon may possibly be related to our finding that MFB electrolytic lesions blocked the adrenocortical response to photic stimulation. In the instance of 6-OHDA the neurotoxin was injected directly into the MFB destroying NE fibers, while the administration of 5,7-DHT in the raphe nuclei affected most probably also the 5-HT axons in the MFB, which is a major projection pathway of this neurotransmitter. If this is the case, then it can be assumed that the neurotoxic lesions of the NE and 5-HT fibers in the MFB,which normally innervate the PVN (Palkovits et al., 1977; Moore and Kromer, 1978) can affect directly the function of the CRF cells in this region.

3. Electrophysiological Correlates of Neuroendocrine Secretion

As previously discussed, the location of the CRF cell bodies within the hypothalamus of the rat appears to be principally within the dorsal medial parvocellular components of the PVN. We have recently made a study, in an acute model, of the activity of PVN neurones following stimulation of central and peripheral neural structures. The secretion of ACTH from the anterior pituitary gland is probably dependent on the electrical activity of hypothalamic CRF-neurones of the tuberoinfundibular system, axons of which terminate in the region of the hypophyseal portal vessels. Our studies have attempted to correlate the electrical activity of PVN neurones in response to peripheral and central stimuli, with changes in adrenocortical secretion following stimulation of the same modalities.

Anatomical studies have demonstrated the presence of preoptic area (POA) efferent projections to the PVN (Conrad and Pfaff, 1975) and stimulation of this area has been shown to cause an increase in adrenocortical secretory activity (Redgate and Fahringer, 1973).

Similarly, projections have been demonstrated as arising from the subiculum (SUB) (Silverman and Oldfield, 1984) although stimulation of this site has been shown to produce variable effects on adrenocortical secretion (Dunn and Orr, 1984). These were therefore two of the sites chosen for stimulation in this study. The choice of nucleus accumbens (ACB) as the third central site of stimulation was from the anatomical evidence of extensive efferent projections from this region terminating in POA, PVN and other hypothalamic structures (Koikegami et al., 1967). Furthermore, Joseph and Knigge,(1983) have demonstrated the presence of substantial numbers of CRF-immunoreactive cell bodies within ACB. Photic stimulation (PHO) and electrical stimulation of the sciatic nerve (ScN)with short trains of stimuli were also employed. Such stimuli, as discussed in a previous section, are able to elicit increases in adrenocortical secretory activity.

In order to ascertain that some of the neurones recorded in our study were presumed neurosecretory cells of the tuberinfundibular system, a transpharyngeal approach to the hypothalamus was employed and a stimulating electrodewas placed on the median eminence (ME) in order to antidromically identify neurones as projecting to this region. Standard testing criteria to obtain this electroanatomical data were employed. In brief, constant latency of the antidromic action potential following the stimulus and the ability of the cell to generate, at constant latency, antidromic action potentials following delivery of short trains of high frequency stimulation (frequency following). A third test criterion for spontaneously active units was also employed, when an orthodromic action potential, used to trigger the stimulator, was tested for the ability to collide with and cancel out the antidromic action potential thus generated. Using this technique of antidromic identification, a measure of success has been achieved in the characterization of tuberoinfundibular neurone function and the correlation of their unit activity during the stimulated release of some anterior pituitary hormones (Dyer and Saphier, 1981; Saphier and Dyer, 1980; 1981). Numerous cell bodies of the PVN magnocellular neurones are known to send axon projections to the neurohypophysis (PIT) and secrete vasopressin and oxytocin, therefore an electrode was also palced in the neural stalk to enable the antidromic identification of such cells. (Fig. 6).

A total of 122 cells, later histologically shown to be primarily within the dorsal medial components of PVN, were recorded from. Of these, seventeen (14%) were antidromically identified as projecting to ME. These cells were found to have a significantly ($p < 0.005$) slower firing rate than those adjacent to them and were also located significantly ($p < 0.002$) closer to the base of the brain than those belonging to the tuberohypophyseal system and antidromically identified as projecting to PIT. ACB stimulation was found to evoke orthodromic inhibitory responses from 42% of the cells tested, seven

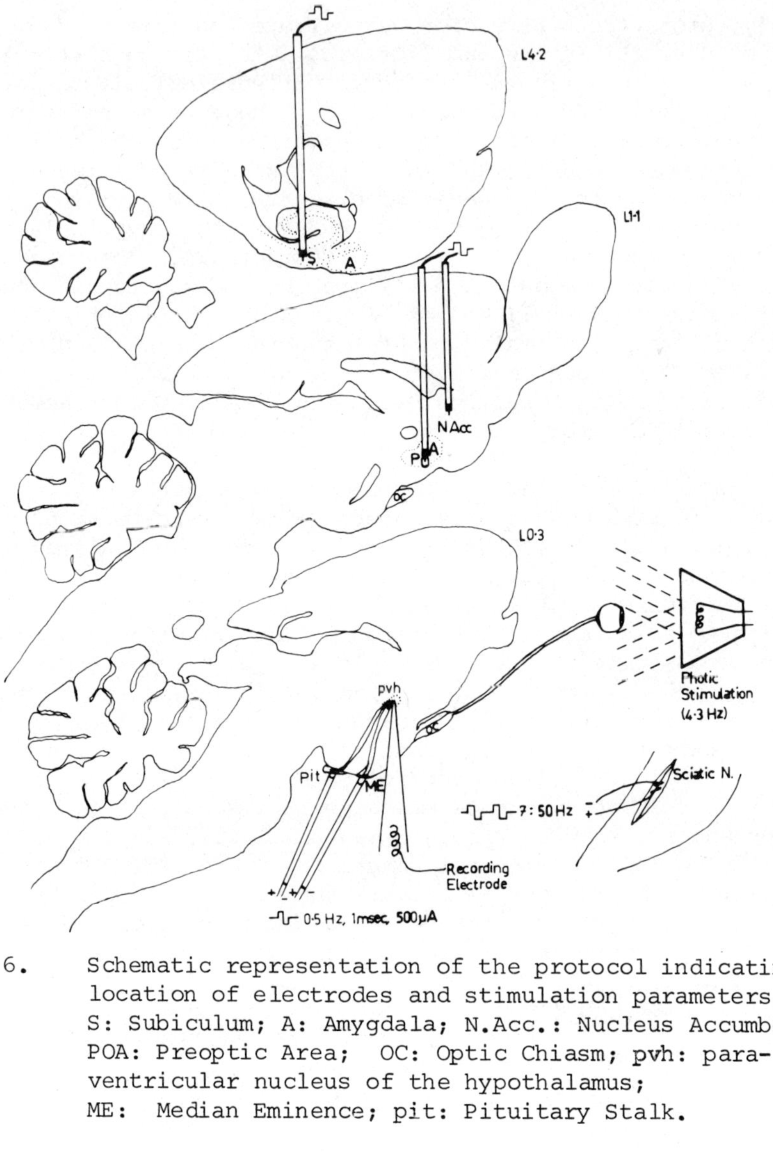

Fig. 6. Schematic representation of the protocol indicating location of electrodes and stimulation parameters. S: Subiculum; A: Amygdala; N.Acc.: Nucleus Accumbens; POA: Preoptic Area; OC: Optic Chiasm; pvh: paraventricular nucleus of the hypothalamus; ME: Median Eminence; pit: Pituitary Stalk.

out of ten responses of the identified cells showing an inhibition. Stimulation of POA evoked equal numbers of inhibitory and excitatory orthodromic responses from the cells tested, all five responsive cells identified as projecting to ME were facilitated by POA stimulation. Stimulation of SUB evoked predominantly (52%) excitatory responses from the unidentified cells, and, once again, only facilitation from identified neurones.

ScN and PHO stimulation were found to evoke excitatory responses from 34% and 45% of PVN neurones, respectively. The proportion of such responses recorded from neurones antidromically identified as projecting to ME following this stimuli was even greater, i.e. eleven out of fifteen responsive units. There was also a high degree of response convergence following these stimuli ($p < 0.001$). Convergence of responses, following stimulation of central brain sites, upon both the identified and unidentified cells, was also significant ($p < 0.001$; $p < 0.025$, respectively). Fig. 7 shows the responses of a typical cell identified as projecting to ME.

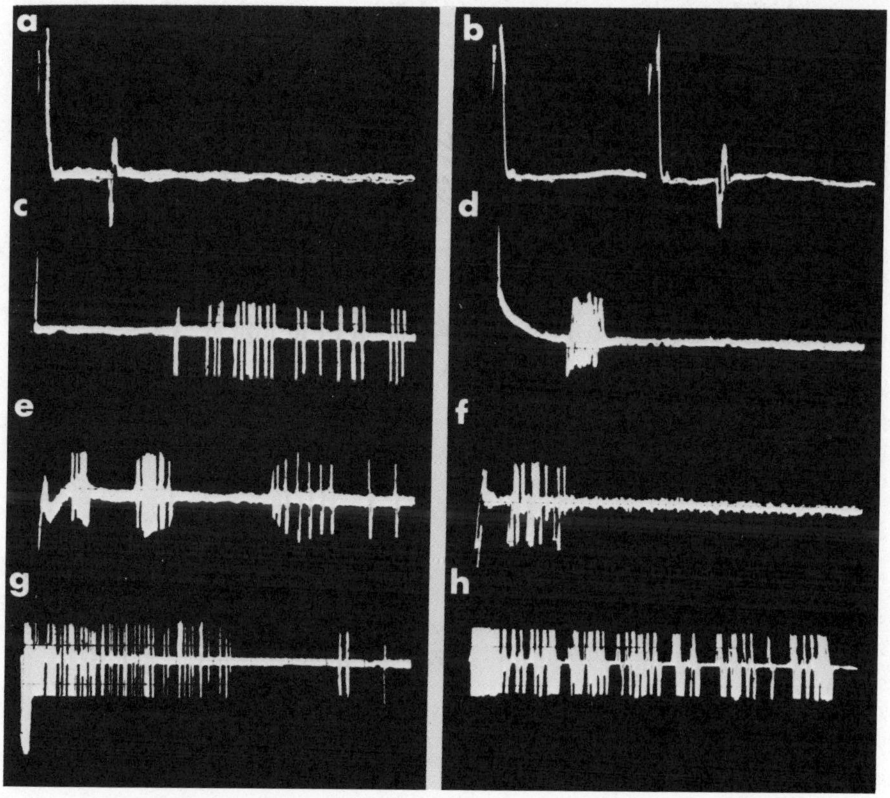

Fig. 7. Cell recorded from the PVN and antidromically identified as projecting to ME by constant latency (a) and collision testing (b). The cell was orthodromically inhibited following stimulation of ACB (c) and excited by POA (d), SUB (e), PIT (f), ScN (g) and Photic (h) stimulation. Full-sweep time bases; a,b,d,e; 50ms; c,f,h: 100ms; g: 2s. Minimum of 15 sweeps per test.

An interesting observation was made concerning PVN cells projecting to ME when recorded following PIT stimulation. This was that orthodromically influenced cells showed more excitatory than inhibitory responses (3:1) following stimulation of this site. For some time it has been known that vasopressin is able to act synergistically to increase release of ACTH from the pituitary gland and it had been suggested that vasopressin was CRF (Gillies and Lowry, 1982). Leng (1981) has suggested that recurrent orthodromic pathways thought to exist within supraoptic nucleus (SON) neurones projecting to PIT and detected following antidromic invasion may instead be due to the antidromic invasion of many SON neurones followed by a complex intranuclear "crosstalk". If this is the case, then the orthodromic reponses recorded from the putative CRF-neurones in our study may be due to such an invasion of magnocellular PVN neurones. This could then be followed by orthodromic communication between these and the antidromically activated vasopressin or oxytocin-secreting neurones. Such a suggestion raises the possibility that the action of vasopressin in effecting ACTH secretion exists not only at the level of the pituitary gland but perhaps also at a neural level.

We were not able to measure the endocrine effects of the various stimuli in the same preparation, as the rats were highly stressed by the surgical procedure. However,in an attempt to correlate the data obtained with any effects upon adrenocortical secretion, electrical stimulation of the same sites was performed in conscious animals. These were chronically implanted with jugular cannulae and electrodes in the relevant sites, i.e. POA, ACB and SUB, Photic stimulation was also employed, the frequency of light flashes being 4.3Hz in a darkened room . Electrical stimulation was as for the electrophysiological tests (bipolar square-wave pulses of lmsec total duration and lmA peak to peak current strength) but delivered at a frequency of 50Hz for ten out of every twenty seconds for a total of 15 mins. The effects of these stimuli on plasma CS concentrations are illustrated in Fig. 8. It can be seen that all the stimuli were able to elicit an increase in plasma CS levels relative to the control, unstimulated, animals with the notable exception of ACB. From the data of the electrophysiological study, it will be recalled that ACB was the only site from which excitatory synaptic inputs were not demonstrated as projecting to the PVN neurones antidromically identified as projecting to ME. The other sites of stimulation producing orthodromic activation of these cells.

Thus, in view of the correlation of effects of stimulation of these sites upon plasma CS levels and the activity of the PVN neurones observed, it is possible that the electrical activity recorded may have been that of CRF-secreting neurones.

In a further attempt to correlate the release of CS with unit activity of neurones in the regions of PVN known to contain

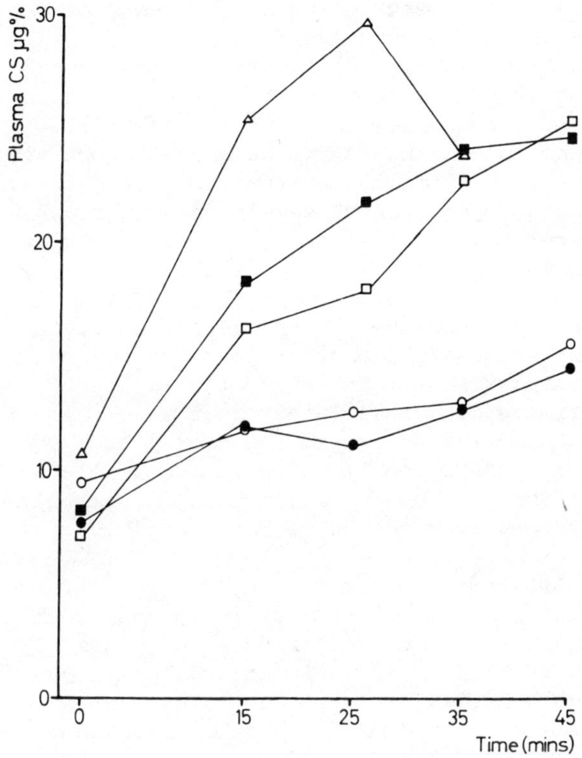

Fig. 8. Plasma corticosterone concentrations in conscious unrestrained male rats following photic stimulation (open triangles) and electrical stimulation of POA (open squares,) SUB (closed squares), ACB (closed circles) or in control animals (open circles). Stimulation applied for 15 min following the first sample.

CRF cells bodies, we have carried out a series of experiments in the conscious animal. Male rats were used for the experiemnts, a stimulating electrode being implanted, under pentobarbitone anaesthesia, into the POA whilst an array of 5-7 fine-wire recording electrodes were lowered into the region of the parvocellular PVN where we previously recorded cells antidromically identified as projecting to ME in the acute electrophysiological study. A chronic indwelling jugular cannula was also implanted to allow for blood sampling stimultaneous with electrophysiological testing. After a suitable recovery period of one to two weeks, with regular injections of heparin to maintain the patency of the cannula, the animals were removed to a conscious-recording cage and the electrode plug attached to a swivelling lead-holder to allow the animal to move about freely. All leads were led to a conventional electronic recording and stimulating system. In this way, we were able to record multi-unit activity. Using differntial recording from two of the wires, 36 records were made of multiple unit activity. After discrimination of a suitable single unit, its spontaneous electrical activity was recorded for up to two hours. A blood sample was then removed from the indwelling cannula and recording continued for a further 30 minutes, when another sample was withdrawn. Stimulation was then delivered for four minutes (50Hz; 1msec pulses; 10sec on: 10sec off) at a low enough current strength not to evoke any behavioral reactions from the animal. During this time the discriminated activity of the selected neurone was recorded and upon cessation of the stimulation another blood sample was removed. Further blood samples were then taken, ten and thirty minutes from the onset of stimulation. Immediately following removal of each blood sample, plasma was separated and stored at -20°C for subsequent estimation of CS concentrations. The cellular fraction of each sample was resuspended in warm physiological saline and reinjected after removal of the subsequent sample.

Of the 36 experiments carried out, 21 (58%) of the records showed an overall increase in unit activity during stimulation of POA, whereas inhibition occurred in only 10 cases (28%). The mean firing rate was doubled during stimulation ($p < 0.005$) and after cessation of the stimulation there was a rebound inhibition, such that the firing rate dropped significantly from that recorded prior to stimulation ($p < 0.05$). These results were even more significant considering just those records in which excitation was recorded, firing rate increasing during stimulation of about 300%. Fig. 9 shows polygraph records of the electrical activity of four PVN neurones excited during the periods of POA stimulation. The level of activation during stimulation being greatest for the unit displayed in the top trace and least for the one in the lower trace. What may also be seen is the tendency for some of the units to discharge in bursting pattern of firing similar to that of mediobasal hypothalamic neurones observed previously(Saphier and Dyer, 1980).

The stimulation was also shown to be effective in causing a release of CS, plasma concentrations rising sharply following the onset of stimulation. Thus, for seven individual animals, the plasma concentrations of CS and the activity of the recorded units are shown in Fig. 10. The activity of units and plasma CS concentrations from a group of control, unstimulated, animals during the same time period is also shown. It is evident that only during the four minutes of stimulation is there a significant rise in the rate of electrical discharge. This is followed by a decrease in firing rate that parallels the measured increases in plasma CS levels. Indeed, at the last point of measurement, 30 min after the onset of stimulation, the firing rate is significantly decreased and this

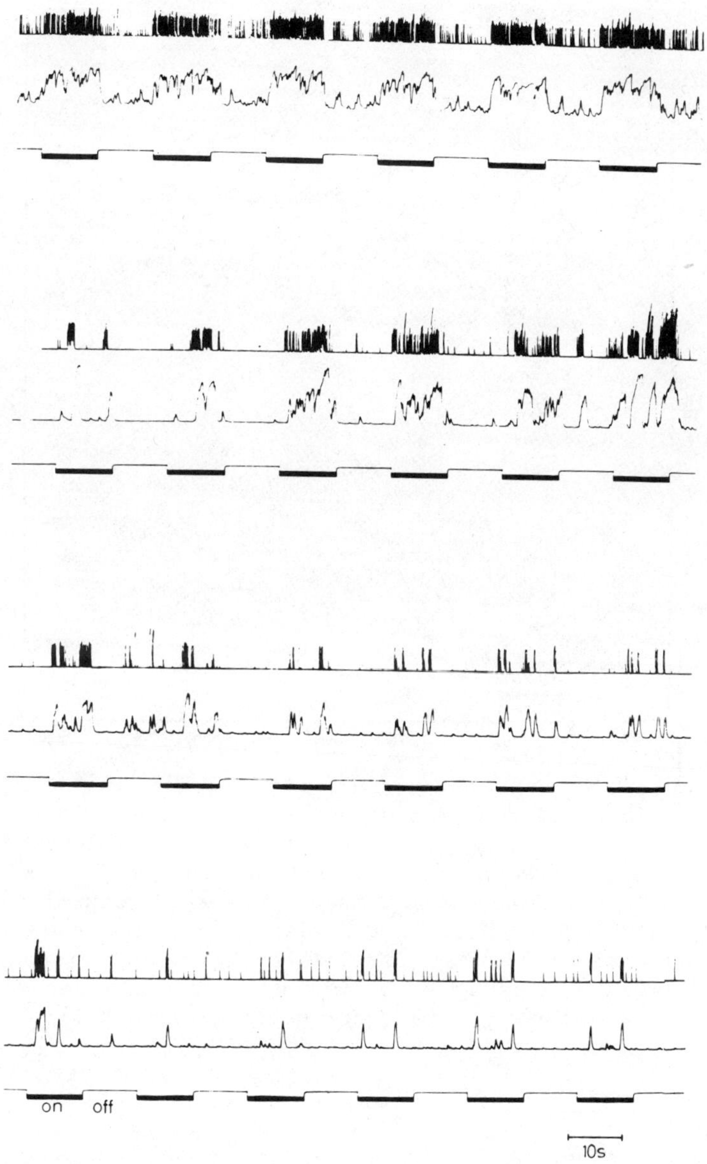

Fig. 9 Polygraph records showing the effects of 50Hz stimulatio of POA on the firing of single PVN neurones in each of four conscious unrestrained rats, Top trace of each record shows unit activity; middle trace shows integrated record of unit activity; lower trace indicates on:off mode of stimulation.

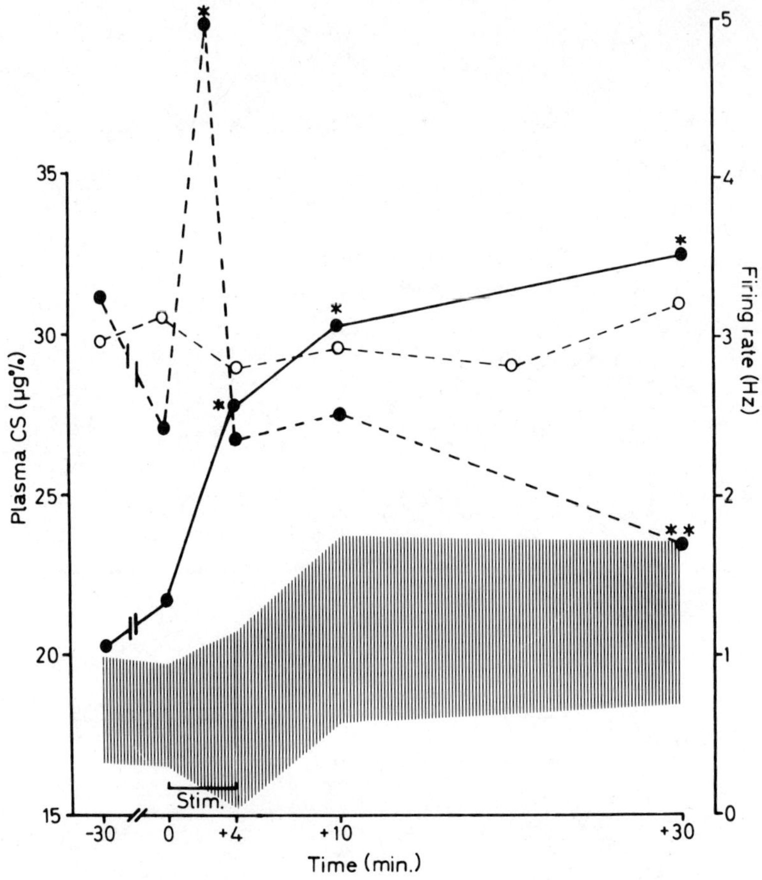

Fig. 10 Effects of four min of electrical stimulation (50Hz; 10s on: 10s off) delivered to POA on firing rate (dotted line, closed circles) of PVN neurones and on plasma CS levels (solid line, closed circles). Control firing rate for the same time period in unstimulated animals (dotted line, open circles) and plasma CS concentratins (mean ± standard error: shaded area) are also shown. *p < 0.05; **p < 0.01 for seven experimental animals.

may represent a negative feedback effect of CS exerted upon the electrical activity of these PVN neurones (Feldman, 1983).

The present experiments demonstrate parallel changes relating increases in PVN unit activity and rises in plasma CS levels. This may represent an electrophysiological correlate of neuroendocrine regulation by CRF-secreting PVN neurones of adrenocortical secretory activity.

4. Electrophysiological Connections of the PVN with Forebrain Limbic Areas: Effects of Adrenocorticoid Hormones

A number of forebrain limbic stuructures have been implicated in the regulation of adrenococtical secretory activity. The involvement of the cingulate cortex (CC) has been evidenced and the stimulation of this and other cortical regions has been shown to elicit an elevation of plasma CS levels, as discussed in section 1. Similarly, the involvement of POA, ACB and the lateral septum (LS) in adrenocortical regulation have also been reported. The precise nature of the neural information arising from these areas has not been examined closely. This experiment was designed in order to improve our knowledge in this area.

Records were made of single unit activity in adrenalectomized male rats anaesthetized with urethane. A bipolar stimulating electrode was placed in the PVN in order to deliver stimuli to this site, as previously detailed. The responses, to single shocks delivered to PVN, of neurones located within CC, LS, POA, bed nucleus of the stria terminalis (BST) and the nucleus proprioris commisurae/nucleus accumbens (BCA/ABC) were recorded from a total of 305 single units. The primary responses of neurones being shown in Table 1. Non-responsive units are not shown.

Table 1. Responses of Neurones Located Within Forebrain Limbic Structures Following Stimulation of PVN.

Location of cells	(No.)	Antidromically identified	Orthodromically excited	Orthodromically inhibited
CC	(72)	19	33	12
LS	(103)	41	45	11
BST	(23)	7	10	6
BCA/ACB	(25)	4	8	11
POA	(83)	33	27	20

The large proportion of antidromically identified neurones indicates that extensive PVN afferent projections arise from all the regions examined, 40% of recorded neurones in LS and POA sending projections to PVN. An extensive PVN efferent projection was also demonstrated and mathematical analysis suggests that many of the orthodromic responses recorded at these sites were monosynaptic. Those of an inhibitory nature blocking the generation of spontaneous action potentials on 1:1 basis. These observations indicate a possible involvement of the recorded areas in the neural regulation of adrenocortical activity, as indicated by the antidromically identified cells. The orthodromic responses indicate that PVN neurones project to and influence the activity of other brain sites. Thus, some of the responses of CC cells, as well as those in other regions, may have been mediated by CRF acting as a neurotransmitter, there being a high density of CRF-receptor sites within this region of cortex (Holmes et al., 1984).

Effects of local or humoral administration of adrenocortical steroid hormones on evoked potentials and the electrical activity of single units in hypothalamic and extrahypothalamic brain sites has been studied in our laboratory for a number of years and has

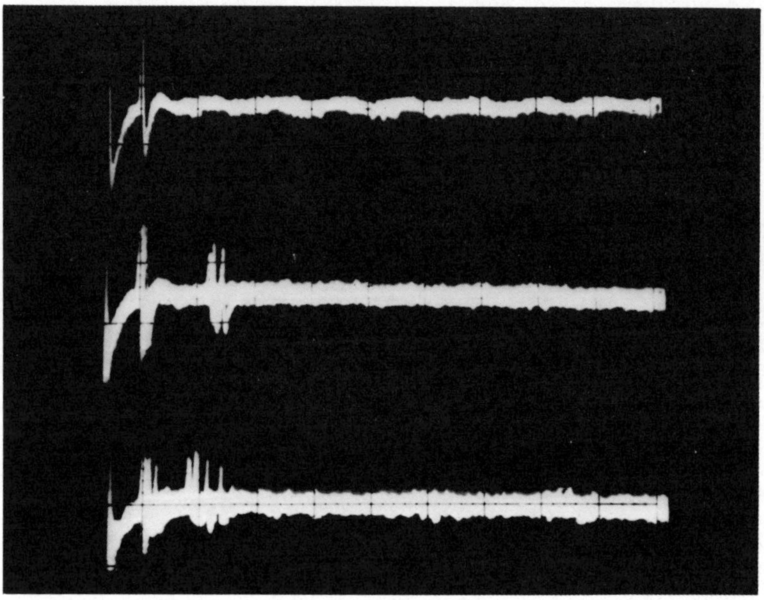

Fig. 11 POA neurone antidromically identified (top trace) as projecting to PVN, recorded in an adrenalectomized rat. Middle trace shows the appearance of orthodromic action potentials 2 mins following i.p. injection of 5 mg Cortisol. Further orthodromic activation and shortening of latency observed 5 mins later in lower trace. Each trace consists of 20 oscilloscope sweeps of 50ms duration.

been reviewed previously (Feldman, 1983). The extrahypothalamic units studied were not identified as projecting to the site of the CRF cell bodies as it was not known where exactly these were to be found. As detailed previously, these have now been shown to be located within the parvocellular components of the PVN. Therefore, we decided to examine the effects of intraperitoneal injection of cortisol on the activity of some of the neurones antidromically identified as projecting to the PVN.

A number of these identified cells also showed orthodromic responses following stimulation of PVN. In the case of four LS and eight POA cells projecting to PVN, examination was made of the activity of such pathways following the i.p. injection of 5 mg cortisol (sodium succinate) to these adrenalectomized animals. Prior to injection, two of the eight POA cells also exhibited an orthodromic excitation following PVN stimulation and two were inhibited orthodromically following the antidromic action potential. Cortisol injection reduced the duration of the inhibition in the latter two cells and increased the post-stimulus excitation in the first two. In a further two examples the appearance of short latency action potentials of synaptic origin, following stimuli delivered to PVN, was observed after the injection. This effect was also recorded for two of the three LS neurones for which stable records were obtained. All cells tested also showed an increase in spontaneous acitivity of up to 500% following injection of cortisol (Fig. 11).

These results suggest that adrenocortical hormones may alter or even activate recurrent synaptic pathways in some POA and LS cells projecting to PVN. Such effects may serve to regulate some aspects of the feedback control of ACTH secretion by glucocorticoid hormones, at a neural level.

REFERENCES

Antoni, F.A., Palkovits, M., Makara, G.B., 1983, Immunoreactive corticotropin releasing hormone in the hypothalamoinfundibular tract. Neuroendocrinology 36:415.

Brownstein, M.J., Palkovits, M., Tappaz, M.L., Saavedra, J.M., and Kizer, S., 1976, Effect of surgical isolation of the hypothalamus on its neurotransmitter content. Brain Res. 117:287.

Bruhn, T.O., Plotsky, M., and Vale, W.W., 1984, Effect of paraventricular lesions on corticotropin-releasing factor (CRF)-like immunoreactivity in the stalk-median eminence: studies on the adrenocorticotropin response to ether stress and exogenous CRF, Endocrinology 114:57.

Conrad, L.C.A., and Pfaff, D.W., 1975, Axonal projections of medial preoptic and anterior hypothalamic neurones, Science,NY 190:1112.

Cuello, A.C., Shoemaker, W.J., and Ganong, W.F., 1974, Effect of 6-hydroxydopamine on hypothalamic norepinephrine and dopamine content, ultrastructure of the median eminence and plasma corticosterone, Brain Res.78:57.

Dunn, J.D., and Orr, S.E., 1984, Differential plasma corticosterone responses to hippocampal stimulation. Exp. Brain Res., 54:1.

Dyer, R.G., and Saphier, D.J., 1981, Electrical activity of antidromically identified tuberoinfundibular neurones during stimulated release of luteinizing hormone and prolactin in prooestrous rats. J. Endocr.89:35.

Feldman, S., 1981, Introduction to The extrahypothalamic structures in neuroendocrine regulation. in: 28th International Congress of Physiological Sciences, E. Stark, G.B. Makara, Ac.Zs. Endroczi, eds., Pergamon Press.

Feldman, S. 1983, Neurophysiological changes in the limbic system related to adrenocortical secretion, in: Integrative Neurohumoral Mechanisms, E. Endroczi, D. de Wied, L. Angelucci, and U. Scapagnini, eds.,Elsevier Science Publishers.

Feldman, S., and Conforti, N., 1976, Inhibition and facilitation of feedback influences of dexamethasone on adrenocortical responses to ether stress in rats with hypothalamic deafferentations and brain lesions, Acta Endocr. Copenh. 82:785.

Feldman, S., and Conforti, N, 1980, Participation of the dorsal hippocampus in the glucocorticoid feedback effect on adrenocortical activity, Neuroendocrinology, 30:52.

Feldman, S., and Conforti, N., 1980a, The role of the medial septal nucleus in mediating adrenocortical responses to somatosensory stimulation, J Neur. Res. 5:19.

Feldman, S., and Conforti, N., 1980b, Inhibition of adrenocortical responses following olfactory stimulation in rats with stria terminalis lesions, Neuroscience, 5:1323.

Feldman, S., and Conforti, N., 1984, Mediation of adrenocortical responses by medial forebrain bundle following frontal cortex stimulation, Isr J Med Sci.,20:449.

Feldman, S., Conforti, N., Chowers, I., and Siegel, R.A., 1981, Effects of sciatic nerve stimulation of ACTH secretion in intact and in variously hypothalamic deafferentated male rats. Exp. Brain Res.42:486.

Feldman, S., Conforti, N., Siegel R.A., 1982, Adrenocortical responses following limbic stimulation in rats with hypothalamic deafferentations. Neuroendocrinlogy,35:205.

Feldman, S., Melamed, E., Conforti, N., and Weidenfeld, J., 1984, Effect of central serotonin depletion on adrenocortical responses to neural stimuli, Exp.Neurol.85: in press.

Feldman, S., Melamed., E., Conforti, N., and Weidenfeld, J, 1984b, Inhibition in corticotrophin and corticosterone secretion following photic stimulation in rats with 6-hydroxydopamine injection into the medial forebrain bundle, J Neurosci.Res. 12:87.

Feldman, S., Siegel, R.A., and Conforti, N., 1983, Differential effects of medial forebrain bundle lesions on adrenocortical responses following limbic stimulation, Neuroscience 9:1.

Feldman, S., Siegel, R.A., Weidenfeld, J., Conforti, N., and Melamed, E., 1983, Role of medial forebrain bundle catecholaminergic fibers in the modulation of glucocorticoid negative feedback effects. Brain Res.260:297.

Feldman, S., Siegel, R.A, Weidenfeld, J., Conforti, N., and Melamed, E., 1984a, Adrenocortical responses to ether stress and neural stimuli in rats following the injection of 6-hydroxydopamine into the medial forebrain bundle. Exp. Neurol.83:215.

Fuxe, K.., Hokfelt, T., Johnsson, G., Levine, S., Lidfriak, P., and Lofstrom., A., 1973, Brain and pituitary-adrenal interactions, studies on central moncamine neurons.in: Brain-Pituitary-Adrenal Interrelationships. Brodish A, and Redgate, E.S., eds., Karger, Basel.

Gillies, G., and Lowry, P.J., 1982, Corticotropin-releasing hormone and its vasopressin component, in: Frontiers in Neuroendocrinology, Ganong, W.F. and Martini, L. eds., Raven Press, New York.

Holmes, M.C., Wynn, P.C., Hauger, R.,L., Millan, MA.., Catt, K.J., and Aguilera, G., 1984, Characterization and localization of corticotropin-releasing factor receptors in the rat brain. Abst#959. 7th Intl. Congr. Endocrinology, Quebec, Canada.

Holzwarth, M., Wilkinson, C.W., Dallman, M.F., 1980, Compensatory adrenal growth in immature and mature male rats. Neuroendocrinology 31:34.

Jones, M.T., Hillhouse, E., and Burden, J., 1976, secretion of corticotropin-releasing hormone in vitro, in: Frontiers in Neuroendocrinology, Martini, L., and Ganong W.F. eds., Raven Press, New York.

Joseph, S.A., and Knigge, K.M., 1983, Corticotropin releasing factor: Immunocytochemical localization in rat brain. Neurosci.Lett. 35:135.

Karteszi, M., Palkovits, M., Kiss, J.Z., Kanyicska, B., Fekete, M.I. K., and Stark, E., 1981, Lack of correlation between hypothalamic serotonin and the ether-induced ACTH secretion in adrenalectomized rats. Neuroendocrinology,32:7.

Koikegami, H., Hirata, Y., and Oguma, J., 1967, Studies on the paralimbic brain structures.Fol.Psych. et Neurol.Jap., 21:151.

Krieger, D.T., 1973, Neurotransmitter regulation of ACTH release, Mt. Sinai J Med.3:302.

Leng.G., 1981, The effects of neural stalk stimulation upon firing patterns in rat supraoptic neurones. Exp. Brain Res.,41:135.

Makara, G.B., Stark, E., and Palkovits, M., 1980, Reevaluation of the pituitary-adrenal response to ether in rats with various cuts around the medial basal hypothalamus, Neuroendocrinology, 30:38.

Moore, R.Y., and Kromer, L.F., 1978, The organization of central catecholamine neuron system,in: Neuropharmacology and Behavior, B. Haber and M.H. Aprison, Eds., Plenum Publishing Corp.

Nieuwenhuys, R.L., Geeraedts, M.G., and Veening, J.G., 1982, The medial forebrain bundle of the rat. I. General Introduction, J. Comp. Neurol. 206:49.

Palkovits, M., Saavedra, J.M., Jacobowitz, D.M., Kizer, J.S., Zaborszky, L., and Brownstein, M.J., 1977, Serotonergic innervation of the forebrain: effect of lesions on serotonin and tryptophane hydroxylase levels, Brain Res.130:121.

Plotsky, O.M., and Vale, W., 1984, Hemorrhage-induced secretion of corticotropin-releasing factor-like immunoreactivity into the rat hypophysial portal circulation and its inhibition by glucocorticoids. Endocrinology 114:164.

Redgate, E.S., and Fahringer, E.E., 1973, A comparison of the pituitary adrenal activity elicited by electrical stimulation of preoptic, amygdaloid and hypothalamic sites in the rat brain Neuroendocrinology, 12:334.

Saphier, D.J., and Dyer, R.G., 1980, Bursting activity in tuberoinfundibular neurones during electrical stimulation of the rostral hypothalamus. Exp. Brain Res.39:113.

Saphier, D.J., and Dyer, R.G., 1981, Effects of neonatal exposure to monosodium glutamate on the electrical activity of neurones in the mediobasal hypothalamus, and on the plasma concentrations of thyroid-stimulating hormone and prolactin, following stimulation of the rostral hypothalamus in adult female rats. J. Endocr.89:379.

Sawchenko, P.E., and Swanson, L.W., 1983, The organization of forebrain afferents to the paraventricular and supraoptic nuclei of the rat. J. Comp. Neurol.218:121.

Siegel,R. A,Chowers, I., Conforti, N., and Feldman, S., 1980, Corticotropin and corticosterone secretory patterns following acute neurogenic stress, in intact and in variously hypothalamic deafferented male rats, Brain Res.188:399.

Siegel, R.A., Chowers, I., Conforti, N., and Feldman, S., 1981, The role of the medial forebrain bundle in the mediation of the hypothalamic-hypophyseal-adrenal reponses to acute neurogenic stress, Brain Res. Bull.6:113.

Silverman, A., J., and Oldfield, B.J., 1984, Synaptic input to vasopressin neurons of the paraventricular nucleus (PVN). Peptides 5 (Suppl.)1:139.

Swanson, L.W., Sawchenko, P.E., Rivier, J., and Vale W.W., 1983, Organization of ovine corticotropin-releasing factor immunoreactive cells and fibers in the rat brain: an immunohistochemical study, Neuroendocrinology 36:165.

Weiner, R.I., Ganong, W.F., 1978, Role of brain monoamines and histamine in regulation of anterior pituitary secretion. Physiol. Rev. 58:905.

ROLE OF BRAIN NORADRENALINE IN THE EFFECTS OF PRE- AND EARLY POSTNATAL STRESS ON THE ADRENOCORTICAL FUNCTION IN ADULTS

Eugene V. Naumenko

Institute of Cytology and Genetics, Academy of Sciences of the USSR, Siberian Branch
Novosibirsk, USSR

INTRODUCTION

Studies of consequences of stress or of an alteration of corticosteroid balance at an early period of the ontogeny have a great fundamental and practical significance. Such effects are capable to modify some physiological functions for as long as months, years, and even permanently. However, specific biochemical and physiological mechanisms, whose alterations during the pre- or neonatal period of life can change the reactivity of the hypothalamic-pituitary-adrenocortical axis in adulthood, are almost unknown.

According to the idea that at the early ontogeny hormones provide for the development of central neuroendocrine mechanisms underlying the hormonal regulation in adulthood (Levine, 1962; Mitskevich, 1974), it may be assumed that it is just these neuroendocrine mechanisms that are altered. Brain neurotransmitters are known to be the main links in the neuroendocrine mechanisms and among them catecholamine neurons have proved to be involved in the control of the hypothalamic-pituitary-adrenocortical axis (Naumenko, 1973).

PRENATAL EFFECTS

Previously it was found that two or four hydrocortisone injections to pregnant rats are followed by a decrease of reactivity of the pituitary-adrenocortical system in their offspring as adults to emotional stress produced by 1h restriction (Naumenko and Dygalo, 1979). Further experiments have shown that even a single prenatal hormone injection resulted in a distinct diminution of adrenocortical response to an emotional stressor in adult offspring (Naumenko and Dygalo, 1980a). The results of the experiments depended largely on the period of hormone administration. Male 3-4 months old progeny born to mothers which had been treated with hydrocortisone on days 16, 18 or 19 of pregnancy exhibited a significantly decreased reaction to the restriction as compared to untreated rats (Fig. 1).

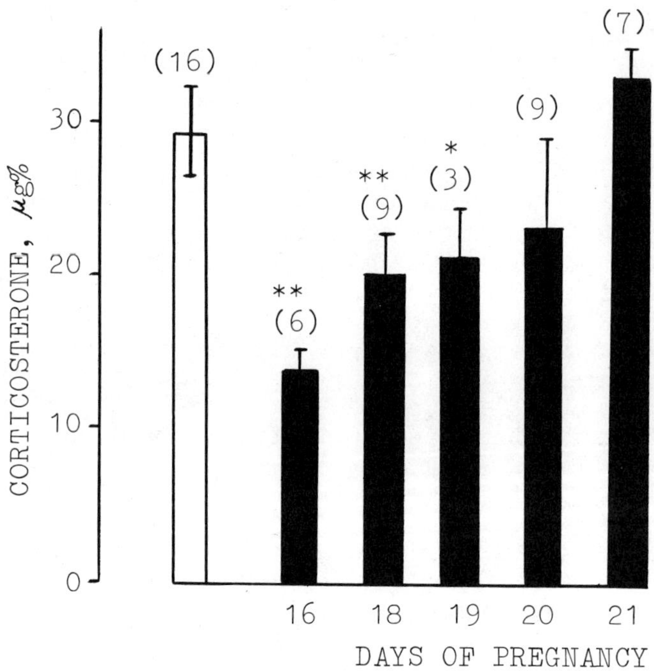

Fig. 1. Levels of plasma corticosterone 1h after emotional stress in male offspring as adults. Mothers were treated with a single hydrocortisone (5 mg/100 g b.w.) or saline injection during pregnancy. The white column represents mean corticosterone level after saline. The black columns represent mean corticosterone levels after hydrocortisone. The vertical bars represent S.E.M. Number of determinations represents in parenthesis. $*p<0.05$, $**p<0.01$ (by Naumenko and Dygalo, 1980a).

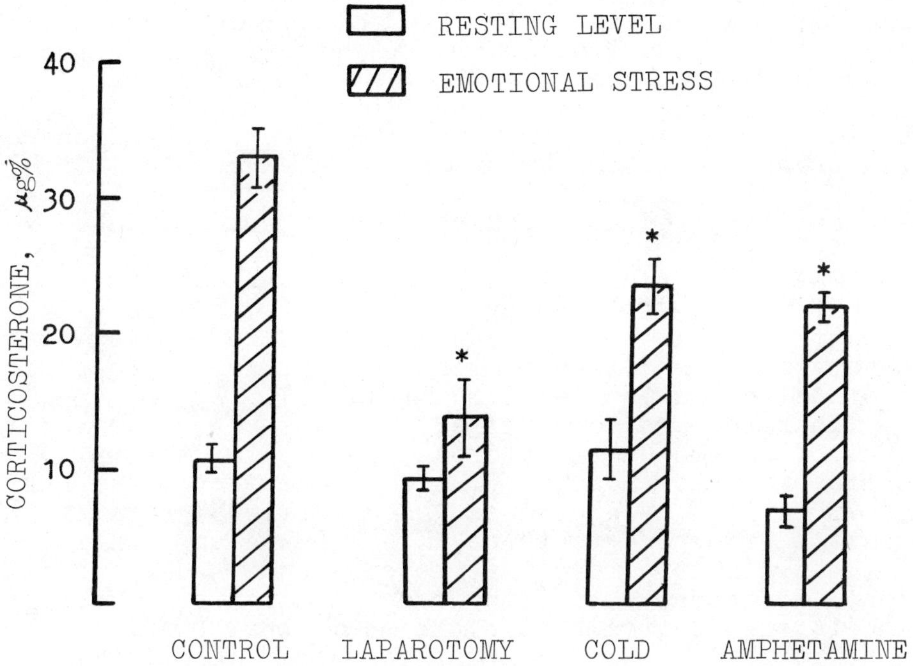

Fig. 2. Levels of plasma corticosterone 1h after emotional stress in male adult offsprings. Mothers were subjected with laparotomy (at 18 day of pregnancy), or with cold (1h exposure at 0°C) or s.c. amphetamine (0.05 mg/100 g b.w.) administration from day 18 to day 21 of gestation. The vertical bars represent S.E.M. *p<0.001 as compared to control level under emotional stress.

Similar changes were found as an effect of a variety of stressors during the last week of pregnancy. The alteration of emotional stress response in adult offspring produced by different kinds of stressors depended largely on the intensity of stressors used. The greatest decrease of the pituitary- adrenocortical response to emotional stress was obtained in adult offspring born to mothers subjected to laparotomy (Fig. 2).

Corresponding experiments have demonstrated that one of the main cause of decreased reactivity of the hypothalamic-pituitary-adrenocortical axis in prenatally treated offspring to emotional stressor was the alteration in the brain noradrenergic mechanism. Thus, injection of noradrenaline into the lateral brain ventricle resulted in an activation of the pituitary-adrenocortical system both in the adult offspring of saline-treated mothers and in adult rats born to mothers treated with hydrocortisone during gestation. However, the adrenocortical response latter group of animals was significantly diminished as compared to the offsprings of mothers which had been injected with saline (Naumenko and Dygalo, 1980a).

The role of brain noradrenaline was confirmed by the experiments with assay of the brain noradrenaline concentration after emotional stress in offspring of mothers which had been administered either hydrocortisone or saline during gestation (Fig. 3).

In rats born to hormone treated mothers the resting level of plasma corticosterone was similar to that in control animals. However, the adrenocortical response was significantly decreased under emotional stress. The results correspond to those which showed an inhibition of the brain noradrenaline response under such conditions. It appeared that the concentration of noradrenaline in the frontal lobe of the hemispheres under emotional stress was reduced markedly only in offspring of mothers which had been administered saline during pregnancy.

Therefore, the revealed differences in the brain noradrenaline reaction of control and hormone treated rats which had underwent an emotional stress, together with the results reflecting diminished response of the pituitary-adrenocortical system after intraventricular noradrenaline injection, can be interpreted as an evidence that the alteration of prenatal corticosteroid balance modifies the brain noradrenaline mechanism, and this is obviously the cause of inhibition of the response of the hypothalamic-pituitary-adrenocortical axis to emotional stressor in adulthood.

In subsequent experiments on adult offspring from female rats intact or adrenalectomized before mating but treated with hydrocortisone, adrenaline or saline during pregnancy it was found that responses of their pituitary-adrenocortical systems under emotional stress were inversely proportional to the concentration of corticosteroids in the blood of their mothers during gestation (Fig. 4).

Besides, it was found that the adrenocortical response to intraventricular noradrenaline injection in adult rats depended also on the corticosteroid contents in the blood of their mothers during gestation. Thus, an increase of corticosteroid level in the blood of pregnant mothers caused by endogenic or exogenic glucocorticoids

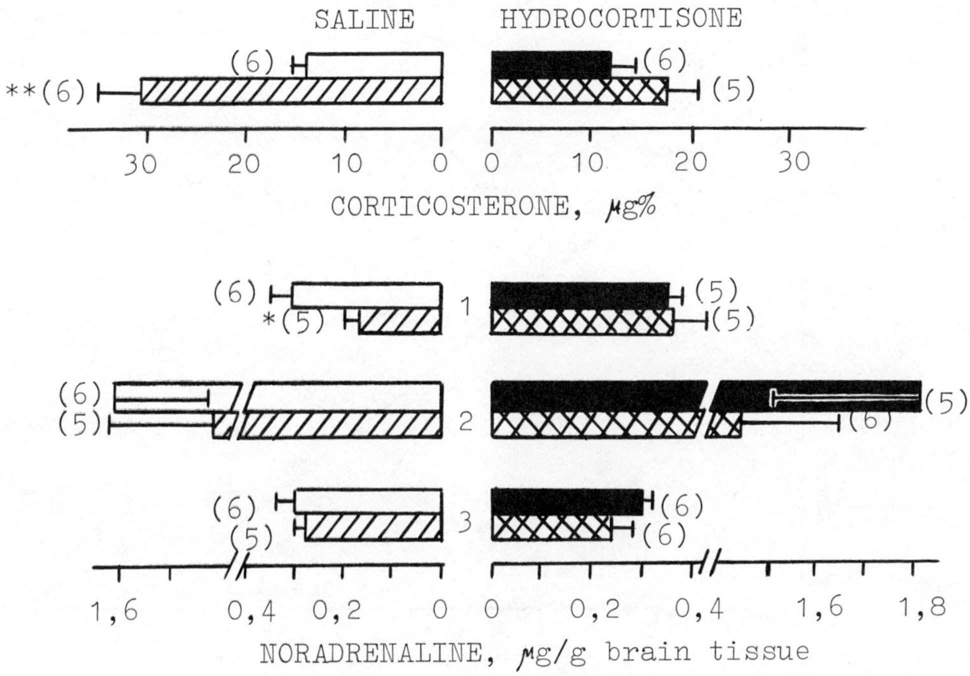

Fig. 3. Levels of plasma corticosterone and brain noradrenaline contents 1h after emotional stress in male adult offspring. Mothers were treated with hydrocortisone (5 mg/kg b.w.) or saline on days 16 and 18 of pregnancy. The white and the black columns represent mean resting corticosterone or noradrenaline contents. The striped columns represent mean corticosterone or noradrenaline contents after emotional stress. The vertical bars represent S.E.M. 1-frontal lobe, 2-hypothalamus, 3-brain stem. Number of determinations in parenthesis. $*p<0.05$, $**p<0.01$ (by Naumenko and Dygalo, 1980a).

was followed by a decrease of the hypothalamic-pituitary-adrenocortical reaction to the central noradrenaline administration in their offspring as adults. A significant inter-group correlation was obtained between the responses of the pituitary-adrenocortical system to noradrenaline injection and to emotional stressor ($\rho=0.83$; $p<0.05$, by Naumenko and Dygalo, 1984).

The formation of low response to central noradrenaline injection or to emotional stress in adult off-

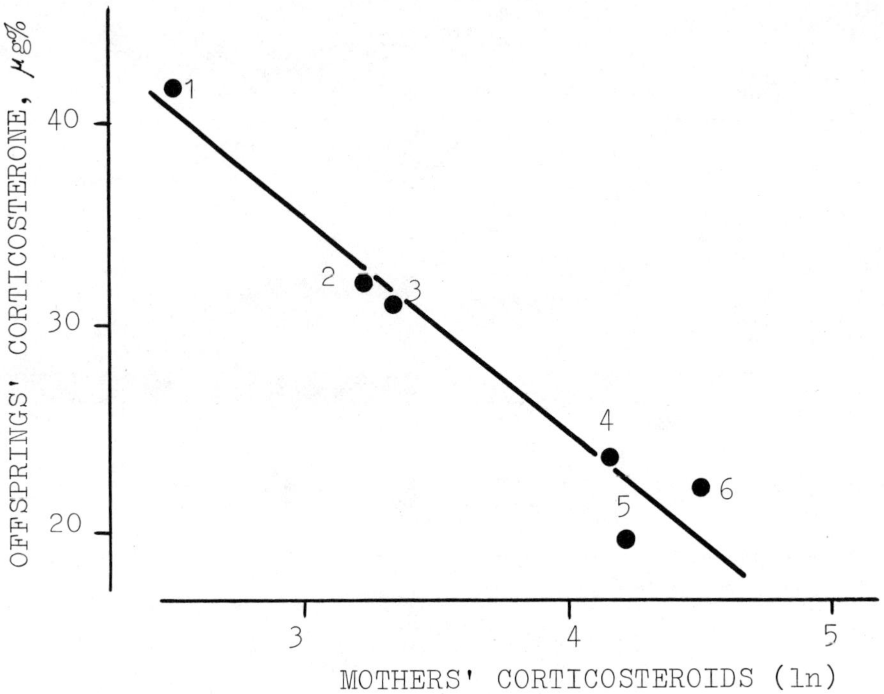

Fig. 4. The line of regression of corticosterone levels in blood of adult offspring after emotional stress on the corticosteroid levels in blood of pregnant mothers. Intact(Int) or adrenalectomized (ADX) before mating female rats were treated with saline, hydrocortisone, or epinephrine at 16 and 18 days of gestation. 1-ADX+saline; 2-ADX+epinephrine; 3-Int+saline; 4-Int+hydrocortisone; 5-ADX+hydrocortisone; 6-Int+epinephrine. On X-axis - natural logarithm of corticosteroid levels in blood of pregnant mothers. On Y-axis - corticosterone content in blood of offspring as adults (by Naumenko and Dygalo, 1984).

spring as a consequence of high adrenocortical hormone level in the blood of their mothers during gestation can be interpreted as one of adaptive reactions to fluctuations of rodent population size in nature.

Indeed, as it has been shown by Christian (1950) and many others (Christian et al., 1965), the endocrines play a very important role in mechanisms of the self-regulation of mammalian populations. Recent studies have shown that zoosocial behavior affects the pituitary-adrenocortical and pituitary-gonadal system in ways that decrease birth rate and increase the mortality rate. It seems that adrenocortical activity is negatively related to zoosocial rank of animals and to population size. It is well documented that the pituitary-adrenocortical system of subordinate animals is activated or even exhausted in overcrowded populations of rodents. This, in its turn, is followed by an increase of mortality among them.

Therefore, it can be assumed that in our experiments the increased level of corticosteroids in the blood of pregnant mothers appears to serve as a signal for development of a low stress response in the offspring. Such kind of reaction may play an important role for animals which live in populations of high density. Such assumption is consistent with the experiments of Belyaev et al.(1977) in which it has been revealed that the animals with diminished stress response exhibited a higher fitness in overcrowded population of the laboratory mice as compared to animals with marked reaction to emotional stressors.

Conseqently, the adaptive value of modification of stress mechanism by hormones during prenatal period of the development appears to be likely.

A number of peculiarites exist concerning brain noradrenergic mechanism changes which were induced by stress or by the alteration of corticosteroid balance during early ontogeny. First of all, the changes in noradrenergic system are general rather than local ones.

After prenatal hydrocortisone injections some alterations in noradrenergic mechanism responsible for the regulation not only of the pituitary-adrenocortical system but also of thermoregulation were found. Data were obtained indicating that noradrenaline injections into the lateral brain ventricle of control animals resulted in a marked decrease of colonic temperature. At the same time, after prenatal hydrocortisone treatment the drop of body temperature was significantly less in adulthood (Fig.5). Taking into account that the central mechanism of thermoregulation and the mechanism of regulation of adrenocortical system are not directly connected it may be suggested that the change of corticosteroid balance during prenatal period of life produces a general alteration of the brain noradrenaline system.

The alteration of noradrenaline mechanism depends on the animal genotype(Naumenko and Dygalo, 1980b). Hydrocortisone administration to pregnant August rats, unlike Wistar ones, did not change the response of the hypothalamic-pituitary-adrenocortical axis to emotional stress or to intraventricular noradrenaline injection

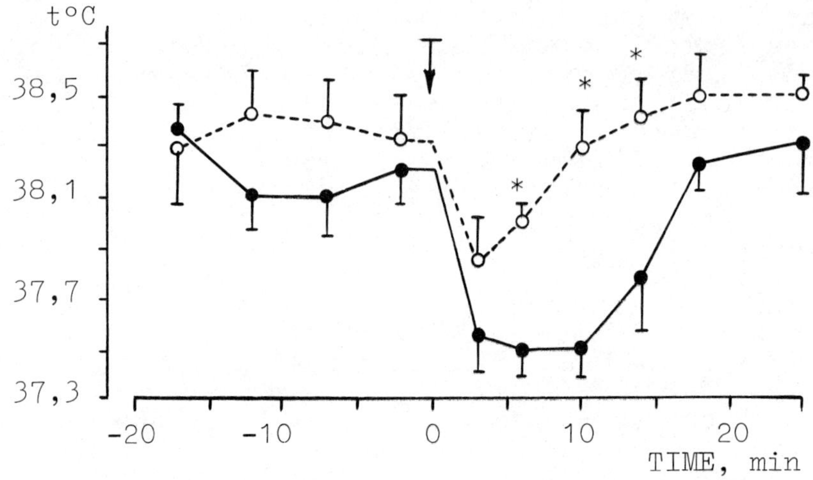

Fig. 5. Body temperature after noradrenaline injection into the lateral brain ventricle of male offspring as adults. Mothers were treated with 5 mg/100 g b.w. of hydrocortisone (the white circles) or saline (the black circles) on days 16 and 18 of pregnancy. Arrow indicate point of noradrenaline (7.5μg) injection. The vertical bars represent S.E.M. *$p<0.05$ (by Naumenko and Dygalo, 1980a).

in adult offspring.

The response of the pituitary-adrenocortical system of the offspring to emotional stress or to central noradrenaline injection in adulthood was decreased not only in Wistar rats but in their reciprocal hybrids with August strain either (Fig. 6). Therefore, the revealed interstrain differences in the sensitivity of fetal adrenergic mechanism of the brain to the hormone treatment are genetically controlled. According to the data obtained on the first generation hybrids the high sensitivity of animals to the hydrocortisone in the prenatal period of life is inherited as a dominant trait.

The causes of the difference in the sensitivity of the embrionic brain noradrenergic system of August and Wistar rats are unknown. At all events, it is not determined by the maternal organism only. An evidence in support of this view is given by experiments with reciprocal hybrids when different mothers gave birth to similar offspring. The reaction to emotional stressor or to intraventricular noradrenaline injection was significantly

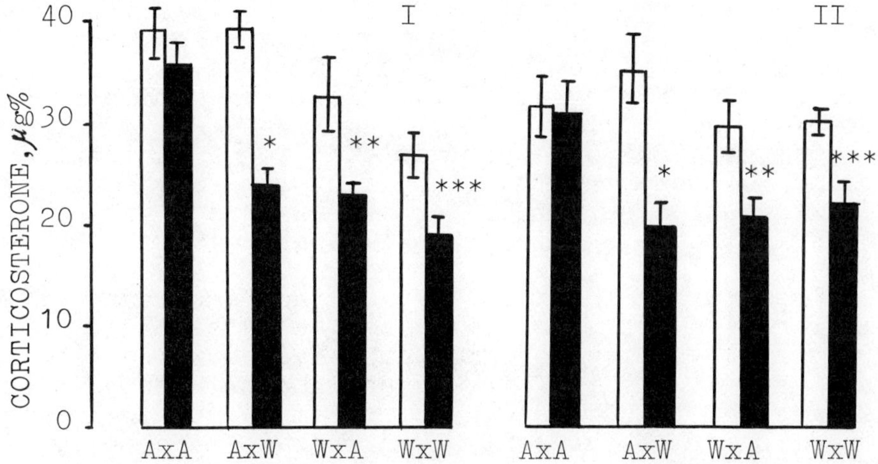

Fig. 6. Levels of plasma corticosterone after emotional stress (I) or noradrenaline injection into the lateral brain ventricle (II) of male offspring as adults of August strain (A), Wistar strain (W), and their reciprocal hybrids F_1 (AxW and WxA). Mothers were treated with hydrocortisone (5 mg/100 g b.w.) or saline on the days 16 and 18 of pregnancy. The white columns represent mean corticosterone level after saline injection. The black columns represent mean corticosterone level after hydrocortisone. The vertical bars represent S.E.M. $*p<0.001$, $**p<0.005$, $***p<0.01$. (by Naumenko and Dygalo, 1980b).

and uniformly decreased both in adult direct and reverse hybrid offsprings, whose mothers had been injected on the 16th and 18th days of pregnancy with hydrocortisone. It has to be mentioned that the resting levels of corticosterone in the peripheral blood plasma did not differ significantly in Wistar, August rats and in their reciprocal hybrids.

Two groups of facts attract attention in the interpretation of difference in the sensitivity of brain noradrenaline system in rats of different genotype.

On the one hand, a chronic stress or glucocorticoid treatment in the early stages of life resulted in an alteration of noradrenaline content (Moyer et al., 1978; Peters, 1982; Simmons et al., 1984) or its metabolism (Nasello and Ramirez, 1978; Simmons et al., 1984), of α-adrenergic receptor binding (Ramirez et al., 1983), of normal synaptic development of biogenic amine system (Slotkin et al., 1979), and, finally, of activity of tyrosine hydroxylase (Nasello and Ramirez, 1978; Nyakas et al., 1980; Markey et al., 1982) in the brain of adult progeny or of pups.

On the other hand, it has been found that the development of the brain adrenergic system (Berger et al., 1979; Touret et al., 1982) or of enzyme activities of catecholamine metabolism (Ozaki et al., 1980) depended on the animal genotype.

Therefore, it may be assumed that the cause of the difference in the sensitivity of the fetal brain noradrenergic system to administered hydrocortisone in Wistar and August rats is a genetic distinction in development of the brain enzyme system of catecholamine metabolism or of the central adrenergic receptors, or both of them.

Probably prenatally administered hormone affected as a genetic inducer the fetal catecholamine mechanism during its development. Such posibility is supported by a number of data available. Thus, in the majority of experiments (Naumenko and Dygalo, 1979, 1980a,b, 1984) hydrocortisone was injected on days 16 and 18 of pregnancy. Apparently, this is the very period of formation in the rat fetus of key enzyme participating in catecholamine metabolism. Tyrosine hydroxylase activity was found firstly in rat brain 3 days before birth (Breese and Traylor, 1972),or according to others authors (Coyle and Axelrod, 1972),as early as the day 15 of the prenatal stage of life, i.e. just before hormone administration in our experiments.

Besides, the inhibiting effect of even a single prenatal hydrocortisone injection on the adrenocortical response to emotional stress persisted for a long time, no less then for 6 months after birth, and as has been shown by Dygalo (in preperation), the activity of tyrosine hydroxilase was changed in the brain of adult offspring born to hormone treated mothers as compared with adult progeny whose mothers had been injected with saline. Finally, some investigations showed that the change of glucocorticoids balance was followed not only by the alteration of the activity but obviously of the rate of synthesis of catecholamine enzymes, too (Wurtman and Axelrod, 1966; Ciaranello and Black, 1971; Thoenen et al., 1973).

Therefore, there are reasons to suggest that prenatal stress or prenatally injected hydrocortisone changes the normal display of the genetic program. This, in turn, is followed by the alteration of the brain noradrenergic neuronal system.

POSTNATAL EFFECTS

The alteration of the central noradrenergic system was observed not only after prenatal disorders but after postnatal stress as well. It was found that daily injections of 0.9% saline from the 7th to the 9th days of postnatal life were not followed by any acute elevation of the corticosterone level in the peripheral blood plasma (Fig. 7). Nevertheless, such animals in adulthood showed, on the one hand, an increase of the pituitary-adrenal reaction to central noradrenaline injection, and, on the other hand, a diminution of the adrenocortical response to emotional stress as compared with animals untreated in the early period of life. Besides, by contrast to the prenatal period stress during 7 to 9 days of the postnatal stage of the ontogeny caused a long-lasting increase of the basal corticosterone level in peripheral blood (Fig. 8).

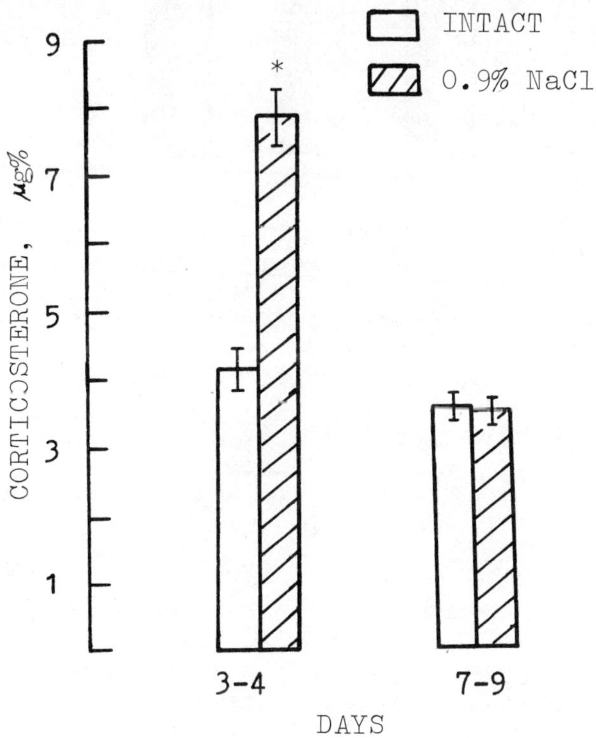

Fig. 7. Levels of plasma corticosterone 30 min after s.c. injections of 0.9% NaCl in 3-4 and 7-9 days old rats. The vertical bars represent S.E.M. $*p<0.001$ as compared to intact.

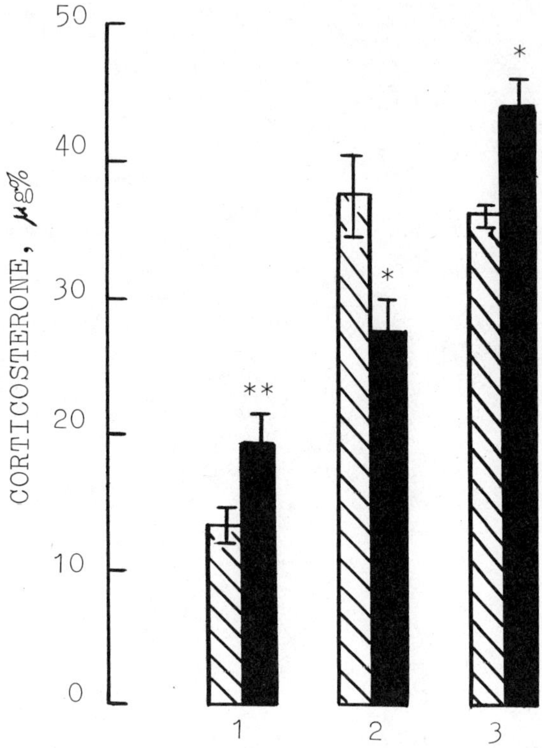

Fig. 8. Levels of plasma corticosterone produced by emotional stress or noradrenaline injection into the lateral brain ventricle in 3-4 months old male rats. Animals were treated with 0.9% NaCl from 7 to 9 days of postnatal life. The striped columns represent mean corticosterone level in untreated animals. The black columns represent mean corticosterone level after NaCl injections. 1 - resting level, 2 - emotional stress (1h restriction), 3 - noradrenaline injection (15 μg). $^{**}p<0.01$, $^{*}p<0.05$.

Even more clear-cut distinctions were revealed between pre- and early postnatal periods of life in the experiments with hydrocortisone administration. In contrast to the stage of fetal development, daily hydrocortisone injections from 7 through 9 days of the postnatal period of life were not followed by any alterations of the pituitary-adrenocortical response neither to intraventricular noradrenaline injection nor to emotional stress in 3-4 months old rats as compared to untreated control (Table 1).

Table 1. Effects of Hydrocortisone Treatment in Pre- and Early Postnatal Stages of Life on the Pituitary-Adrenal Function in Adult Rats

Series of Experiments	Stages of Ontogeny	
	Prenatal	Postnatal
Resting Level	No Changes	No Changes
Emotional Stress	Decrease	No Changes
Noradrenaline	Decrease	No Changes

The differences of stress or corticosteroid effects during embryogenesis and the postnatal period of life are determined by the stage of development of the hypothalamic-pituitary-adrenocortical axis as well as of the development of the noradrenergic mechanism participating in the regulation of this neuroendocrine system. Though definite mechanisms of the distinctions are unknown, some hypothesis can be discussed.

During the prenatal period of life the mother's adrenocortical hormones participate in stress-reactions, and the fetus is influenced by high glucocorticoid concentrations. As it has been demonstrated, elevated blood corticosterone level during the late stage of the fetal development results in a long-lasting modification in the regulation of the pituitary-adrenocortical function under emotional stress or after intraventricular noradrenaline injection.

The maternal corticosteroid influence stops immediately after delivery. However, the development of the hypothalamic-pituitary-adrenocortical axis and its regulating mechanisms is not yet completed after birth in the rats. Therefore,the pituitary-adrenocortical system is not capable to respond for the first few days with a high increase of the blood corticosterone level to stress stimuli. Moreover, as shown above daily subcutaneous injections of 0.9% saline solution for 7 to 9 days of postnatal period were not followed by any elevation of the corticosterone level in the peripheral blood plasma. That is why some conditions can occur under stress for the development of the relative hormonal deficiency during this stage of the postnatal ontogeny.

The data Butte et al.(1973) testify that a clear-cut dissociation exists between the necessity of the brain for corticosterone and the available hormone content in the blood under stress during 7-9 days of life.

Therefore, a corticosteroid insufficiency can, evidently, result in a deficit of brain development and appears to be the cause of a long-lasting alteration of the regulating mechanisms of the hypothalamic-pituitary-adrenocortical axis. If that is the case, the damaging effect of stress induce by saline administration from 7 through 9 days of life must be able to be prevented by injection of additional amount of the adrenocortical hormones.

Indeed, as it shown above repeated saline injections for 7 to 9 days did not change the blood corticosterone level but were accompanied by a long-term modification of the hypothalamic-pituitary-adrenocortical function. At the same time, the injections of the hydrocortisone solution in the same volume as saline were not followed by any alterations of the adrenocortical response either to emotional stress or to intraventricular noradrenaline administration in adult rats.

The idea about the cause of distinctions between stressor or hormone action during the early postnatal period of life is consistent with the experimental data available. Thus, stress at the early postnatal stage of life is followed, as a rule, by a decrease of the adrenocortical response to emotional stressors (Levine et al., 1967; Ader, 1968; Denenberg et al., 1969; Weiner and Levine, 1983). At the same time, glucocorticoid injections in such period of the individual development is accompanied only by a transitory effect (Nyakas and Endröczi, 1972; Krieger, 1974; Ulrich et al., 1976; Erskine et al., 1979) and do not influence stress response of the pituitary-adrenocortical system in adult animals (Nyakas and Endröczi, 1972; Miyabo and Hizada, 1973; Krieger, 1974).

It has to be noted that the stress consequences differ from those produced by a specific alteration of catecholamine metabolism at the early stage of postnatal ontogeny. Thus, daily intraperitoneal administrations of α-methyl-d,l-thyrosine (α-MT) from day 5 to day 7 resulted in a long-lasting diminution of the resting corticosterone level in the peripheral blood plasma. At the same time, α-MT injections were not followed by any alterations of the adrenocortical response to emotional stress in adulthood as compared with untreated animals (Maslova et al., 1984). Besides, in α-MT treated rats a decrease of noradrenaline concentration in the hypothalamus and the midbrain was found (Fig. 9).

CONCLUSION

Stressors or disturbance of corticosteroid equilibrium during the early stages of the individual development yields long-lasting alterations of the brain noradrenergic mechanism participating in the control of the hypothalamic-pituitary-adrenocortical axis. The character of modification of the noradrenergic system depends on the stage of the ontogeny, on the agent used, on the animal genotype, and caused, in its turn, different alterations of the hypothalamic-pituitary-adrenocortical function.

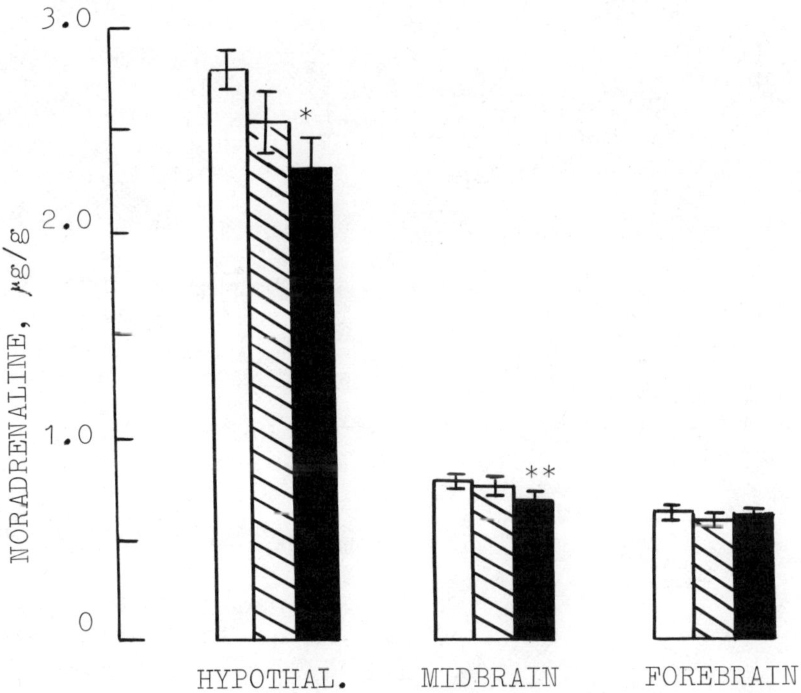

Fig. 9. Noradrenaline concentration in the brain of adult rats. Animals were injected with distilled water (striped columns) or with α-MT (150 mg/kg b.w.)(black columns) during 5-7 days of postnatal period of life. The white columns-intact animals. The vertical bars represent S.E.M. *$p<0.05$ vs intact, **$p<0.01$ vs intact and distilled water.

REFERENCES

Ader, R., 1968, Effects of early experiences on emotional and physiological reactivity in rat, J. Comp. Physiol. Psychol., 66:264.

Belyaev, D. K., Schüler, L., and Borodin, P. M., 1977, Problems of stress genetics. III.Differential effect of stress on the fertility of mice of different genotypes, Genetika, 13:52 (in Russian).

Berger, B., Herve, D., Dolphin, A., Barthelemy, C., Gay, M., and Tassin, J. L., 1979, Genetically determined differences in noradrenergic input to the brain cortex: a histochemical and biochemical study in two inbred strains of mice, Neuroscience, 4:877.

Breese, G. R., and Traylor, T. D., 1972, Developmental characteristics of brain catecholamines and tyrosine hydroxylase in the rat: effect of 6-hydroxydopamine, Brit.J. Pharmacol., 44:210.

Butte, J. C., Kakihana, R., Fornham, M. L., and Noble, E. P., 1973, The relationship between brain and plasma corticosterone stress response in developing rats, Endocrinology, 92:1775.

Christian, J. J., 1950, The adreno-pituitary system and population cycles in mammals, J. Mammal., 31:247.

Christian, J. J., Lloyd, J. A., and Davis, D. E., 1965, The role of endocrines in the self-regulation of mammalian populations, in:"Rec. Progr. Hormone Res", G. Pincus, ed., Acad. Press, N.Y. and Lond.

Ciaranello, R. D., and Black, I. B., 1971, Kinetics of the glucocorticoid-mediated induction of phenylethanolamine N-methyltransferase in hypophysectomized rat, Biochem. Pharmac., 20:3529.

Coyle, J. T., and Axelrod, J., 1972, Tyrosine hydroxylase in rat brain: developmental characteristics, J. Neurochem., 19:1117.

Denenberg, V. H., Rosenberg, K. M., and Zarrow, M. X., 1969, Mice reared with rat ants: effects in adulthood upon plasma corticosterone and open-field activity, Physiology and Behavior, 4:705.

Erskine, M. S., Geller, E., and Yuwiler, A., 1979, Effects of neonatal hydrocortisone treatment on pituitary and adrenocortical response to stress in young rats, Neuroendocrinology, 29:191.

Krieger,D.T., 1974, Effect of neonatal hydrocortisone on corticosteroid circadian periodicity, responsiveness to ACTH and stress in prepubertal and adult rats, Neuroendocrinology, 16:355.

Levine, S., 1962, Plasma-free corticosteroid response to electric shock in rats stimulated in infancy,

Science, 135:795.
Levine, S., Haltmeyer, L. C., Koras, L. L., and Denenberg, V. H., 1967, Physiological and behavioral effects of infantile stimulation, Physiology and Behavior, 2:55.
Markey, K. A., Towle, A. C., and Sze, P. Y., 1982, Glucocorticoid influence on tyrosine hydroxylase activity in mouse locus coeruleus during postnatal development, Endocrinology, 111:1519.
Maslova, L.N., Nikulina, E. M., Popova N. K., and Naumenko E. V., 1984, Alteration of catecholamine synthesis in early ontogeny and pituitary-adrenocortical system in adult rats, Ontogenes, 15:327 (in Russian).
Mitskevich, M. S., 1974, Some problems of the development of humoral regulation in prenatal period, Ontogenes, 5:557 (in Russian).
Miyabo, S., and Hisada, T., 1973, Sex difference in ontogenesis of circadian adrenocortical rhythm in cortisone-primed rats, Nature (Lond.), 256:590.
Moyer, J. A., Herrenkohl, L. R., and Jacobowitz, D. M., 1978, Stress during pregnancy: effect on catecholamine in discrete brain regions of offspring as adults, Brain Res., 144:173.
Naumenko, E. V., 1973, "Central Regulation of the Pituitary-Adrenal Complex", Plenum Publ.Corp., N.Y.
Naumenko, E. V., and Dygalo, N. N., 1979, Hypothalamo-pituitary-adrenal reactivity in adult rats after hydrocortisone administration to their mothers during pregnancy, Ontogenes, 10:476 (in Russian).
Naumenko, E. V., and Dygalo, N. N., 1980a, Noradrenergic brain mechanisms and emotional stress in adult rats after prenatal hydrocortisone treatment, in: Biogenic Amines in Development", H. Parvez, and S. Parvez, eds., Elsevier/North-Holland, Inc., N.Y.
Naumenko, E. V., and Dygalo, N. N., 1980b, Brain noradrenaline mechanisms and emotional stress in adult rats after prenatal hydrocortisone treatment, in: Catecholamines and Stress: Recent Advances", E. Usdin, R. Kvetnanský, and I. J. Kopin, eds., Elsevier North -Holland, Inc., N.Y.-Amsterdam-Oxford.
Naumenko, E. V., and Dygalo, N. N., 1984, Role of maternal corticosteroids and epinephrine changes during pregnancy in alteration of pituitary-adrenal reactivity of adult offspring, in: Stress: The Role of Catecholamines and Other Neurotransmitters", E. Usdin, and R. Kvetnanský, eds., Gordone and Breach, Science Publ., Inc., N.Y.
Nasello, A. G., and Ramirez, O. A., 1978, Brain catecholamines metabolism in offspring of amphetamine

treated rats, Pharmac. Biochem. Behav., 9:17.

Nyakas, C., and Endroczi, E., 1972, Effect of neonatal corticosterone administration on behavioral and pituitary-adrenocortical responses in the rat, Acta Physiol. Acad. Sci. Hung., 43:231.

Nyakas, C., Viltsek, J., and Endroczi, E., 1980, Sensitivity of catecholamine neuron system to corticosterone and ACTH 4-10 in newborn rats. Studies on brain and adrenal tyrosine hydroxylase, in:"Catecholamine and Stress: Recent Advances," E. Usdin, R. Kvetnansky, and I. J. Kopin, eds., Elsevier/ North Holland, Inc.,N.Y.-Amsterdam-Oxford.

Ozaki, M.,Sugawara, K., Takami, N., Mayemura, S.-J., and Niwa, M., 1980, Development of hypertension and metabolism of biogenic amines in spontaneously hypertensive rats, in:"Biogenic Amines in Development," H. Parvez, and S. Parvez, eds., Elsevier/ North-Holland, Inc.,N.Y.-Amsterdam-Oxford.

Peters, D. A., 1982, Prenatal stress: effect on brain biogenic amine and plasma corticosterone levels, Pharmac.Biochem.Behav., 17:721.

Ramirez, O. A., Keller, E. A., and Orsingher, O. A., 1983, Prenatal amphetamine reduces alpha but not beta adrenergic receptor binding in brain of adult rats, Life Sci.,32:1835.

Simmons, R. D., Kellog, C. K., and Miller, R. K., 1984, Prenatal diazepam exposure in rats: long-lasting, receptor-mediated effects on hypothalamic norepinephrine-containing neurons, Brain Res., 293:73.

Slotkin, T. A., Whitmore, W. L., Salvaggio,M.,and Seidler,F. J.,1979, Perinatal methadone addiction affects brain synaptic development of biogenic amine systems in the rat, Life Sci.,24:1223.

Thoenen, H., Otten, U., and Oesch, F., 1973, Transsynaptic regulation of tyrosine hydroxylase, in:"Frontiers in Catecholamine Research", E.Usdin, and S.H. Snyder, eds., Pergamon Press, Oxford.

Touret, M., Valatx, J.- L., and Jouvet, M., 1982, The locus coeruleus: a quantitative and genetic study in mice, Brain Res., 250:353.

Ulrich, R., Yuwiler, A., and Geller, E., 1976, Neonatal hydrocortisone: effect on the development of the stress response and the diurnal rhythm of corticosterone, Neuroendocrinology, 21:49.

Weiner, S. G., and Levine, S., 1983, Influence of perinatal malnutrition and early handling on the pituitary-adrenal response to noxious stimuli in adult rat, Physiology and Behavior,31:285.

Wurtman, R.,and Axelrod,J.,1966, Control of enzimatic synthesis of adrenaline in the adrenal medulla by adrenal cortical steroids, J.Biol.Chem.,241:2301.

MODIFIED DEVELOPMENT OF THE HYPOTHALAMO-PITUITARY-ADRENOCORTICAL (HPA) AXIS RESPONSE TO STRESS IN YOUNG RODENTS WITH EXPERIMENTALLY ALTERED THYROID STATUS

Lee A. Meserve

Department of Biological Sciences, Bowling Green State University, Bowling Green, Ohio 43403 USA

INTRODUCTION

The study of development of the stress-adaptive hypothalamo-pituitary-adrenocortical (HPA) axis in young rodents is of interest because of the considerable degree of maturation which occurs postnatally. When first described by Schapiro et al. (1962), the so-called stress non-responsive (SNR) period was felt to be absolute, with the HPA axis of rats unable to respond to a stress between approximately postnatal days 3 and 12. With the advancement of technological methods it has been demonstrated that the SNR period is relative rather than absolute, and that HPA axis response during this time is dampened rather than prevented (Schoenfeld et al., 1980; Milkovic et al., 1982). Nonetheless, significant maturation of HPA axis components must occur before response levels approach those of adults, after the third postnatal week (Guillet et al., 1980).

The influence of pre- and early postnatal alteration of thyroid status on development and maturation in general has been widely studied and reported (see Greenberg et al., 1974, for review). Appropriate thyroidal input appears to be particularly important for proper brain development with either an excess or a deficiency of thyroid hormone being detrimental. For example, an excess of thyroid hormone accelerates developmental measures such as time of eye opening and righting reflex in rats (Eayrs, 1964), but this early acceleration leads to deficiencies in brain mechanisms in adult life (Pelton and Bass, 1973). The possible importance of thyroxine in the maturation of HPA stress response was recognized by Schapiro (1968) who found thyroxine injection on postnatal days 1, 2, and 3 to result in a stress-induced increase in the adrenal corticosterone content of 5 day old animals, but injection of saline did not cause such an increase. More recent studies have found maternal ingestion of thyroid powder during gestation and lactation to increase the stress response of rat pups, as measured by elevated circulating corticosterone levels, at 12 days (Meserve and Leathem, 1974) but not at 30 days of age (Meserve and Scriffignano, 1984), and chronic injection of pups with thyroxine to increase stress response between 4 and 18 days of age (Poland et al., 1979).

The primary focus of the studies reported herein is the effect of depressed thyroid status on development of the HPA axis response to stress. Infantile hypothyroidism continues to be an important clinical concern in undeveloped countries (Vanderpas et al., 1984) as well as in developed nations (Larson, 1980). Thus the influence of perinatal depression of thyroid status on development of endocrine control mechanisms, such as the HPA axis, is of clinical as well as experimental interest. Although the understanding of the interplay of thyroid hormones with HPA axis development is far from complete, the following in vivo and in vitro studies suggest that the deficiency of these hormones has a greater influence upon the hypothalamic component than upon pituitary or adrenal cortex.

MATERIALS AND METHODS

Animals

Rats used in these experiments were derived from outbred Sprague-Dawley parents, and were bred and reared in the laboratory of the investigator. Virgin females were mated at an initial body weight of 150-175 g with sexually experienced males of the same strain. Sexually mature female Swiss-Webster mice were mated to sexually experienced males of the same strain to produce most of the mice used in these studies. Recent experiments with congenitally hypothyroid animals used C·RF/J mice obtained from the Jackson Laboratory (Bar Harbor, ME, USA). Phenotypically normal *hyt*/+ mice were mated to the hypothyroid *hyt*/*hyt* animals of the opposite sex. Desiccated thryoid powder (Sigma Chemical Co., St. Louis, MO, USA) was incorporated into the diet of these animals during cohabitation to ensure reproductive competence (Beamer and Cresswell, 1982) and during gestation to guarantee success of the pregnancy.

Alteration of Thyroid Status

The thyroid status of pregnant rats and mice and of their offspring was chemically depressed by incorporation of 2-thiouracil (0.25%, w/w, Sigma Chemical Co.) into their diet from the day of conception as previously reported (Meserve, 1976; Meserve and Leathem, 1973, 1981). Thiouracil inhibits the iodination of tyrosyl residues in thyroglobulin (Taurog, 1976) and decreases peripheral deiodination of thyroxine (T_4) to triiodothyronine (T_3) (Oppenheimer et al., 1972), thus resulting in the cretinoid characteristics of hypothyroidism in the offspring of animals so fed. Congenitally hypothyroid (hyt/hyt) young mice were provided, as noted above, from matings of C·RF/J stock. These animals are hypothyroid as a result of an autosomal recessive gene on chromsome 12, producing a hypoplastic thyroid gland which is insensitive to thyroid stimulating hormone (TSH) (Beamer et al., 1981).

Tests of HPA Axis Function

In vivo tests:

Rats made hypothyroid chemically were tested for HPA axis function at 15, 20, 25, 30, and 35 days of age. This was done by fluorometric determination (Hilf et al., 1960) of corticosterone concentration in adrenals and serum of animals which were unstimulated (controls), and 15 min after stimulation in those stressed by exposure to ether fumes (1 min), subcutaneously injected with depot adrenocorticotropin (ACTH, 4 IU in 0.1 ml), or subcutaneously injected with physiological saline (0.1 ml). These results were compared with those of euthyroid pups at 15, 20, and 25 days of age. Normal and chemically hypothyroid mice were similarly tested at 15 days of age and their circulating corticosterone levels were determined by the method of Glick et al. (1964). Additionally, electron microscopic analyses were made of adrenocortical cells from the zona fasciculata in euthyroid and chemically hypothyroid rats at 15 and 20 days of age, using standard morphometric techniques (Weibel et al., 1966).

In vitro tests:

The activity of two adrenal enzymes involved in steroidogenesis and in steroid degradation was determined in euthyroid and chemically hypothyroid adult male mice. Adrenocortical 3β-hydroxysteroid dehydrogenase (3β-HSD) activity was determined by the method of Davenport and Mallette (1966), and that of steroid 5α-reductase as reported by Kitay et al. (1970).

Bioassays of response of adrenals from 15 day old normal and chemically hypothyroid rats to a standard ACTH stimulus, and of the ACTH content of their pituitaries, was accomplished using the flowing system of Saffran et al. (1971). Corticotropin-releasing factor (CRF) content of hypothalamic extracts was initially measured by the semi-automated bioassay of Pearlmutter et al. (1974), and after extract purifications (Angwin and Barchas, 1982) by radioimmunoassay (RIA) using a commerically available kit (Peninsula Laboratories, Inc., San Carlos, CA, USA). This RIA kit is based on the recently characterized and synthesized rat CRF_{1-41} peptide (Rivier et al., 1983). The CRF RIA kit has also been used in preliminary studies of the hypothalamic CRF content of 15 and 30 day old, and adult, congenitally hypothyroid (hyt/hyt) mice.

RESULTS AND DISCUSSION

In Vivo Studies

Exposure of developing rats to thiouracil from conception by its incorporation into the diet of the mother prevented a measureable increase in adrenal corticosterone concentration in response to ether fumes at 15 days of age, but not at 20, 25, or 35 days of age, and did not prevent an adrenal response to ACTH at any age tested (Fig. 1. a,c). Further, thiouracil did not modify unstimulated serum corticosterone levels at the ages tested (Fig. 1. b,c). On the other hand, ether fumes did not cause an increase in circulating corticosterone in hypothyroid rats until 30 days of age, and the increase in response to injected ACTH was subnormal after 15 days of age. It should be noted that euthyroid young were not included in the study past 25 days of age because the mother rats would not abide the presence of older offspring in the same cage: hypothyroid pups still relied upon the mother for nutrition through 35 days of age, and could not be weaned successfully. Therefore, weaned euthyroid rats separated from the mother would have been exposed to different conditions than unweaned hypothyroid animals, confounding interpretation of the results.

The HPA response data provided by the above experiments can be interpreted in a number of ways. It would appear that basal release of ACTH is not modified by thiouracil exposure, since basal corticosterone levels were not altered. The adrenals of hypothyroid rats seem to be responsive to exogeneous ACTH, albeit their production of corticosterone was subnormal after 15 days. Thus, by the process of exlcusion, the hypothalamic component of the HPA axis of the rat appears to be suppressed at 15 days by thiouracil exposure (Meserve and Leathem, 1973). A subsequent study demonstrated a similar pattern of response in 15 day old thiouracil fed mice (Meserve, 1976). With advancing age, the hypothalamic component of hypothyroid rodents may develop sufficiently to allow, first, adrenal synthesis of corticosterone by 20 days, and, second, adrenal secretion of corticosterone by 30 days in response to ether stress (Meserve and Leathem, 1981). On the other hand, it could be argued that the responsiveness of the adrenocortical component of the axis is depressed by thiouracil, and that its obvious responsiveness to exogeneous ACTH (and not to the endogeneously produced peptide) is merely a result of the large dose administered. Indeed, structural alterations of the

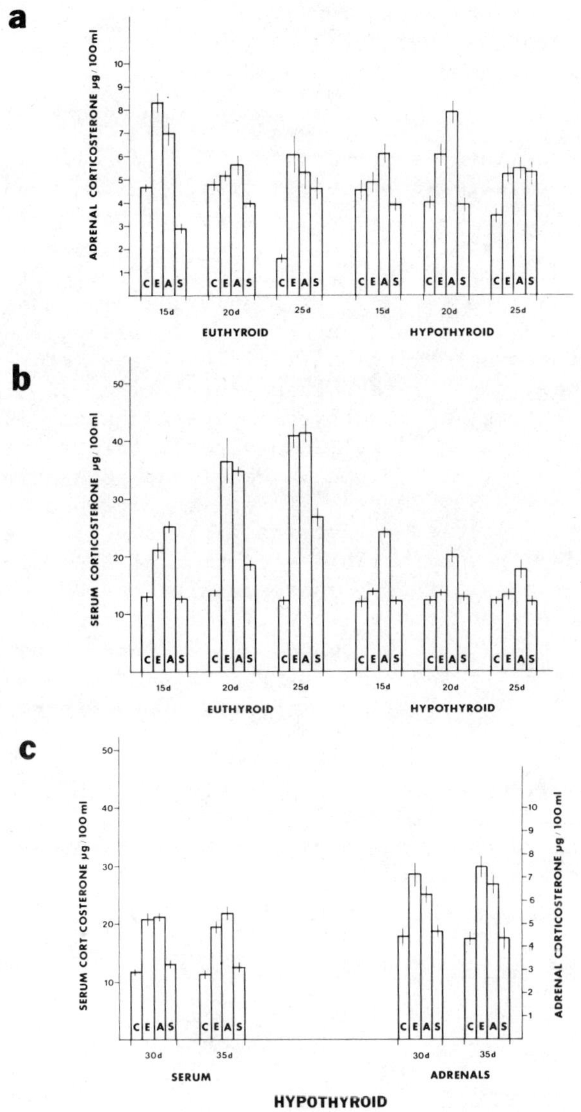

Fig. 1. Response of serum and adrenal corticosterone levels to stimulation in 15, 20, and 25 day old euthyroid rats and in 15, 20, 25, 30, and 35 day old chemically hypothyroid (thiouracil-induced) rats. a. Adrenal corticosterone concentrations at 15, 20, and 25 days. b. Serum corticosterone concentrations at 15, 20, and 25 days. c. Serum and adrenal corticosterone concentrations in chemically hypothyroid 30 and 35 day olds. C - control, E - ether stressed, A - ACTH injected, S - saline injected. Each bar represents mean ± SEM for 10 rats.

adrenal cortex of adult rats are caused by propylthiouracil (Callas, 1971) which may alter function. Consequently, electron microscopic observations were made of zona fasciculata from the adrenals of stimulated and unstimulated young euthyroid and hypothyroid rats.

The primary organelles of zona fasciculata cells which are involved with steroidogenic processes are the lipid droplets, the smooth endoplasmic reticulum (SER), and the mitochondria (Nussdorfer et al., 1984). Therefore, volume fractions of these organelles were determined in zona fasciculata cells of 15 and 20 day old normal and hypothyroid rats (Table 1). The most striking differences between 15 day old euthyroid and thiouracil exposed rats are a deficiency of volume of lipid droplets before stimulation and an accumulation, rather than a depletion, of lipid in response to ether fumes in hypothyroid pups (Schulte, 1980). Although somewhat more equivocal, exposure to thiouracil may also result in elevation of SER volume in basal and ACTH stimulated conditions (Table 1). By 20 days of age, the influence of thiouracil on lipid droplet volume fraction is eliminated (Klak and Meserve, 1983), and a possible elevation of SER volume persists only in the basal state. These results may be interpreted to indicate that any obvious structural effects upon adrenocortical cells of hypothyroidism induced by perinatal exposure to thiouracil occur before two weeks of postnatal development, can be over-ridden by administration of a large dose of exogeneous ACTH, and largely disappear by 20 days of age.

Table 1. Volume fraction of lipid droplets, smooth endoplasmic reticulum (SER), and mitochondria of adrenal zona fasciculata cells from 15 and 20 day old euthyroid (Eu) and hypothyroid (Hypo) rats before and after stimulation.*

Stimulus	Age	Lipid Droplets		SER		Mitochondria	
		Eu	Hypo	Eu	Hypo	Eu	Hypo
None							
	15d	2.35	0.15	6.97	8.96	9.74	10.07
	20d	2.18	3.06	5.51	8.96	11.29	10.94
Ether	15d	0.33	4.83	7.00	6.55	7.90	10.07
	20d	2.73	3.57	6.70	6.27	11.98	8.47
ACTH	15d	2.38	2.23	5.22	7.75	9.65	9.92
(4 IU)	20d	3.98	3.22	7.30	7.61	11.94	11.16

* Expressed as m^3 of organelle per 33.3 m^3 of adrenal cell.

The above studies do not provide evidence as to whether the functional alterations of HPA axis response and the alterations caused in adrenal ultrastructure are direct effects of thiouracil, direct effects of hypothyroidism, or indirect effects of either of these conditions. It is important to differentiate between these influences, since Steinetz and Beach (1963) reported differences in response of adrenal glands from adult rats made hypothyroid by surgical thyroidectomy and those fed thiouracil. Furthermore, thiouracil induced hypothyroidism is known to depress pituitary growth hormone content in mice (Meserve and Rhodes, 1979) and in rats (Froelich and Meserve, 1982), and growth hormone is required to minimize the 5α-reduction of corticosterone within the adrenal cortex (Colby et al., 1973). Thus, is became necessary to perform in vitro studies to determine activity of selected adrenal enzymes and reactivity of HPA axis components from chemically and congenitally hypothyroid animals.

In Vitro Studies

The activity of 3β-HSD and 5α-reductase was determined in adrenocortical homogenates from normal and chemically hypothyroid male mice to ascertain whether alterations could cause the effects on HPA axis response seen in vivo. Although circulating T_4 levels were significantly depressed, alterations of enzyme activity of the sort required to prevent cortiosterone synthesis and/or release did not occur (Table 2). Since 3β-HSD is a rate limiting enzyme in steroidogenesis, catalyzing the conversion of pregnenolone to progesterone, a decrease in corticosterone synthesis brought about by alteration of this enzyme would require that its activity be decreased (Meserve and Ting, 1982). If there was any change in the activity of 3β-HSD in response to thiouracil exposure, it was an increase (Table 2). Conversely, thiouracil would be required to cause an increase in the activity of 5α-reductase if this enzyme were to be responsible for decrease release of corticosterone from the adrenal (Meserve and Rahman, 1984). However, activity of 5α-reductase decreased, if it changed at all, in the thiouracil fed mice. Given the minimal modification of activity of 3β-HSD and 5α-reductase in thiouracil fed mice, and given that the possible direction of change of activity of both enzymes would increase corticosterone synthesis and release, rather than decrease it, it would seem unlikely that such modification of activity would importantly hamper HPA axis function.

Alteration of a number of physiological processes by induction of chemical or congenital hypothyroidism could confound results of in vivo measurements of HPA axis function. For example, modifications of rate of circulation, permeability of capillaries, or concentration of plasma carrier proteins, could provide results interpretable as changes in HPA axis function.

Table 2. Thyroxine (T_4) levels, and adrenal 3β -hydroxysteroid dehydrogenase (3β -HSD) and 5α-reductase activities, in euthyroid and chemically hypothyroid (thiouracil-induced) adult male mice.

	Euthyroid	Hypothyroid	Significance
n	20	20	-
T_4 μg/dl	2.8 ±0.1	1.8 ±0.1	P<0.05
3β-HSD*			
μU/g	3.81 ±0.21	5.26 ±0.18	P<0.01
U/pair	19.3 ±1.0	22.0 ±1.7	N.S.
5α-reductase**			
U/10mg	3.37 ±0.20	3.50 ±0.57	N.S.
U/pair	1.12 ±0.04	0.85 ±0.11	P<0.05

*1U = 1 mol NADH formed per min.
**1U = 1 μg corticosterone reduced per hr.
N.S. - not significant.

Thus, assessement of the functional potential of HPA axis components after removal from the animal is important to the understanding of functional alterations. As previously reported (Meserve and Pearlmutter, 1983), the response of adrenals to a standard ACTH stimulus, and the ACTH content of pituitary glands from 15 day old rats was not modified by thiouracil when measured by bioassay using the flowing system of Saffran et al. (1971). On the other hand, bioassay (Pearlmutter et al., 1974) of hypothalamic CRF content from the same animals revealed a severe deficit as a result of thiouracil feeding (Table 3). With the advent of RIA components for CRF_{1-41}, the bioassay experiment was repeated to determine the levels of immunoactive peptide in hypothalamic extracts. While the results provide the same general trend as those obtained by bioassay, there are important differences which cannot be ignored (Table 3). A comparison of adult CRF reactivity with that from 15 day old normal rats shows the bioactivity to be similar, but the immunoactivity to be significantly (3X) greater in the adult. Furthermore, the large difference between euthyroid

Table 3. Bioactive and immunoactive corticotropin-releasing factor (CRF) in the hypothalamus of normal adult, 15 day old euthyroid, and 15 day old chemically hypothyroid rats

	Bioactive CRF		Immunoactive CRF	
	n[a]	% of adult	n[a]	μg/hypothalamus
Adult	17	100.0[b]	6	1038.5 ± 91.6
15D Euthyroid	8	84.0 ± 7.6	6	355.6[d] ± 52.0
15D Hypothyroid	9	4.0[c] ± 1.4	6	139.9[d,e] ± 45.0

a. Number of hypothalamic pools assayed.
b. Adult bioactivity set at 100%.
c. Significantly different from euthyroid ($P<0.001$).
d. Significantly different from adult ($P<0.001$).
e. Significantly different from euthyroid ($0.01<P<0.02$).

and hypothyroid pups relative to bioactivity of CRF is decreased, but still significant, when immunoactivity is measured. It is hypothesized that these discrepancies are the result of immunologically active precursors of CRF in the hypothalamus of the adult which are not bioactive, and to deficiencies of molecules in the hypothalamus of hypothyroid pups which interact with immunoactive CRF_{1-41} to confer greater biological activity (Meserve, 1984).

The availability of congenitally hypothyroid mice (<u>hyt/hyt</u>) as described by Beamer et al. (1981) has obviated the necessity of administration of thiouracil to induce hypothyroidism. This allows the removal of confounding influences of thiouracil which are non-specific to thyroid function. To date, only preliminary in vitro studies have been done using these animals to determine hypothalamic content of CRF by RIA (Table 4). Interpretation of these data suggests that congenital hypothyroidism also depresses hypothalamic CRF content. It should be noted that the only difference of significance was found in 30 day old animals in which very small numbers of data points were analyzed. The variability of CRF content at 15 days and in adult mice, which prevented significance at $P<0.05$, may be the result of failure to control for the genotype of the mother. After birth of the young, diet containing thyroid powder, which was fed to ensure mating and pregnancy (Beamer and Cresswell, 1982), was withdrawn. Normal thyroid hormone levels would be maintained in the phenotypically

Table 4. Hypothalamic CRF immunoreactivity in hyt/+ and hyt/hyt mice

Age	pg CRF per hypothalamus	
	hyt/+	hyt/hyt
15d	304.9 (6) ±25.5	248.2 (6) ±13.6
30d	±320.3 (2)* 14.6	213.9 (2)* ±43.9
Adult (5-7 mo)	±331.6 (5) 57.3	250.7 (5) ± 43.9

Mean ± SEM (number of hypothalamic pools)
* Different at $P<0.05$

normal hyt/+ dams, but the resulting drop in thyroid hormone levels of hyt/hyt mothers might alter postnatal development of the pups. This suggestion is strengthened by the decrease in CRF levels of hyt/hyt pups between 15 and 30 days (Table 4).

Further in vivo studies of the functional development of the HPA axis in hyt/hyt mice and comparisons of these animals with chemically hypothyroid mice remain to be done. Now that these animals are readily available for experimentation the beginning of a literature base of studies related to the HPA axis in this animal model is being generated. For example, Noguchi and Sugisaki (1984) have described hypomyelination in cerebral tissue of 40 day old hyt/hyt mice. Such modifications of brain development might parallel alterations in CRF production. Additionally, Shire and Beamer (1984) have found the X-zone to be poorly developed in the adrenal cortices of female hyt/hyt mice. While the X-zone may be more important in female mice, its modification by hypothyroidism may be indicative of alteration of other adrenocortical steroidogenic zones as well.

SUMMARY AND CONCLUSIONS

Taken together, the studies reported above provide evidence that hypothyroidism modifies development of the HPA axis response to stress. When hypothyroidism is induced chemically with thiouracil, ultrastructural changes in adrenocortical cells may occur, but these alterations appear to have little influence on adrenal function and are largely returned to normal by 20 days of age. A more severe deficit in bioactivity and immunoactivity of hypothalamic CRF is caused by thiouracil in 15 day old rats. In vivo studies indicate that this deficit is overcome, with HPA axis functionality achieved, by 30 days of age. Preliminary experiments with genetically hypothyroid hyt/hyt mice indicate that these animals display depressed hypothalamic CRF content as well. More detailed comparisons of development of the HPA axis in chemically and congenitally hypothyroid animals remain to be determined.

ACKNOWLEDGEMENTS

The above research was supported in part by NIH grants HO 09533 and AM 18393, by Biomedical Research Support grants to Bowling Green State University and the Medical College of Ohio, by Grants-In-Aid-of-Research from Sigma Xi Research Honor Society, and by grants from the Faculty Research Committee, Bowling Green State University.

The author is indebted to the following for their input and their support of this research: Arlene (Klak) Hall, Denise (Schulte) Knox, James H. Leathem (deceased), A. Frances Pearlmutter, Zia-Ur Rahman, Murray Saffran, Joseph S. Scriffignano, and Shu-Mei Ting. Jane Trumbull is thanked for preparation of the manuscript.

REFERENCES

Angwin, P., and Barchas, J.D., 1982. Analysis of peptides in tissues and plasma: use of silicic acid extraction and reverse-phase columns for rapid purification prior to radioimmunoassay, J. Chromatogr., 231: 173-177.

Beamer, W.G., and Cresswell, L.A., 1982, Defective thyroid ontogenesis in fetal hypothyroid (hyt/hyt) mice, Anat. Rec., 202: 387-393.

Beamer, W.G., Eicher, E.M., Maltais, L.J., and Southard, J.L., 1981, Inherited primary hypothyroidism in mice, Science, 212: 61-63.

Callas, G., 1971, Changes in the fine structure of the adrenal cortex in the albino rat following the administration of propylthiouracil, Anat. Rec., 169: 474.

Colby, H.D., Caffrey, J.H., and Kitay, J.I., 1973, Interaction of growth hormone and ACTH in the regulation of adrenocortical secretion in rats, Endocrinology, 93: 188-192.

Davenport, G.R., and Mallette, L.E., 1966, Some biochemical properties of rabbit ovarian hydroxysteroid dehydrogenases, Endocrinology, 78: 672-678.

Eayrs, J.T., 1964, Effect of neonatal hyperthyroidism on maturation and learning in the rat, Anim. Behav., 12: 195-199.

Froelich, P.A., and Meserve, L.A., 1982, Altered growth patterns and depressed pituitary growth hormone content in young rats: effects of pre- and postnatal thiouracil administration, Growth, 46: 296-305.

Glick, D., von Redlich, D., and Levine, S., 1964, Fluorometric determination of corticosterone and cortisol in 0.02-0.05 milliliters of plasma or submilligram samples of adrenal tissue, Endocrinology, 74: 653-655.

Greenberg, A.M., Naijar, S., and Blizzard, R.M., 1974, Effects of thyroid hormone on growth, differentiation, and development, in "Handbook of Physiology, Endocrinology, Thyroid," M.A. Greer and D.H. Solomon, eds., American Physiological Society, Washington, D.C., USA.

Guillet, R., Saffran, M., and Michaelson, S.M., 1980, Pituitary-adrenal response in neonatal rats, Endocrinology, 106: 991-994.

Hilf, R., Burnett, F.F., and Borman, A., 1960, The effect of sarcoma 180 and other stressing agents upon adrenal and plasma corticosterone in mice, Cancer Res., 20: 1389-1393.

Kitay, J.I., Coyne, M.D., and Swygert, N.H., 1970, Influence of gonadectomy and replacement with estradiol or testosterone on formation of 5α-reduced metabolites of corticosterone by the adrenal gland of the rat, Endocrinology, 87: 1257-1265.

Klak, A.T., and Meserve, L.A., 1983, Effects of thiouracil-induced hypothyroidism on adrenal ultrastructure, Micron Microsc. Acta, 14: 275-276.

Larsen, P.R., 1980, Hypothyroidism: a common endocrine disease in all age groups, Med. Times, 108: 47-60.

Meserve, L.A., 1976, The influence of thiouracil-induced hypothyroidism upon hypothalamo-hypophyseal-adrenal axis response in the 15 day old mouse, Sci. Biol. J., 2: 200-206.

Meserve, L.A., 1984, Depressed hypothalamic CRF immunoreactivity in 15 day old thiouracil-treated rats, Hormone Metab. Res., In press.

Meserve, L.A., and Leathem, J.H., 1973, Hypothyroidism and the maturation of the hypothalamo-hypophyseal-adrenal axis, Develop. Psycholbiol., 6: 123-129.

Meserve, L.A., and Leathem, J.H., 1974, Neonatal hyperthyroidism and maturation of the rat hypothalamo-hypophyseal-adrenal axis, Proc. Soc. Exp. Biol. Med., 147: 510-512.

Meserve, L.A., and Leathem, J.H., 1981, Development of hypothalamic-pituitary-adrenal response to stress in rats made hypothyroid by exposure to thiouracil from conception, J. Endocrinol., 90: 403-409.

Meserve, L.A., and Pearlmutter, A.F., 1983, Perinatal thiouracil exposure depresses corticotropin-releasing factor activity in 15 day old rats, Hormone Metab. Res. 15: 488-490.

Meserve, L.A., and Rahman, Z.-U., 1984, Adrenal 5α-reductase activity in normal male and female and thiouracil fed male mice, Ohio J. Sci. 84: 28.

Meserve, L.A., and Rhodes, A.B., 1979, Influence of pre- and postnatal thiouracil on pituitary growth hormone content in mice, Ohio J. Sci., 79: 267-271.

Meserve, L.A., and Scriffignano, J.S., 1984, Thyroid feeding from conception and hypothalamo-pituitary-adrenal axis response in 30 day old rats, Ohio J. Sci., In press.

Meserve, L.A., and Ting, S.-M., 1982, Response of adrenal 3β-hydroxy-Δ^5-steroid dehydrogenase to adrenocorticotropin treatment in thiouracil-fed male mice, Can. J. Physiol. Pharmacol., 60: 83-87.

Milković, K., Peruzović, M., and Paunović, J., 1982, Pituitary and adrenal glands in neonatal rats studied by metopirone (SU 4885), Biol. Neonate. 41: 32-37.

Noguchi, T., and Sugisaki, T., 1984, Hypomyelination in the cerebrum of the congenitally hypothyroid mouse (*hyt*), J. Neurochem., 42: 891-893.

Nussdorfer, G.G., Meneghelli, V., and Mazzocchi, G., 1984, Fine structure of the adenal cortex, *in*: "Ultrastructure of Endocrine Cells and Tissues," P.M. Motta, ed., Martinus Nijhoff Publishers, The Hague, Netherlands.

Oppenheimer, J.H., Schwartz, H.L., and Surks, M.I., 1972, Propylthiouracil inhibits the conversion of L-thyroxine to L-triiodothyronine. An explanation of the antithyroid effect of propylthiouracil and evidence supporting the concept that triiodothyronine is the active thyroid hormone, J. Clin. Invest., 51: 2493-2497.

Pearlmutter, A.F., Rapino, E., and Saffran, M., 1974, A semi-automated in vitro assay for CRF: activities of peptides related to oxytocin and vasopressin, Neuroendocrinology, 15: 106-119.

Pelton, E.W., and Bass, N.H., 1973, Adverse effects of excess thyroid hormone on the maturation of the rat cerebrum, Arch. Neurol., 29: 145-150.

Poland, R.E., Weichsel, Jr., M.E., and Rubin, R.T., 1979, Post-natal maturation patterns of serum corticosterone and growth hormone in rats: effect of chronic thyroxine administration, Hormone Metab. Res., 11: 222-227.

Rivier, J., Spiess, J., and Vale, W., 1983, Characterization of rat hypothalamic corticotropin-releasing factor, Proc. Natl. Acad. Sci. USA, 80: 4851-4856.

Saffran, M., Matthews, E.K., and Pearlmutter, A.F., 1971, Analysis of the response to ACTH by rat adrenal in a flowing system, Recent Prog. Hormone Res., 27: 607-630.

Schapiro, S., Geller, E., and Eiduson, W., 1962, Neonatal adreno-cortical response to stress and vasopressin, Proc. Soc. Exp. Biol. Med., 109: 937-941.

Schoenfeld, N.M., Leathem, J.H., and Rabii, J., 1980. Maturation of adrenal stress responsiveness in the rat, Neuroendocrinology, 31: 101-105.

Schulte, D., 1980, Effect of hypothyroidism on adrenal ultra-structure in stressed and unstressed young rats, Ohio J. Sci., 80: 12.

Shire, J.G.M., and Beamer, W.G., 1984, Adrenal changes in genetically hypothryoid mice, J. Endocrinol. 102: 277-280.

Steinetz, B.G., and Beach, V.L., 1963, Some influences of thyroid on the pituitary adrenal axis, Endocrinology, 72: 45-58.

Taurog, A., 1976, The mechanism of action of the thioureylene antithyroid drugs, Endocrinology, 98: 1031-1046.

Vanderpas, J., Bordoux, P., Lagasse, R., Rivera, M., Dramaix, M., Lody, D., Nelson, G., Delange, F., Ermans, A.M., and Thilly, C.H., 1984, Endemic infantile hypothyroidism in a severe endemic goitre area of central Africa, Clin. Endocrinol., 20: 327-340.

Weibel, E.R., Kistler, G.S., and Scherle, W.F., 1966, Practical stereological methods for morphometric cytology, J. Cell Biol. 30: 23-38.

IMMUNOLOGICAL STRESS INDUCES SEVERE CARDIAC MYOLYSIS:

MEDIATION BY LEUKOTRIENES

*U. Zor, *S. Moshonov, **A. Meshorer and ***N. Kauli

Depts. of Hormone Research* and Experimental Animals**
The Weizmann Institute of Science, Rehovot 76100
***Heart Institute, Kaplan Hospital, Rehovot, Israel

INTRODUCTION

In this review we bring evidence that immunological stress can lead directly to severe cardiac myolysis, which in turn could result in acute myocardial infarction (AMI). This kind of stress results from the reaction following antigen-antibody (Ag-Ab) complex formation on various cell surfaces. The chain of events includes an increase in intracellular Ca^{2+} concentration in certain cells which results in leukotriene (LT) generation. Leukotrienes are the principal mediators of anaphylatic shock, and cardiac anaphylaxis. A possible mechanism by which psychological (emotional) stress causes AMI will also be discussed. This is based on the hypothesis that stress-induced neurotransmitter release (acetylcholine, noradrenaline, dopamine) can stimulate LT production in the heart.

The most alarming and unexplained feature of an AMI is that it strikes suddenly and unexpectedly. Atherosclerosis may have been present for years, yet why the AMI should occur at the particular moment when it does is quite unknown. It has been generally accepted that thrombotic occlusion of a coronary artery is responsible for AMI, although a significant number do occur in the absence of thromboses. Roberts et al. (1) have also raised the question whether the thrombotic occlusion is a cause or result of the AMI.

An AMI may be initiated by spasm of the coronary arteries, and indeed the importance of the coronary spasm in inducing fatal AMI in the atherosclerotic patient has been emphasized in recent years (2). A spasm raises the local coronary resistance, which is largely under the control of locally produced vasoactive substances such as LTs. Whichever mechanism is responsible for initiating AMI, whether spasm and/or thrombus, the cardinal question is, why, at a particular time, is there a precipitous release of chemical mediators, which can lead to AMI and coronary sudden death (CSD). It is well known that both psychological (3) and physical stress, can trigger AMI, and we suggest that a third type of stress, immunological, has this same property. During the expression of each of these three types of stress there may be an elevation of intracellular Ca^{2+} in LT-producing cells, thereby stimulating LT formation (see Fig. 1). Since LTs are extremely potent vasoconstrictors and have spasmogenic activity, we are examining the possibility that they are intimately involved in AMI and CSD.

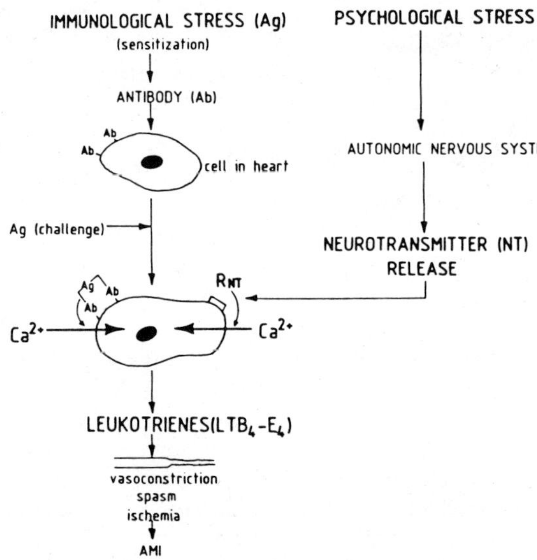

Fig. 1. Suggested chain of events and mechanism by which immunological and psychological stress can lead to AMI. Leukotrienes are generated in the heart vasculature following either a cellular immune response, or neurotransmitter release.

Characterization and spectrum of actions of LTs

Some years ago, Samuelsson and his colleagues in Sweden, Austen, Corey and colleagues in the U.S.A. and Piper and colleagues in the U.K. elucidated the chemical structure of a group of newly discovered metabolites of arachidonic acid, catalyzed by lipoxygenase, and named them leukotrienes. Some members of the LT family are constituents of "slow reacting substance of anaphylaxis" (SRS-A) which for many years was suspected as the predominant mediator of bronchoconstriction in asthma.

LTs are far more potent (on a molar basis) than histamine, thromboxane A_2, bradykinin and angiotensin, which are variously implicated in asthma and cardiovascular pathology. LTs have a variety of effects on different tissues: 1) they cause migration (chemotaxis) of leukocytes and enhance their adhesion to the endothelium of post capillary venules; 2) they increase blood vessel permeability; 3) they cause sustained contraction of smooth muscle, especially bronchial and vascular (4). As a result, LTs are responsible for a decrease in circulating leukocytes, and for their accumulation at the site of "injury" and inflammation, where edema is also present. Endogenous LTs, which are formed and released in response to a specific stimulus, such as Ag-Ab complexing, cause chronotropic and inotropic changes in the heart and reduce coronary blood flow (5). On exogeneous application to the heart there is a prolonged coronary vasoconstriction leading to ischemia and cardiac dysfunction. Like PGs, LTs are a family of compounds each of which has its own defined spectrum of actions.

The role of free intracellular calcium ions in stimulation of LT formation and action

Under resting conditions, the intracellular concentration of free Ca^{2+} is several orders of magnitude lower than the extracellular concentration. A large number of biological responses are dependent on an increase in the level of free intracellular calcium ion concentration. These include, for example, smooth muscle contraction, cellular adhesion, stimulus-secretion coupling, neurotransmitter release, enzyme activation, and other biological effects. As a result of Ag-Ab complexing, intracellular free calcium ion concentration rises, and mediators which produce the symptoms of anaphylaxis are synthesized and/or released. A high level of free calcium stimulates the activity of the intracellular enzyme, phospholipase A_2. This enzyme catalyzes the formation of free arachidonic acid and LTs appear finally among the mediators of anaphylaxis. Both phospholipase A_2 and free arachidonic acid are rate limiting factors for LT formation.

The Ca^{2+} antagonists, such as Mg^{2+} or calcium-channel-blocking agents are potent inhibitors of high blood pressure, vasoconstriction and CSD. These symptoms could possibly be attributed partially to LTs, in which case some of the effect of the calcium antagonists may result from inhibiting LT formation and action.

Immunological stress: Cardiac anaphylaxis

Cardiac anaphylaxis, which results from Ag-Ab cellular complexing in the heart itself, is one of the events which can take place during an allergic reaction both *in vitro* and *in vivo* (6). It is an immediate hypersensitivity reaction and comparable with lung anaphylaxis. There is an enhanced release of several mediators, including LTs, prostaglandins, thromboxane A_2, histamine and platelet activating factor (PAF) which separately and severally contribute to the reduced coronary flow, contractile failure and conduction arrhythmias characteristic of cardiac anaphylaxis. The LTs are probably derived in part from the adventitial layer of coronary vascular tissue, since this was recently shown to be a rich source of LTs (4), and possibly also from the leukocytes which accumulate in the heart following the primary immune response.

We are in fact suggesting that AMI is the climax of severe cardiac anaphylaxis. As such it would be triggered by the same factors which precipitate any other immune response. LTs are among the most important mediators of anaphylaxis (7), so treatment with LT synthesis inhibitors or LT receptor antagonists, would be expected to prevent an AMI if given before the immune response has time to erupt.

Antigenic factors which could trigger an AMI might be reinfection with a mild viral disease such as influenza. There would be a generalized immune reaction to the virus, and this would include cardiac anaphylaxis. This hypothesis is supported by preliminary reports which have appeared recently in which young patients with normal coronary arteries and no risk factors for coronary artery disease developed myocardial infarction two weeks after an acute viral illness (3). Also, in a recent prospective study involving 2 matched groups of 150 patients each, there was a history of acute respiratory symptoms in twice as many patients in the group with AMI as in the control group (9). These reports strengthen the basis for the correlation which has been found between influenza and mortality from AMI in epidimiological studies (10).

METHODS

Sensitization of guinea pigs with antigen

Guinea pigs of either sex, strain DH, weighing about 300 g were injected subcutaneously (s.c.) with 10^8 plaque-forming-units (pfu) of vesicular stomatitis virus (VSV).

Challenge with antigen *in vivo*: histological examination of heart

Two weeks after sensitization, the guinea pigs were challenged intraperitoneally (i.p.) with the virus (10^8 pfu). The animals were sacrificed between one and six hours after challenge and the heart removed for histological examination. In some experiments, the LT synthesis inhibitor, BW-755C was given (10 mg/kg) 1 h before challenge. The heart sections were stained in such a way as to distinguish morphological changes and identify infiltrating blood cell types.

Challenge with antigen *in vitro*: LT production in Langendorff preparation

Two to 4 weeks after sensitization, guinea pigs were sacrificed and the heart immediately removed. The coronary vasculature was perfused with warmed Tyrode solution and, after a half-hour stabilization period, the perfusate was collected for periods of 15 minutes. The challenge, 10^8 pfu VSV, was injected directly into the perfusion fluid. Coronary outflow rate was estimated by determination of perfusate volume per collection period.

Bioassay of LT on guinea pig ileum strip

Naive guinea pigs (DH) were sacrificed and the ileum was removed. Strips, two cm long, were cut and suspended in an organ bath containing Tyrode solution to which inhibitors of prostaglandin synthesis (indomethacin) had been added. In addition atropine and diphenhydramine, were added to the Tyrode to prevent contractions due to extraneous acetylcholine and histamine, respectively. Responses to standard doses of LTD_4 were obtained, and the perfusates from the isolated hearts assayed against them.

At the end of the experiment, standard and each unknown that had produced an LT-like response was given again, together with FPL 55712 1 µg/ml, at which concentration it is a specific LT receptor blocking agent.

RESULTS

Our study demonstrates in the guinea pig, that re-infection with a mild virus causes severe cardiac myolysis *in vivo*, cardiac anaphylaxis *in vitro*, and shows that LTs have an important role in the expression of these symptoms.

No detectable amounts of LT (< 0.5 ng/heart/15 min) were observed in the perfusion fluid from hearts isolated from naive guinea pigs or from those given either sensitizing or challenging dose of antigen alone. On the other hand, *in vitro* challenge of the hearts from 7 animals sensitized with VSV released 12.7±2.7 ng LTD_4-equivalent/heart/15 min within 15 min of challenge.

Cardiac Myolysis

A marked cardiac myolysis characterized by atrophy of the cytoplasm while the cell wall remains intact, was observed in VSV-sensitized animals, already 1 h after *in vivo* challenge (Fig. 2). The myolytic areas occurred as islands mainly in the auricular but also scattered in the ventricular region of the heart.

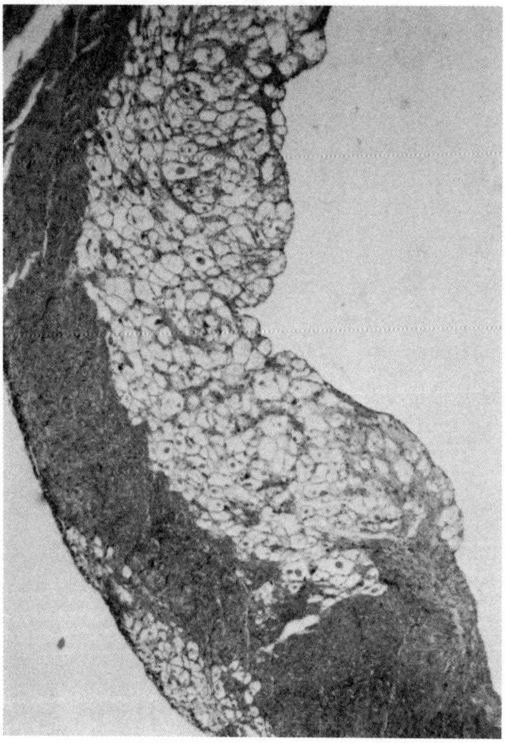

Fig. 2. Section of heart from guinea pig sensitized and challenged with VSV; animal sacrificed 6 h after challenge. Note severe myolysis, which occurs in islands.

Infiltration of leukocytes into myocardium

In many hearts taken from challenged animals, there was a strong inflammatory response already 1 h after challenge. Neutrophils and eosinophils accumulated especially in the auricles; lymphocytes and monocytes were not usually observed (Figs. 3A and B).

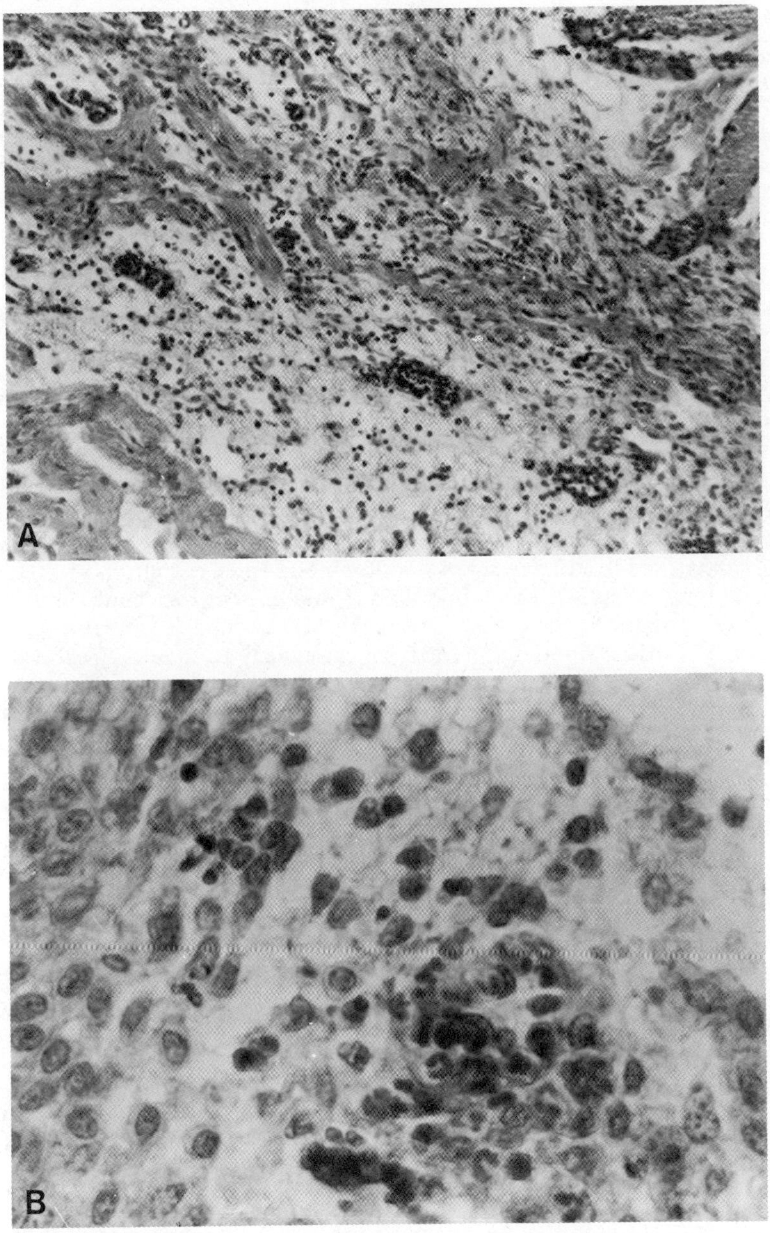

Fig. 3. Infiltration of leukocytes into the heart. Section of guinea pig heart removed 1 h after challenge with antigen. A. Magnification X 150; B. Magnification X 1000. These figures show many capillaries and small blood vessels packed with granulocytes. The same cells have infiltrated into the surrounding tissue.

DISCUSSION

A most important finding in our study was the appearance of myolysis in the heart tissue following recurrent mild viral infection. To the best of our knowledge this phenomenon has not been previously described in association with an immune response. In general, it was accompanied by infiltration of neutrophils and eosinophils. The process was remarkably fast and destruction of all intracellular organelles, including nuclei, was often complete within 2 hours of the challenge. The mechanism by which the recurrent viral infection causes damage to the heart is not clear. However, it is probably related to the immunological response since neither the sensitizing nor challenging dose of VSV alone induced myolysis or cell infiltration. Furthermore, a similar and more severe response was noted following immunization with albumin. It is suggested that due to enhanced production of LTs following challenge with VSV antigen (Fig. 1), the coronary vasculature undergoes spasm which leads to ischemia of the cardiac muscle, and this could account directly for the myolysis. Indeed oxygen deprivation has been found to induce focal myocytolysis in the cat heart (11). The fact that in our experiments the myolysis occurred in islands with clearly defined borders strongly favours the interpretation that the damage results from local ischemia. The main difference between myolysis and necrosis (which occurs in AMI in humans) is that in the latter case the cell destruction is total, including the cell wall, but both can result from ischemia. That the myolysis is a direct result of an abrupt cessation of the coronary blood supply may be inferred from the speed with which it develops and from the observation that all the myolytic cells are at the same stage of disintegration.

As in our immunologically-stimulated model, neutrophils (and eosinophils) appear in the myocardium, following infarction both in man and experimental animals (12,13). These leukocytes are a rich source of LTs (7), which, as mentioned earlier, are strongly chemotactic and chemokinetic for leukocytes, and, in addition, increase blood vessel permeability. Thus a positive feedback system seems to be engendered. A stimulus, immunological stress in this study, in the coronary blood vessels causes them to release LTs which in turn produce powerful local vasoconstriction and ischemia. Polymorphonuclear leukocytes are attracted to the region, themselves producing yet more LTs which exacerbate the damage to the myocardium. Indeed, when LT synthesis was inhibited, by administering BW755C to dogs, leukocyte infiltration into the occlusion-infarcted myocardium was attenuated (12). The importance of neutrophils themselves in the expression of infarct in experimental animals has also been demonstrated. When their number was reduced, by treatment with hydroxyurea or giving antibodies against neutrophils, or their accumulation limited by LT synthesis inhibitor, the infarcted area was smaller (12,13).

During cardiac anaphylaxis induced by challenge with albumin, several mediators are released in the heart, including histamine, PAF, prostaglandins, thromboxanes and LTs, which are responsible, at different stages and to varying degrees, for most of the symptoms of anaphylaxis (6). In our study, the antigen used was a virus which is not generally known to produce immunoglobulin E type antibodies. Nevertheless, in an immune system designed to produce immunoglobulin G antibodies, LTs were released and partially mediated the anaphylactic bronchoconstriction in guinea pigs (14). Thus complexes on the cell surface comprised of antigen with immunoglobulin G antibody could be responsible for the enhanced release of LT in our experiments following viral reinfection.

In order to verify the connection between the observed pathological changes and enhanced production of LTs during immunological response, one should show that the major changes can be mimicked by direct injection of LTs into the heart or coronary vasculature. On the other hand, when inhibitors and/or antagonists of LTs are given with the viral challenge, the pathological changes should be attenuated. It is probable that the combination of histamine, LTs, prostaglandins and thromboxanes may be necessary for full development of the pathological processes in the heart. Indeed, glucocorticosteroids, which among their other actions, prevent formation of all arachidonic acid metabolites, reduced infarct size and animal mortality in animals with experimentally-induced MI (15).

Psychological Stress

AMI occurs to a much greater extent in subjects whose coronary arteries are atherosclerotic than those with healthy arteries (16). Similarly, CSD rarely occurs when the heart is histologically normal (17).

Individuals exhibiting Type A behaviour (competitive, impatient, with excessive drive) are much more prone to AMI than their more relaxed Type B counterpart. Interestingly, these people also have a higher incidence and severity of atherosclerosis (3). This in turn is probably related to their exaggerated response to stress, when the Type A person inclines to a faster rise in blood pressure, increased platelet aggregation, more rapid clotting time, and excessive adrenal medullar activity (18).

In the shock ensuing a major catastrophe, the Athens earthquake of 1981, it was found that the stress-related CSD tended to occur in a background of atherosclerotic heart disease (19). This means that, equating atherosclerosis with AMI and not other causes of CSD, the immediate fatal response to this emotional stress was AMI. Other types of emotional stress, for example acute grief, or loss of a close relative or personal danger, are all well known to be liable to precipitate an AMI.

The mechanism by which emotional stress gives rise to an AMI is not clear. Our working hypothesis suggests that this type of stress stimulates areas in the CNS which control the autonomic nervous system, and thus neutrotransmitter release (noradrenaline, acetylcholine, dopamine) in the coronary vasculature (Fig. 1). Some neurotransmitters increase free intracellular calcium, and might therefore be responsible for LT generation and coronary spasm.

Neurotransmitters and generation of leukotrienes

According to our hypothesis LTs are the principal spasmogenic agents when an AMI results from coronary arterial vasoconstriction. Transmitter or hormone release during stress would not usually involve a single agent alone, but other hormones and mediators which can modify LT activity would be released alongside.

The vasomotor tone of coronary arteries, both large and small, is controlled by α-adrenergic sympathetic innervation (noradrenaline release) (20). During stress the sympathetic nervous system is activated so it has been suggested that these arteries could go into spasm, and trigger an AMI. At the same time, the sympathetic stimulation releases adrenaline from the adrenal medulla which acts in an opposing direction, and this is of greater importance during stress than adrenergic nerve activity (21). Coronary arterial spasm is the cause of Prinzmetal's variant angina, an illness which often develops into AMI. An attack was found to be brought on by adrenaline stimulating α-receptors, since phenoxybenzamine, an α-adrenoceptor antagonist, but not propranolol, a β-adrenoceptor antagonist, could suppress the attack (22). Furthermore, α-adrenergic stimulation by noradrenaline (NA) activated arachidonic acid formation and PG production in the rabbit iris (23). Thus NA might be expected to induce LT formation, should it similarly stimulate LT-producing cells. This suggestion is supported by evidence that α-adrenergic stimulation enhances the antigen-induced release of mediators of the immune response in the lung (24).

On the other hand β-adrenergic agonists tend to attenuate, and antagonists, such as propranolol, aggravate the constrictor response to LTs. This is found both in naive and antigen-sensitized tissues. Thus when stress activates the sympathetic system, the β-receptors in the heart are stimulated, cardiac function improves, and the deleterious effects of LT on myocardial contraction may be compensated (25-27). This indeed has been demonstrated in immunologically-stressed mice. Thyrotropin-releasing-hormone, a centrally acting sympathetic nervous system stimulant, caused an 80% reduction in mortality of these animals, and its probable mode of action was shown to be via release of adrenaline from the adrenal medulla. This selectively stimulated the β_1-adrenergic receptors in the heart and overcame the lethal effect of the Ag-Ab reaction (21).

Dopamine (DA) has not yet been proven to be a peripheral neurotransmitter, but two types of DA receptor exist in the cardiovascular system. If DA has a role in LT-induced coronary spasm it should be to oppose its effect since DA both causes vasodilation (post-junctional receptor stimulation), and inhibits release of NA (prejunctional receptor stimulation). During stress it is not known whether there are changes in DA activity (28).

Parasympathomimetic agents, such as methacholine and pilocarpine, cause an attack of Prinzmetal's variant angina in susceptible subjects (22,29). The action is via muscarinic receptors since atropine prevents the attack, but as there is little parasympathetic innervation in coronary arterioles, these agents could be acting indirectly. Indeed in the rabbit aorta acetylcholine (ACh) does appear to release a LT-like substance (30).

In antigen-sensitized animals there is an enhanced response to ACh-mediated reactions (31). This may be related to the finding that rat mast cells have muscarinic receptors, and very low doses of ACh do release histamine (32). It is reasonable to assume that the mechanism is Ca^{2+}-dependent, in which case LT-production would also be stimulated by ACh (see Fig. 1).

Thus, both α-adrenergic stimulation by NA and cholinergic muscarinic stimulation by ACh, systems which frequently work in opposition, are capable of releasing LT, and this potential is enhanced in antigen-immunized animals. NA and ACh can raise the level of free intracellular Ca^{2+} and so each neurotransmitter could activate phospholipase A_2 and LT synthesis.

<u>Viral infection (immunological stress) in humans associated with AMI</u>

In guinea pigs, which do not naturally develop AMI, we have seen that recurrent infection with a mild virus leads to LT production, myolysis and cell infiltration in the heart. In the same way, the immunological reactions following recurrent respiratory infection in man might also induce LT formation in the heart. These could cause spasm of the coronary vasculature, and ischemia of the area of heart nourished by those vessels, resulting finally, in atherosclerotic subjects, in an AMI. There are indeed subjects in whom the allergic response to ampicillin and ragweed pollen is expressed as myocardial ischemia, rather than asthmatic bronchoconstriction (33). Furthermore, in young human patients with healthy coronary arteries, viral infection was found to be associated with AMI and myocarditis (8,34); and epidemiologically, the incidence of AMI is significantly greater following respiratory illness than in the absence of infection (9,10). More epidemiological studies should be carried out to discern both the incidence of influenza and other viral infections in patients with AMI, and the incidence of AMI following viral infection. The role of LTs under these circumstances has also to be more clearly defined. Should a causal relationship be revealed between viral infection and AMI, an anti-leukotriene drug might prove useful in preventing AMI in virus-infected atherosclerotic subjects.

SUMMARY AND CONCLUDING REMARKS

Ever since the remarkably potent spasmogenic effect of leukotrienes (LTs) on coronary blood vessels was observed, these hormones have been invoked as important mediators for cardiac ischemia and consequently, acute myocardial infarction (AMI). We have suggested a mechanism which could explain the sudden onset of a spasm-induced AMI in terms of immunologically-induced LT release within the heart. LTs themselves are a family of compounds derived from arachidonic acid, and formed on demand via lipoxygenase enzymes. While several cell types, including those within the coronary vasculature, have the potential to generate LTs, the pathological trigger(s) for the formation of LTs in AMI remains unidentified. It is possible to induce LT production artificially with calcium ionophore (A23187), or naturally, as a result of Ag-Ab reaction on the cell surface; both of these treatments increase intracellular free calcium. We have suggested that stress, whether physical (exercise or injury), psychological (emotional) or immunological sets into motion a series of events which ultimately leads to LT release. Physical stress and emotional shock are both considered "risk factors" for AMI, so there is good reason to assume that the third type of stress, immunological, would fall into the same category. It is proposed that emotional stress directly causes release of neurotransmitters which elevate the intracellular calcium level and induce LT generation (Fig. 1).

Leukotrienes are known to be formed and released during immediate hypersensitivity reactions, and in the heart they induce cardiac anaphylaxis. In our study the severe pathological responses in the heart, following administration to guinea pigs, of a mild virus, occurred only on reinfection, with the same virus - an immunological reaction. We observed the development of cardiac myolysis and infiltration of granulocytes *in vivo* into the myocardium, and LT release *in vitro* from the isolated heart. It is suggested, therefore, that LT production, stimulated by Ag-Ab complexing on certain cell membranes, is, possibly in conjunction with other mediators, the immediate cause of these pathological findings.

The sympathetic nervous system is activated under all conditions of stress and so catecholamines, whether originating at nerve endings or in the adrenal medulla, may be involved in regulation of LT release and/or action. Thus, our hypothesis postulates that a) an important stimulus for LT release in the heart is immunological stress, which can result from viral, or other, infection. b) LTs are agents responsible for spasm-induced AMI. c) Emotional stress could induce neurotransmitter release which may increase LT formation or action in the coronary vasculature. Thus it follows that triggering of any immunological reactions in susceptible persons should as far as possible be prevented, since it would increase the risk of AMI.

A potential new treatment for AMI could be to increase the serum magnesium ion concentration (antagonist of Ca^{2+}) and thereby relax the coronary arterial spasm. Alternatively, Ca^{2+} antagonist drugs could be used prophylactically to prevent the increase of intracellular free Ca^{2+}. They are already in use for the treatment of hypertension and angina pectoris, and recently have actually been found to prevent allergic reactions.

It can be anticipated that in the near future, a drug will be introduced for clinical use which specifically blocks the synthesis and/or action of LTs. This kind of drug would be expected to prevent stress-induced AMI.

Acknowledgements

We are grateful to Dr. S. Moncada, Wellcome Research Laboratories, England, Dr. J. Rokach, Merck Frosst, Canada, and Mr. P. Sheard, Fisons, England, for supplying us with BW 755C, leukotrienes and FPL 55712, respectively; to Mrs. Doria Nathan for superb technical assistance in preparation of the histological slides; and to Mrs. Malka Kopelowitz for typing this manuscript.

REFERENCES

1. W.C. Roberts and B. M. Buja, The frequency and significance of coronary arterial thrombi and other observations in fatal acute myocardial infarction, Am. J. Med. 52:425 (1974).
2. H.R. Hellstrom, Coronary artery vasospasm: the likely immediate cause of acute myocardial infarction, Br. Heart J. 41:426 (1979).
3. C.D. Jenkins, Recent evidence supporting psychologic and social risk factors for coronary disease, New Eng. J. of Med. 294:987 (1976).
4. P.J. Piper, Pharmacology of leukotrienes, Brit. Med. Bull. 39:255 (1983).
5. G. Feuerstein, Leukotrienes and the cardiovascular system, Prostaglandins 27:781 (1984).
6. R. Levi, J.A, Burke and E.J. Corey, SRS-A, leukotrienes, and immediate hypersensitivity reactions of the heart, in: "Leukotrienes and Other Lipoxygenase Products", B. Samuelsson and R. Paoletti, eds., Raven Press, New York, pp. 215-222 (1982).

7. B. Samuelsson, Leukotrienes: Mediators of immediate hypersensitivity reactions and inflammation, Science 220:568 (1983).
8. C.L. Miklozek and W.H. Abelmann, Viral myopericarditis presenting as acute myocardial infarction, Circulation 64:IV-25 (1982).
9. D.H. Spodick, A.P. Flessas and M.M. Johnson, Association of acute respiratory symptoms with onset of acute myocardial infarction: Prospective investigation of 150 consecutive patients and matched control patients, Am. J. Cardiol. 53:481 (1984).
10. D. Bainton, G.R. Jones and D. Hole, Influenza and ischaemic heart disease - a possible trigger for acute myocardial infarction? Intl. J. Epidemiology 7:231 (1978).
11. M.J. Schlesinger and L. Reiner, Focal myocytolysis of the heart, Amer. J. Pathol. 31:443 (1955).
12. K.M. Mullane, N. Read, J.A. Salmon, and S. Moncada, Role of leukocytes in acute myocardial infarction in anesthetized dogs: Relationship to myocardial salvage by anti-inflammatory drugs, J. Pharm. Exp. Ther. 228:510 (1984).
13. J.L. Romson, B.G. Hook, S.L. Kunkel, G.D. Abrams, M.A. Schork, and B.R. Lucchesi, Reduction of the extent of ischemic myocardial injury by neutrophil depletion in the dog, Circulation 67:1016 (1983).
14. P. Andersson, Effects of inhibitors of anaphylactic mediators in two models of bronchial anaphylaxis in anaesthetized guinea-pigs, Br. J. Pharmac. 77:301 (1982).
15. P. Libby, P.R. Maroko, C.M. Bloor, B.E. Sobel and E. Braunwald, Reduction of experimental myocardial infarct size by corticosterone administration, J. Clin. Invest. 52:599 (1973).
16. W.P. Newman III, R.E. Tracy, J.P. Strong, W.D. Johnson and M.C. Oalmann, Pathology of sudden coronary death, Ann. N.Y. Acad. Sci. 382:39 (1982).
17. R.S. Eliot and J.C. Buell, Role of the central nervous system in sudden cardiac death, In: "Biobehavioral Bases of Coronary Heart Disease", T.M. Dembroski, T.H. Schmidt, G. Blümchen, eds., S. Karger, Basel pp. 257-270 (1983).
18. J.C. Buell and R.S. Eliot, Behavior and the pathophysiology of coronary heart disease in humans, in: "Biobehavioral Bases of Coronary Heart Disease", T.M. Dembroski, T.H. Schmidt, G. Blümchen, eds., S. Karger, Basel pp. 237-247 (1983).
19. D. Trichopoulos, K. Katsouyanni, X. Zavitsanos, A. Tzonou and P. Dalla-Vorgia, Psychological stress and fatal heart attack: The Athens (1981) earthquake natural experiment. The Lancet, February 26, 441 (1983).
20. S.F. Vatner, Alpha-adrenergic regulation of the coronary circulation in the conscious dog. Am. J. of Cardiol. 52:15A (1983).
21. S. Amir, Anti-anaphylactic action in the mouse of thyrotropin-releasing hormone (TRH) is mediated through β_1-adrenoceptive

22. H. Yasue, M. Touyama, M. Shimamoto, H. Kato, S. Tanaka and F. Akiyama, Role of autonomic nervous system in the pathogenesis of Prinzmetal's variant form of angina, Circulation 50:534 (1974).
23. A.A. Abdel-Latif, J.P. Smith, S.Y.K. Yousufzai and R.K. Dover, Effects of catecholamines and their metabolites and other pharmacological agents on arachidonic acid metabolism and prostaglandin release by rabbit iris muscle and iris microsomes, in: "Neural Membranes", G.Y. Sun, N. Bazan, J-Y Wu, G. Porcellati and A.Y. Sun, eds., The Humana Press, Inc., Clifton, N.J. pp. 97-122 (1983).
24. M. Kaliner, R.P. Orange and F.K. Austen, Immunological release of histamine and slow reacting substance of anaphylaxis from human lung, J. Exp. Med. 136:556 (1972).
25. D.I. Alexander, P. Eyre and V.P. Gordon, Anaphylactic contraction (Schultz-Dale reaction) of the bovine bronchial artery in vitro, Br. J. Pharmac. 80:7 (1983).
26. S. Bongrani, G.C. Folco, R. Razzetti and P. Schiantarelli, β_2-adrenoceptor blockade is the basis of guinea-pig bronchial hyper-responsiveness to leukotriene C_4 and other agonists, Br. J. Pharmac. 79:839 (1983).
27. T. Kirchner and B.M. Weichman, Propranolol potentiates leukotriene D_4-induced bronchoconstriction and enhances antagonism by FPL 55712, Prostaglandins 27:119 (1984).
28. B.A. Berkowitz, Dopamine and dopamine receptors as target sites for cardiovascular drug action, Fed. Proc. 42:3019 (1983).
29. M. Endo, K. Hirosawa, N. Kaneko, K. Hase, Y. Inoue and S. Konno, Prinzmetal's variant angina. Coronary arteriogram and left ventriculogram during angina attack induced by methacholine, New Eng. J. of Med. Jan. 294:252 (1976).
30. U. Förstermann and B. Neufang, C-6-sulfidopeptide luekotrienes are unlikely to be involved in the endothelium dependent relaxation of rabbit aorta by acetylcholine, Prostaglandins 27:181 (1984).
31. M. Halonen and M. Kaliner, Heightened cholinergic responsiveness in IgE-producing rabbits, Int. J. Immunopharmac. 6:351 (1984).
32. R. Fantozzi, E. Masini, P. Blandina, P.F. Mannaioni and T. Bani-Sacchi, Release of histamine from rat mast cells by acetylcholine, Nature 273:473 (1978).
33. L.H. Criep and T.R. Woehler, The heart in human anaphylaxis, Ann of Allergy 29:399 (1971).
34. J. Heikkilä, and J. Karjalainen, Evaluation of mild acute infectious myocarditis, Br. Heart J. 47:381 (1982).

RELATIONSHIPS BETWEEN THE AMOUNT OF SLEEP, STRESS, AND OVARIAN FUNCTION IN WOMEN

Robert T. Chatterton, Jr.,* Alice J. Dan,**
Frank A. DeLeon-Jones,*** Gerald A. Hudgens,****
John N. Haan,* Sara D. Cheesman,* and Kerry L. Cheesman*

*Department of Obstetrics and Gynecology
Northwestern University Medical School
Chicago, IL
**Department of Medical and Surgical Nursing
College of Nursing
University of Illinois at the Medical Center
Chicago, IL
***Research and Development Office
West Side Veterans Administration Hospital
and Department of Psychiatry
University of Illinois at the Medical Center
Chicago, IL
****U.S. Army Human Engineering Laboratory
Aberdeen Proving Ground, Maryland

ABSTRACT

The incidence of ovulation was studied in a group of 33 normal young women by means of changes in basal body temperature (BBT) and by the pattern of pregnanediol glucuronide and LH concentrations in morning urine specimens. Blood was also drawn for progesterone and LH assays on 10 consecutive days of one cycle in each of 15 of these women. Perceived stress and hours of sleep were recorded daily. Ovulation occurred by hormonal criteria in only 22 of 33 cycles studied, and only 14 of the ovulatory cycles had a detectable midcycle rise in BBT. Anovulatory subjects had significantly less sleep than subjects in the ovulatory groups. The frequency of ovulation was not influenced by the stress of blood withdrawal, nor was it related to the level of perceived stress. However, the perception of stress was significantly reduced during the luteal phases of ovulatory cycles in subjects having a clear rise in BBT.

INTRODUCTION

The usefulness of measurements of daily concentrations of LH and pregnanediol (PD) in urine has been demonstrated in a number of recent studies (1-4). Our own method has been validated by comparison of early morning urinary PD concentrations with PD measured in 24 h urine specimens by RIA, with PD measured by gas chromatography, and with progesterone (P) measured in serum of the same subjects (1). Daily morning urine specimens may be collected for the complete menstrual cycle without inconvenience or trauma to the subject, and the results are much more reliable for estimation of the occurrence and precise time of ovulation than basal body temperature (BBT) (5, 6).

Previous investigators of hormone patterns in the normal menstrual cycle have screened subjects primarily on the basis of regularity and length of previous menstrual cycles and absence of contraceptive steroid use (7-18). Even after initial screening, as many as 30% of subjects chosen for the studies have been found to be anovulatory by hormonal criteria (7-18). Among factors that we have considered that might be responsible for anovulatory cycles is the daily blood drawing necessary for measurement of hormones in serum. Other factors such as psychosocial stresses or amount of sleep may be factors leading to anovulation especially in a group of students. In the present study ovulation and duration of luteal function was assessed by measurement of urinary LH and PD, by daily BBT recordings, and by serum LH. Several stress-related factors were monitored daily throughout the study.

MATERIALS AND METHODS

Subjects. Recruitment was from among the students and staff at the University of Illinois Health Sciences Center. Twenty four subjects completed the study in the first year and nine in the second year. All volunteers were women who had regular menstrual periods of from 27 to 33 days during the previous year. They also denied having used oral contraceptives or other drugs chronically during the previous 3 months. The ages of the subjects ranged from 19 to 33 with a median age of 22. Of 33 women in the study, 21 were undergraduate students, 6 were graduate students, and 7 were staff members. Only 5 were married at the time of the study.

Subjects collected morning urine specimens daily. In the first year urine voided between 2300 h and 0700 h was collected. In the second year only an early morning specimen of about 4 oz was collected. Subjects took and recorded basal body temperature daily, and filled out a daily form on which hours of sleep and a stress score were recorded. The subjects recorded their perception of the stress they had experienced during the previous 24 h period by checking one of the following responses: (a) unusually low stress, (b) mild stress, (c) moderate stress, (d) high stress, or (e) unusually severe stress. For purposes of tabulating responses, these were given scores of 1-5, respectively. The actual events considered stressful by the subjects were examinations, upsetting movies and plays, visits to therapists, unexpected good or bad news, etc. Complex psychosomatic states, such as arousal or stress responses, are difficult to assess reliably across subjects, because various physiological indicators may differ in their salience for different individuals. With such differences in the modality of response, it has been found that subjective reports of internal states give a better overall estimate of the strength of the response for most subjects (19). The subjective stress measure has been validated in the context of these study conditions (20). Correlations between overall subject means for perceived stress and a standardized anxiety scale (21), a daily listing of negative events, and hours of sleep/day were 0.50, 0.44, and -0.57, respectively. All correlations were significant at $P < 0.05$.

Specimens and data including BBT values were turned in daily. In the first year subjects were scheduled to participate in the study for two complete menstrual cycles in order to test the effect of the stress of blood drawing on ovulation. Each of 15 subjects was assigned to have 10 ml of blood drawn from the antecubital vein for 10 consecutive days starting on day 9 of one menstrual cycle (first day of menstrual bleeding was day 1). The cycle for blood drawing was selected by random drawing. Blood samples were not collected in the study conducted in the second year.

Assays. RIA for PD glucuronide in urine was carried out as previously described after dilution of urine with buffer (1). The buffer was 0.02 M sodium phosphate, pH 7.0, containing 1.0 mg/ml of gelatin and 1.0 mg/ml of sodium azide. Purification of PD glucuronide prior to RIA was shown to be unnecessary (1).

LH was also measured in urine and serum without purification essentially as described by Schalch et al. (22). Antiserum and reference material (LER-907) were supplied by the National Pituitary Agency.

Progesterone (P) was measured by RIA as described earlier with an antiserum against an 11α-hydroxyprogesterone hemisuccinate-thyroglobulin conjugate (23).

All urine specimens were assayed for PD and all serum samples were assayed for P. The five urine and serum samples that were estimated to encompass the preovulatory period were then assayed for LH. The temporal correspondence between LH in serum and urine

TABLE I

Factors associated with the occurrence of ovulation in the first menstrual cycle studied on each subject.

	Group	No. of first Cycles		Cycle Length (days ± SE)	Proportion of cycles in which blood was drawn	Mean Stress Scores ± SE	Sleep (h/day ± SE)
		yr 1	yr 2		(yr 1 only)		
I	Ovulatory by all criteria	7	7	30.1 ± 1.9	4/12	2.48 ± 0.13	7.32 ± 0.16
II	Ovulatory by hormones but not BBT	7	1	28.1 ± 0.4	5/13	2.42 ± 0.22	7.25 ± 0.21
III	Anovulatory by hormones, but with BBT rise	2	0	25.5 ± 0.5	1/4	2.15 ± 0.23	7.68 ± 0.25
IV	Anovulatory by all criteria	8	1	28.8 ± 1.4	5/17	2.51 ± 0.25	6.53 ± 0.16

has already been reported in these subjects as has the correspondence between the appearance of increases in serum P and urinary PD (1).

Analysis of data. After determination of the day of the greatest concentration (peak) of LH in serum and/or urine, this day of the menstrual cycle was then designated day zero for purposes of analysis. Variables of BBT, hours of sleep, stress scores, and PD concentrations in urine were plotted daily in relation to the LH peak. Statistical analyses were carried out by Analysis of Variance. Because of the lack of independence between first and second consecutive cycles on each subject, only the first cycles were used to evaluate effects of sleep and perceived stress on ovulation. However, second cycles analyzed separately showed no systematic difference from first cycles.

RESULTS

Based on the presence of a midcycle peak of LH in urine exceeding 10 mIU/ml and urinary PD concentrations on 3 consecutive days exceeding 1.5 μg/ml (8-hr collection) or 2.0 μg/ml (early morning specimens) and a luteal phase (day after LH peak through the day before menses) of 11 days or more , 22 women had ovulatory cycles and 11 did not. However, among the cycles that appeared to be ovulatory, only 14 (Group I) had a biphasic BBT pattern indicative of ovulation. The remaining 8 (Group II) individually did not have a discernable increase in BBT, although the mean values of the group tended to increase somewhat with time after the LH peak. The average length of the luteal phase in Group II was significantly less ($P < 0.05$) than that of Group I, 11.9 ± 1.5 and 13.3 ± 1.4 days, respectively. The average PD concentration during an middle 5 days of the luteal phases of these two groups, however, was not different when 8-h specimens are compared. Higher concentrations of PD were found in early morning specimens than in specimens collected during an 8 h interval, as reported previously (1), and therefore data from the second year cannot be averaged with the first. Two women had menstrual cycles with BBT shifts typical of ovulation, but had PD values that showed only sporadic increases during the second half of the cycles (Group III). Serum P, when measured after the BBT rise in subjects of this group was less than 2 ng/ml. Group IV consisted of 9 women with menstrual cycles that had no characteristics of ovulation, including consistently low serum LH and P in all 4 subjects in which blood was drawn. The number of menstrual cycles in each group and cycle length are shown in Table 1. Pregnanediol excretion patterns during the menstrual cycle of Groups I, II, and IV in year 1 are shown in Figure 1. Data were too few in Group III to establish a pattern. The data from year 2 were similar, but were uniformly higher for reasons described above. The patterns of BBT during these cycles are presented in Figure 2.

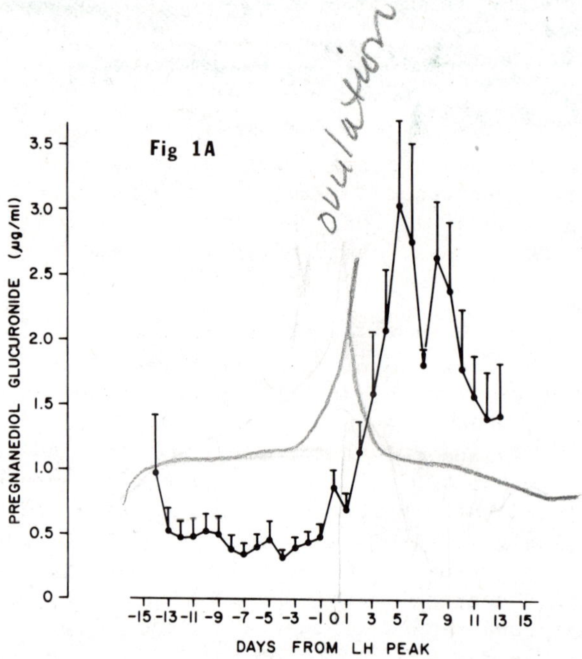

Fig. 1 Mean ± SE pregnanediol glucuronide concentrations in urine during the menstrual cycle. (7 subjects, year 1) Data is plotted from the day of the LH peak, which was designed day zero

A. Group I, subjects that were ovulatory by all criteria

B. Group II, subjects that were ovulatory by hormones but not by BBT

C. Group IV, subjects that were anovulatory by all criteria

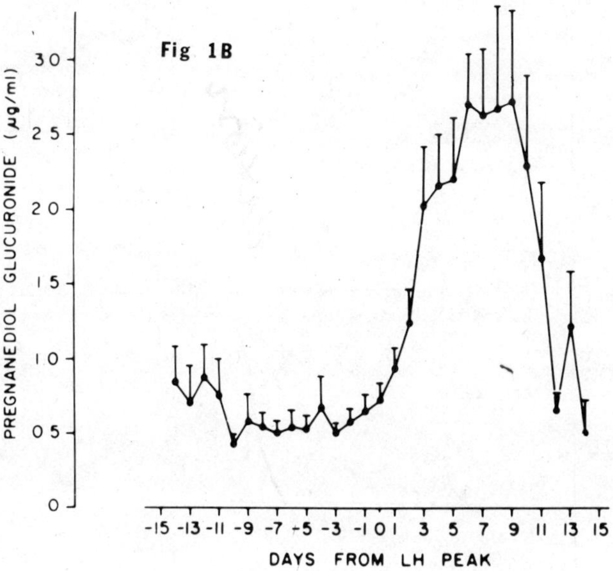
Fig 1B
PREGNANEDIOL GLUCURONIDE (μg/ml)
DAYS FROM LH PEAK

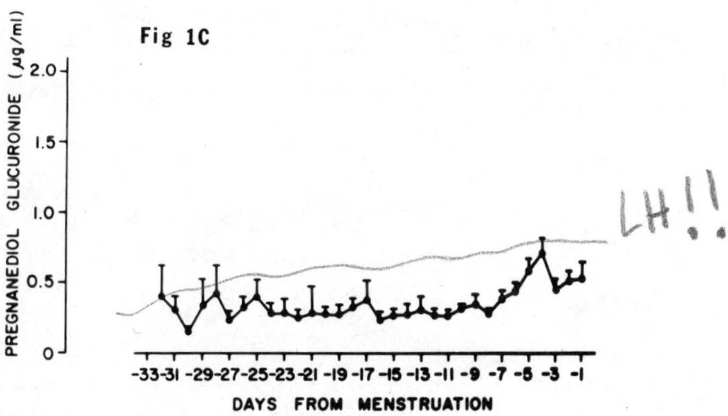
Fig 1C
PREGNANEDIOL GLUCURONIDE (μg/ml)
DAYS FROM MENSTRUATION

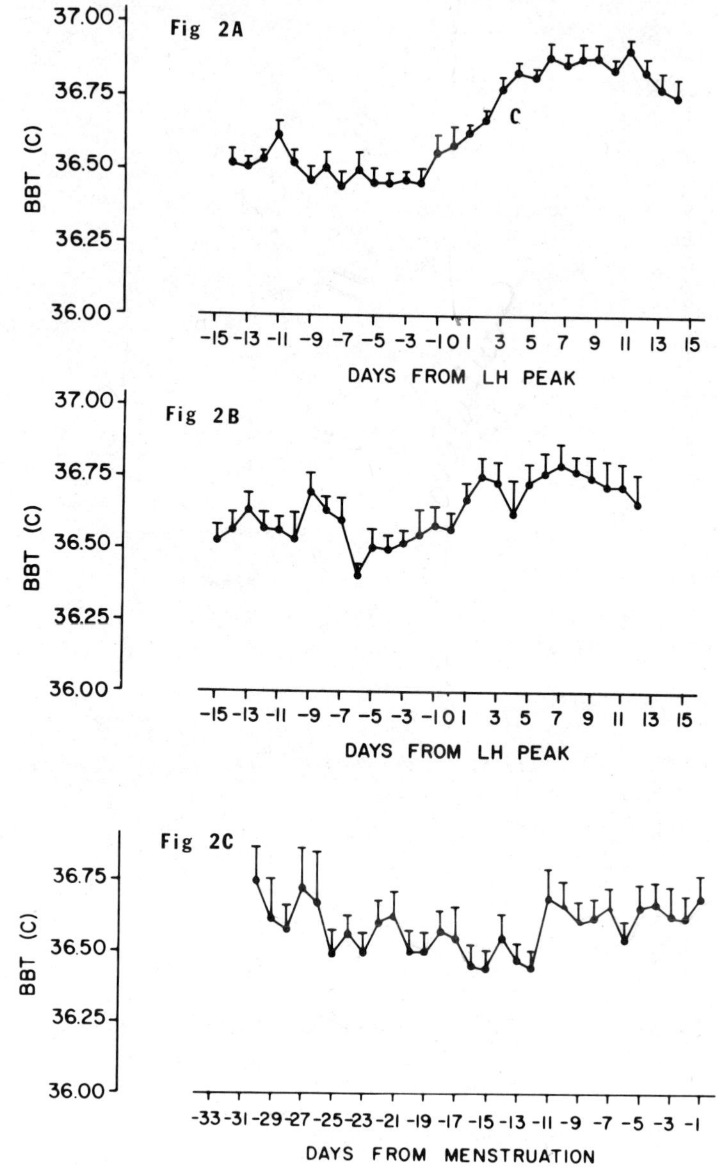

Fig. 2 Mean ± SE basal body temperature (BBT) for 14 subjects during the menstrual cycle.
A. Group I B. Group II C. Group IV

Mean stress scores were calculated for each subject for first menstrual cycles. Group means are shown in Table 1. Differences among Groups I through IV were not significant by Analysis of Variance.

Stress scores for all subjects within Groups I, II, and IV were averaged for each day of the menstrual cycle with the day of the LH peak being designated day zero (Fig 3). A comparision of stress scores in follicular vs. luteal phases of the cycle in ovulatory subjects (Groups I and II) revealed a lower perception of stress during the luteal phase of Group I, but not of Group II. The interaction between Groups and phases was significant (P = 0.01) by Analysis of Variance. Group I was further analyzed by year, as shown in Table 2. The mean levels of perceived stress in each phase of the menstrual cycle were similar, with lower values in the luteal phase both years. Group III had too few subjects for statistical evaluation. For the anovulatory subjects (Group IV) in which no midcycle LH peak from which to date the cycle occurred, dating was done by counting back from the first day of the subsequent cycle. Synchronizing the cycles in this way was done to maximize the probability of detecting luteal or premenstrual changes in stress scores in these women whose menstrual cycles varied considerably in length. However, no changes in stress scores between the two periods, days -1 to -12 and -13 to -24 were detected.

Table 2

Perceived Stress Scores ± SE in Follicular and Luteal Phases of Ovulatory Menstrual Cycles in Subjects During the 1st and 2nd Year of the Study.

Yr	No. Subjects	Follicular		Luteal	
1	7	2.69	0.17	2.39	0.18
2	7	2.83	0.34	2.25	0.15

To evaluate blood drawing itself as a potential stressor, 10 ml of blood was drawn for 10 consecutive days from 15 subjects, from five subjects during the first cycle of the study, and from 10 during the second cycle. Anovulatory cycles were not associated with blood drawing (Table 1). That is, the proportion of ovulatory to anovulatory cycles in which blood had been drawn was not less than the proportion in which it was not drawn.

The mean hours of sleep (first cycles) for subjects was different among Groups ($P < 0.025$) by Analysis of Variance with

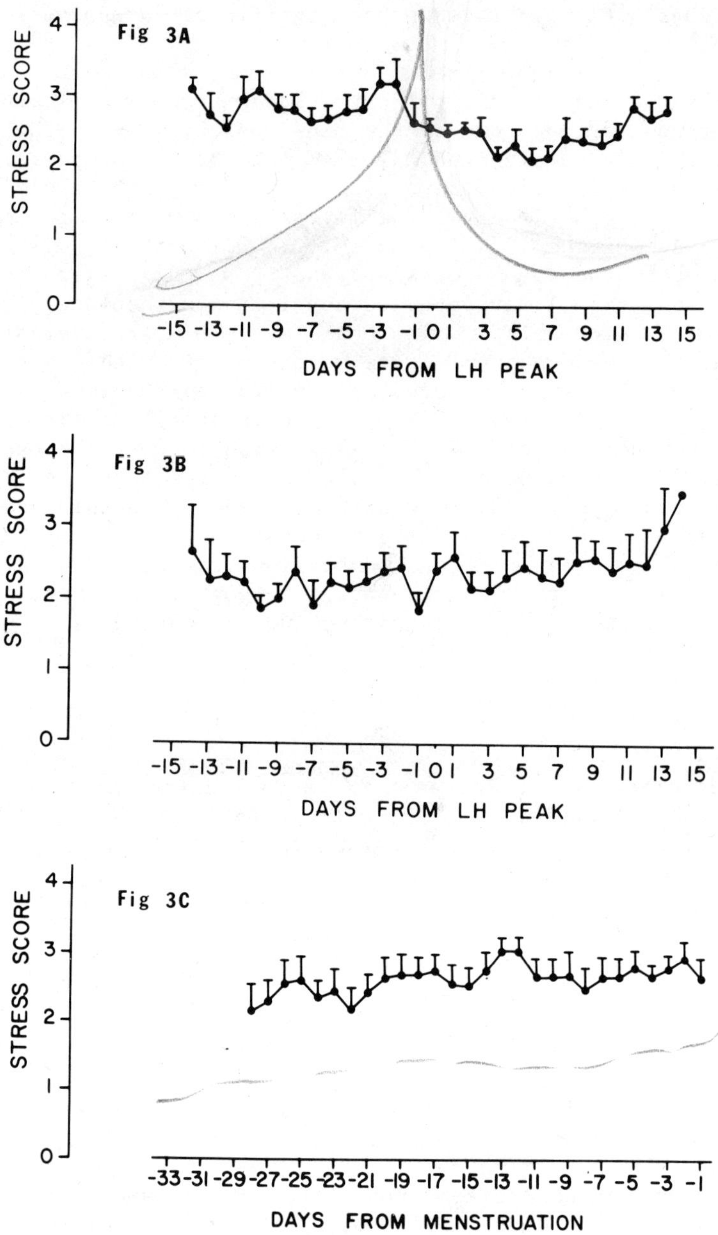

Fig. 3 Mean ± SE subjective stress scores of 14 subjects during the menstrual cycle.
A. Group I B. Group II C. Group IV

the mean being clearly less in anovulatory subjects (Group IV) than in the other groups. Group means are shown in Table 1. There were no significant trends in duration of sleep during the menstrual cycle in any of the groups when group means for each day were plotted in relation to the LH peak. There was, however, a significant negative correlation between stress scores and hours of sleep among subjects (r = -0.57).

DISCUSSION

A surprising lack of correspondence between hormonal criteria of ovulation and occurrence of biphasic BBT occurred in this study. Collecting the BBT data daily from the subjects may have been a contributing factor for two reasons. First, the opportunity for the subjects to observe first-hand the variability caused by failure to comply exactly with the instructions for taking BBT was absent, and thus they did not learn by observation how to improve their technique. Second, no bias was incorporated in the results as a consequence of expected patterns unless the subjects kept separate daily records for themselves. Nevertheless, others (5, 6) have pointed out the inability of even experienced physicians to detect the occurrence of ovulation from traditional BBT records in 20-30% of menstrual cycles that were ovulatory by hormonal criteria.

Even when ovulation was assessed by hormonal criteria, a relatively high percentage (approximately 30%) of menstrual cycles were anovulatory in this study. In part, this may be because of the young age of the subjects (22 yr). Döring (24) found that the frequency of ovulatory cycles increased steadily from the age of menarche to about 26 yr of age.

The stress associated with phlebotomy was clearly not a factor in the incidence of ovulation, and other stresses, as they were perceived by the subjects, had no effect on ovulation. The relatively low percentage of women ovulating, and, when luteal function is considered, the even greater percentage of abnormal cycles, may be a consequence of a high degree of external stress on all subjects that is not recognized by measuring changes in perceived stress. Certainly an absolute level of stress cannot be assessed by the instrument used to assess stress in this study.

If length of the luteal phase is used as a criterion for selection of normal cycles and 13 or more days is considered normal in accordance with criteria employed by Newton *et al*. (15) and Ross *et al*. (17), then only 48% of subjects had normal ovarian function in first cycles studied. The average age of ovulatory (Groups I and II) and anovulatory (Group IV) subjects was 23.6 and 21.9 yr, respectively. Thus, age was not an important determinant in the occurrence of ovulation in this group, probably because of the relatively narrow range of ages represented.

We assume that external stress is exerted randomly throug... the cycle and daily scores will reflect only the subjects' perception of stress. Perceived stress levels were relatively constant throughout anovulatory cycles. Changes in perception of stress were associated with ovulation, but only in cycles in which a biphasic BBT pattern was detected. The reason for the failure to find differences in mean stress scores among the groups was in part because the lower stress scores associated with the luteal phase in Group I were counterbalanced by higher follicular phase stress scores in the same women.

The finding that stress perception was less during the luteal phase of ovulatory cycles is consistent with the known anesthetic-analgesic effects of P (25). That physiological concentrations of P may reduce one's perception of stress is somewhat surprising. If the relation between the time of the menstrual cycle and attempted suicide is considered a reflection of hormonally influenced perception of stress in extreme (26-29), then the premenstrual period should also show some increase in stress perception in normal subjects. In subjects ovulatory by all criteria (Group I) stress scores were not higher in the 5 days before menses than those recorded in the preovulatory phase of the cycle. However, the premenstrual period was a time in which stress perception was increasing from its lowest point. In this group there was a nadir in stress scores that corresponded to the peak concentrations of P in serum. Higher stress perception at midcycle and premenstrually than at midluteal phase is consistent with the findings of Tonks *et al*. (28). Unfortunately, most work in this area has not been directed toward daily changes throughout the menstrual cycle, focusing only on a comparison of 2 or 3 different times in the cycle (27, 29, 30).

The finding that stress scores were uniform throughout menstrual cycles in which ovulation occurred by hormonal criteria, but in which BBT was monophasic is most interesting. It suggests that there may be a reason other than poor technique in taking body temperature that is the cause of the failure to detect a postovulatory rise in BBT. The fact that primarily one metabolite of P, 3α-hydroxy-5β-pregnan-20-one, is a potent thermogenic compound as well as an anesthetic-analgesic agent (25) may account for the findings. If for some reason the formation or retention of this metabolite is decreased, the BBT rise as well as the presumed analgesic effect would be lost simultaneously.

Acknowledgement: Studies described in this report were supported by a contract with the U.S. Army Human Engineering Laboratory, Aberdeen Proving Ground, Maryland.

References

1. Chatterton RT Jr, Haan JN, Jenco JM, Cheesman KL Radioimmunoassay of pregnanediol concentrations in early morning urine specimens for assessment of luteal function in women. Fertil Steril 37:361, 1982
2. Collins WP, Collins PO, Kilpatrick MJ, Manning PA, Pike JM, Tyler JPP The concentrations of urinary oestrone-3-glucuronide, LH and pregnanediol-3α-glucuronide as indices of ovarian function. Acta Endocrinol (Copenh) 90:336 1979
3. Denari JH, Farinati A, Figueroa-Casas PR, Oliva A Determination of ovarian function using first morning urine steroid assays. Obstet Gynecol 58:5, 1981
4. Stanczyk FZ, Miyakawa I, Goebelsmann U Direct radioimmunoassay of urinary estrogen and pregnanediol glucuronides during the menstrual cycle. Am J Obstet Gynecol 137:443, 1980
5. Bauman JE Basal body temperature: unreliable method of ovulation detection. Fertil Steril 36:729, 1982
6. Moghissi KS Accuracy of basal body temperature for ovulation detection. Fertil Steril 27:1415, 1976
7. Aedo A-R, Landgren B-M, Cekan SZ, Diczfalusy E Studies on the pattern of circulating steroids in the menstrual cycle: 2. Levels of 20 alpha-dihydroprogesterone, 17-hydroxyprogesterone and 17-hydroxypregnenolone and the assessment of their value for ovulation prediction. Acta Endocrinol 82:600, 1976
8. Baird DT, Guevara A Concentration of unconjugated estrone and estradiol in peripheral plasma in non-pregnant women throughout the menstrual cycle, castrate and postmenopausal women and in men. J Clin Endocrinol Metab 29:149, 1969
9. Burger HG, Catt KJ, Brown JB Relationship between plasma luteinizing hormone and urinary estrogen excretion during the menstrual cycle. J Clin Endocrinol Metab 28:1508, 1968
10. Cargille CM, Ross GT, Yoshimi T Daily variations in plasma follicle stimulating hormone, luteinizing hormone and progesterone in the normal menstrual cycle. J Clin Endocrinol Metab 29:12, 1969
11. Faiman C, Ryan RJ Serum follicle-stimulating hormone and luteinizing hormone concentrations during the menstrual cycle as determined by radioimmunoassays. J Clin Endocrinol Metab 27:1711, 1967
12. Guerrero R, Aso T, Brenner PF, Cekan Z, Landgren B-M, Hagenfeldt K, Diczfalusy E Studies on the pattern of circulating steroids in the normal menstrual cycle: I. Simultaneous assays of progesterone, pregnenolone, dehydroepiandrosterone, testosterone, dihydrotestosterone, androstenedione, oestradiol and oestrone. Acta Endocrinol 81:133, 1976

13. Johansson EDB, Wide L, Gemzell C Luteinizing hormone (LH) and progesterone in plasma and LH and estrogens in urine during 42 normal menstrual cycles. Acta Endocrinol 68:502, 1971
14. Mishell DR Jr, Nakamura RM, Crosignani PG, Stone S, Kharma K, Nagata Y, Thorneycroft IH Serum gonadotropin and steroid patterns during the normal menstrual cycle. Am J Obstet Gynecol 111:60, 1971
15. Newton J, Joyce D, Pearce B, Revell C, Tyler J Hormone levels in the normal menstrual cycle. J Reprod Fert 27:481, 1971
16. Nunez M, Aedo AR, Landgren BM, Cekan SZ, Diczfalusy E Studies on the pattern of circulating steroids in the normal menstrual cycle. Acta Endocrinol 86:821, 1977
17. Ross GT, Cargille CM, Lipsett MB, Rayford PL, Marshall JR, Strott CA, Rodbard D Pituitary and gonadal hormones in women during spontaneous and induced ovulatory cycles. Rec Progr Hormone Res 26:1, 1970
18. Shaaban MM, Klopper A Plasma oestradiol and progesterone concentration in the normal menstrual cycle. J Obstet Gynecol Br Comm 80:776, 1973
19. Thayer RE Activation states as assessed by verbal report and four psychophysiological variables. Psychophysiology 7:86, 1970
20. Dan AJ (in preparation) Construct validity of a subjective stress measure.
21. Spielberger CD, Gorsuch RL, and Lushene RE Manual for the state-trait anxiety inventory. Publ., Consulting Psychologist Palo Alto, 1970
22. Schalch DS, Parlow AF, Boon RC, Reichlin S Measurement of human luteinizing hormone in plasma by radioimmunoassay. J Clin Invest 47:665, 1968
23. Casper RC, Chatterton RT Jr, Davis JM Alterations in serum cortisol and its binding characteristics in anorexia nervosa. J Clin Endocrinol Metab 49:406, 1979
24. Doring GK The incidence of anovular cycles in women. J Reprod Fert Suppl 6:77, 1969
25. Kappas A, Palmer RH Selected aspects of steroid pharmacology. Pharmacol Rev 15:123, 1963
26. Holding TA, Minkoff K Parasuicide and the menstrual cycle. J Psychosomatic Res 17:365, 1973
27. Pallis DJ, Holding TA The menstrual cycle and suicidal intent. J Biosocial Sci 8:27, 1976
28. Tonks CM, Rack PH, Rose MJ Attempted suicide and the menstrual cycle. J Psychosomatic Res 11:319, 1978
29. Wetzel RD, McClure JN Jr Suicide and the menstrual cycle: A review. Comp Psychiatry 13:369, 1972
30. Wilcoxon LA, Schrader SL, Sherif CW Daily self reports on activities, like events, moods, and somatic changes during the menstrual cycle. Psychosomatic Med 38:399, 1976

HORMONAL RESPONSES TO EXERCISE IN NON-ATHLETIC WOMEN

Robert T. Chatterton, Jr.*, Frank A. DeLeon-Jones**, Gerald A. Hudgens***, Alice J. Dan**** and Kerry L. Cheesman*

*Department of Obstetrics and Gynecology
Northwestern University School of Medicine
Chicago, IL
**Research and Development Office
West Side Veterans Administration Hospital
and Department of Psychiatry
University of Illinois at the Medical Center
Chicago, IL
***U.S. Army Human Engineering Laboratory, Aberdeen Proving Ground
Maryland
****Department of Medical and Surgical Nursing
College of Nursing,
University of Illinois at the Medical Center
Chicago, IL

ABSTRACT

Women who had a history of regular menstrual cycles and who had not participated in a regular exercise or sports program for at least six months were recruited for a study of the effects of initiation of an exercise program on ovulation. After a control menstrual cycle during which basal hormone levels and the occurrence of ovulation were assessed, exercise on a treadmill was begun on the first day of the second menstrual cycle; exercise was continued at 85% of maximum heart rate for three sessions per week of from 15 to 30 minutes. The effect of this program on ovulation, luteal function, and on levels of cortisol, testosterone, prolactin and growth hormone measured 10 minutes after cessation of exercise was studied during the month of exercise and at the same times of day in pre- and postexercise control months. Initiation of the exercise program resulted in a shortening of the follicular phase of the menstrual cycle with no effect on luteal phase length or on progesterone levels or pregnanediol excretion during the luteal phase. Testosterone and growth hormone were significantly elevated after exercise by comparison with values obtained during the control months, but cortisol and prolactin were not. Cortisol levels may have been measured too soon after exercise began to detect an elevation. However, the complete absence of a prolactin elevation may be the reason for the failure of the brief exposure to exercise of this intensity to affect ovulation.

INTRODUCTION

Subsequent to the study described in the previous chapter in which hormonal and ovulatory responses were measured in relation to recorded life events and to the stress of a blood drawing protocol, we chose to investigate the influence of an imposed stress, that of a treadmill exercise program, on ovulation and hormone levels. Since our primary objective has been to evaluate the effect of acute stresses on ovulation in women, we sought a group of women who had not participated in a regular exercise program in the past and who had normal endocrine function including regular menstrual cycles. This is in contrast to most other studies of the effect of exercise on hormone levels and reproductive function in which athletic women were compared with non-athletes or in which athletes were compared with their own performance under conditions of differing intensities of exercise (1,2).

Since we were primarily interested in effects of stress on ovulation rather than effects of cumulative metabolic changes associated with long-term endurance training, we examined the influence of initiation of a vigorous exercise training program on ovulation. Schwartz and associates (3) observed that those runners who found running most stressful were most likely to be amenorrheic. Effects of this type of stress, however, would be confounded by nutritional factors (2,3) and loss of body fat (4) when comparing women of whom some may have been in training for a year or more. That the long-term metabolic effects of endurance training are not the only cause of anovulation and amenorrhea in runners is supported by the occurrence of amenorrhea in runners of normal body composition (5,6).

MATERIALS AND METHODS

Subjects. Recruitment was from among the students and staff at the University of Illinois Health Sciences Center. Eighteen subjects completed the study. All volunteers were women who said they had menstrual cycles of between 26 and 33 days during the previous year. They denied having used oral contraceptives or other drugs chronically during the previous 3 months. The ages of subjects ranged from 21 to 38 with a mean age of 26.8 years; they had between 13 and 21 years of education with a mean of 16.4. Three were married, 13 single, and 2 were divorced. Racially, 10 were white, 5 black, 2 hispanic, and 1 Asian. Before being accepted in the study, each of the subjects who was qualified on the basis of an initial questionnaire was given a medical examination, and an exercise tolerance test was administered by a cardiac exercise technician certified by the American College of Sports Medicine. At this time maximum heart rate was established.

Subjects collected morning urine specimens daily in 120 cc screw-cap specimen cups containing 200 mg of sodium metabisulfite as a preservative. These were stored at 4°C for up to 2 weeks before aliquots were assayed for pregnanediol and LH. Subjects took and recorded basal body temperature daily, recorded hours of sleep, and answered a daily questionnaire designed to evaluate stress and anxiety. Three times per week the subjects were given a test to evaluate their skills and risk-taking behavior on a simulated automobile-driving video game (performance task). The results of psychological and performance measures will be reported in a separate publication.

Subjects entered the study on the first day of a menstrual cycle. The subjects were told to continue their current level of physicial activity which in no case included more than occasional mild exercise of not more than one hour per week. Blood samples (15 ml) were drawn in heparinized tubes from the antecubital vein twice each week after the performance task was completed (usually Monday and Friday). Subjects were scheduled to take the performance task and have blood samples drawn at the same time of day, within one hour of the designated time, throughout the study; some subjects were scheduled for morning and some for afternoon hours. Hematocrit was determined on all blood samples, cells were sedimented by centrifugation, and plasma was stored frozen in sealed vials.

Starting on the first day of the second menstrual cycle, subjects were scheduled to begin the exercise program. Exercise was scheduled for 3 times per week just after the performance task was completed. The inclination of the treadmill was adjusted such that heart rate, which was monitored continuously, was maintained at 85% of maximum. Subjects ran on the treadmill for 15 minutes at each session during the first week. The duration was increased by 5 min each week thereafter. This is sufficient to produce a training effect in untrained individuals (7,8). Blood was drawn twice per week at exactly 10 min after the treadmill exercise was completed during the exercise month. The two hour period after the noon meal was avoided because of the cortisol response to food intake at this time of day (9).

During the subsequent menstrual cycle, the protocol was the same as in the first month; i.e., all measurements were made except that exercise was not performed.

Assays. Pregnanediol was assayed directly on diluted urine specimens as described previously (10). LH was also assayed in urine without purification essentially as described by Schalch et al. (11) using materials obtained from the National Hormone and Pituitary Program (NHPP) of the NIH. The standard of reference was LER 907.

Serum growth hormone and prolactin were measured by radioimmunoassay using materials and procedures obtained from NHPP. Chloramine T was used for iodination of the purified hormones for all of the protein hormone radioimmunoassays. The standards for prolactin and growth hormone were NIAMDD-hPRL-RP-1 and NIAMDD-hGH-RP-1, respectively.

Cortisol was measured by a method employing [1,2-^{3}H] cortisol and an antiserum developed against cortisol 11-hemisuccinate conjugated to bovine serum albumin. Fifty μl of serum was added to 4.95 ml of 0.1 M phosphate buffer, pH 7.0. This was heated for 20 min at 98°C to denature corticosteroid-binding globulin; 100 μl of the supernatant solution was then incubated with tracer and antiserum. Unbound tracer was separated from bound by adsorption to dextran-coated charcoal (0.5 g dextran and 5 g of charcoal per liter). The amount of cortisol in the sample was calculated by interpolation from a logit-log plot of bound radioactivity in standards of cortisol ranging from 0.01 to 1.0 ng. The accuracy of measuring known amounts of cortisol added to charcoal-stripped (steroid free) serum was 101.8% ± 5.8% SD. The intraassay C.V. was 8.7%; the interassay C.V. was 13.9%.

Testosterone was measured in ether extracts of serum using [1,2-^{3}H] testosterone and antiserum to testosterone-3-oxime conjugated to human serum albumin as described previously (12).

Progesterone was measured by RIA as described earlier using [1,2-^{3}H] progesterone and an antiserum againist an 11α-hydroxyprogesterone hemisuccinate - thyroglobulin conjugate (12).

Analysis of data. After determination of the day of the greatest concentration of LH in urine, this day of the menstrual cycle was designated day zero for purposes of analysis. Concentrations of urinary pregnanediol were plotted daily in relation to the LH peak. A paired t-test was used to compare the first control cycle with the second control cycle (the cycle after the exercise cycle). For hormones in which there was no difference between the two control cycles, the data on each subject were averaged to obtain a mean control value before comparing the exercise and control data by a paired t-test. Differences among frequencies were tested by Chi Square.

RESULTS

Menstrual cycle length (first day of menstrual bleeding through the day before menstruation of the next cycle) ranged from 25 to 38 days in subjects during the control month (Fig. 1). The distribution was bimodal with highest frequencies occurring on days 27 and 29. The distribution of cycle lengths in the subjects in the postexercise control cycle was similar to that of the preexercise cycles with a mode of 28 days. In the exercise cycles there was a tendency for shorter cycles; 6 of 18 cycles were less than 26 days long compared to only one cycle in each of the control months shorter than 26 days. This difference is significant ($P<0.05$) by Chi Square analysis.

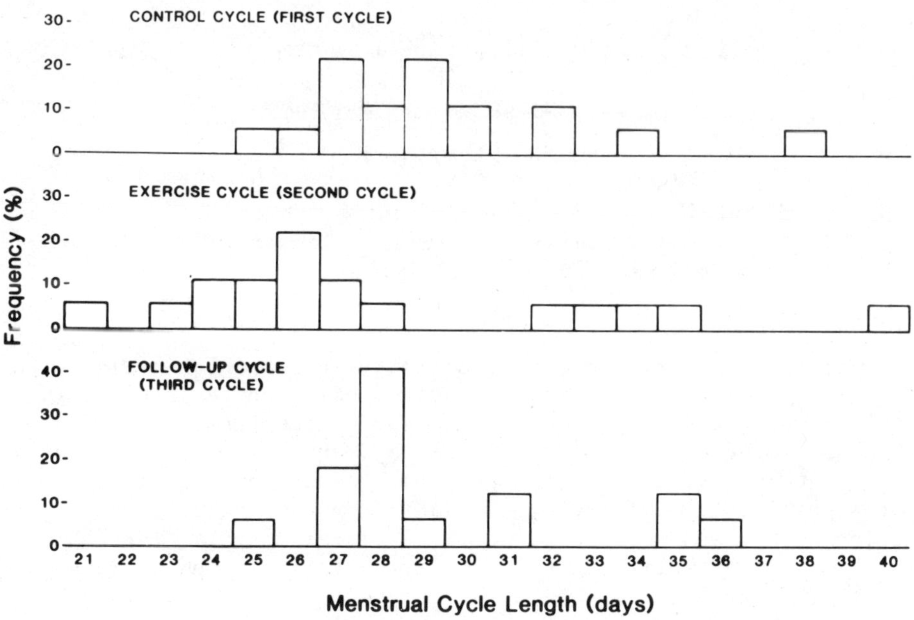

FIG. 1. Distribution of subjects' menstrual cycle lengths in the cycle in which exercise was performed and in the pre- and postexercise control cycles.

Luteal phase length, defined as the day after the LH peak through the day before the beginning of the next menses, was also determined in these subjects. As can be seen in Fig. 2 there was no difference in the distribution of luteal phase lengths. The modal length in each of the control cycles and in the exercise cycle was 11 days. Therefore, we must conclude that the difference in menstrual cycle length is due to a shortening of the follicular phase of the cycle.

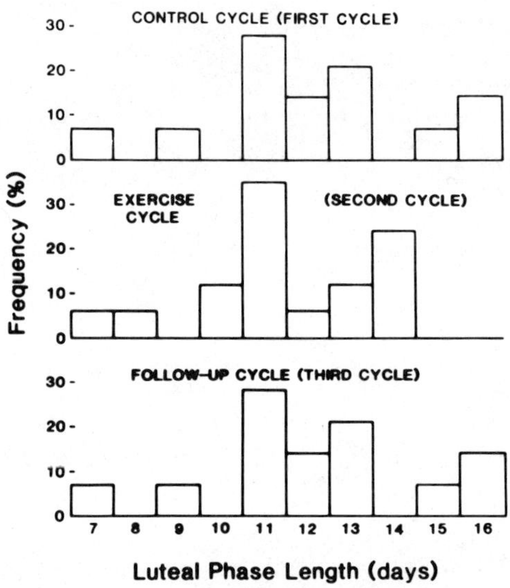

FIG. 2. Distribution of subjects' luteal phase lengths in the cycle in which exercise was performed and in the pre- and postexercise control cycles.

To further evaluate luteal activity in menstrual cycles with and without exercise we measured pregnanediol concentrations in early morning urine specimens. The sum of the μg/ml of pregnanediol over the 10 days preceding menses in shown in Fig. 3. Since the mean values for the pre- and postexercise cycles were not significantly different, the data from the control groups were pooled. The means of the control and exercise cycles were almost identical, substantiating the similarity in luteal phase length. To see whether there may be a shortening of the luteal phase pregnanediol excretion pattern attributable to a delayed appearance of pregnanediol in the periovulatory period we also determined the mean values for the 12 days before menses. As can also be seen in Fig. 3, the mean values for exercise and control cycles were identical.

Since serum had been collected twice weekly during the study, serum progesterone concentrations were measured to ascertain any differences in the excretion of pregnanediol which might reflect differences in the metabolism of progesterone with exercise. Midluteal phase progesterone concentrations were compared to the 12-day sum of pregnanediol concentrations. The combined mean

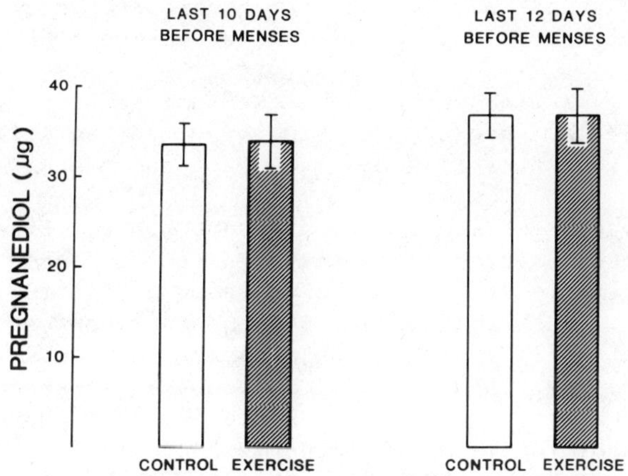

FIG. 3. Pregnanediol excretion in daily urine specimens (means ± standard errors). The concentrations (μg/ml) in early morning urine specimens were summed over the last 10 days before menses and the last 12 days before menses in exercise cycles. The corresponding sums for pre- and postexercise control cycles were not significantly different and were averaged for comparison with exercise cycles.

progesterone concentration for all control cycles was 10.0 ± 1.2 (SE) ng/ml; for exercise cycles it was 12.4 ± 2.3 (SE). The corresponding pregnanediol values were 36.5 ± 1.4 (SE) μg/ml and 35.3 ± 3.5 μg/ml (SE). It is evident that pregnanediol reflects the serum progesterone concentrations from one experimental condition to the other.

In order to assess the stress produced by the exercise regimen, we measured growth hormone, prolactin, cortisol, and testosterone in serum samples that were collected 10 min after cessation of exercise. Hematocrits were not affected by the exercise regimen. During most menstrual cycles, 8 blood samples were obtained. Serum from each sample was assayed for each of the above hormones. Mean values of each hormone were then calculated for each menstrual cycle. Growth hormone was most responsive to the exercise regimen. One subject who was more than 20% over ideal body weight according to Metropolitan Life Insurance standards, however, did not respond at all. Data from this subject was omitted from the means and standard errors shown in Fig. 4. Since the growth hormone response was so great, we also plotted values chronologically during the exercise cycle to see if there were any trends as the subjects progressed in the exercise program. No trends were observed during the month of exercise.

Prolactin was also measured in the same samples as growth hormone. The data, presented in Fig. 5, reveal no difference in the prolactin concentrations among control and exercise cycles.

Cortisol and testosterone were also compared (Figs. 6 and 7). By a paired t-test testosterone was significantly greater 10 min after exercise periods than in the corresponding times during the control months. Cortisol was not quite significant at this level, even though variability within subjects was much less than among subjects. Here also data was pooled from the two control months on each subject for the comparison since pre- and postexercise months did not differ from each other. Each subject was sampled at the same time of day throughout the study, whereas different subjects were sampled at different times of day. The SD of cortisol in the exercise group was $\pm$ 43.4 ng/ml but the standard deviation of differences between the pooled control and exercise sessions was only $\pm$ 12.5 ng/ml.

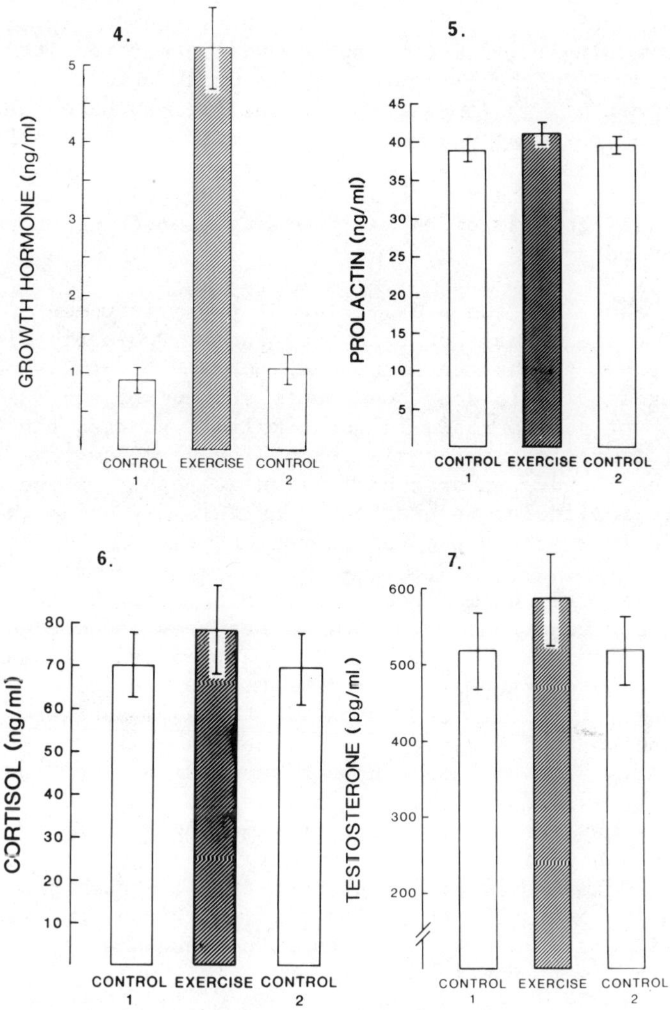

FIG. 4, 5,6, & 7 Blood samples were collected 10 min after the cessation of exercise each time the subjects exercised. Serum from these samples was assayed for growth hormone, prolactin, cortisol and testosterone. The means ± standard errors are shown for the exercise cycle and both control cycles for each hormone.

DISCUSSION

The observation that exercise shortens the menstrual cycle is not new. However, investigatons of the effect of endurance training on ovarian function have centered primarily on ovulation and luteal activity. Several studies have shown that either long distance running (1,13,14) or swimming (15) may result in a short luteal phase. In the present study in which untrained subjects ran on a treadmill 3 times per week for one month beginning on the first day of the menstrual cycle no effect on the luteal phase of the cycle occurred, nor was the following control cycle affected. The shortening of the menstrual cycles observed during the month in which subjects exercised was due to a shortening of the follicular phase.

The reason for the shorter luteal phase in women engaged in endurance training has not been explained. Prolactin elevation has been shown to shorten the luteal phase (17), and some degree of hyperprolactinemia does occur with running (5,16). A deficiency of gonadotropin is not likely to shorten the luteal phase unless gonadotropins are reduced to very low levels (18). On the other hand, a shortened follicular phase must be due to more rapid follicular maturation. Why this may occur in women engaged in an exercise program is not known.

The exercise regimen resulted in a significant increase in serum testosterone concentrations as has been documented in runners by others (5,19,20,21). Cortisol concentrations, however, at the 10 minute interval after cessation of exercise were not significantly increased over those in the same subjects in the preexercise month. Baker et al (21) obtained similar results in women runners. Others have shown that cortisol increases from the immediate preexercise period to postexercise (5,20). These differences may reflect the time of sampling and the control groups with which the runners were compared. In the study by Cummings and Rebar (5) it is apparent that although a significant elevation in cortisol occurred in both untrained and trained runners after a 15-min bicycle test, the levels were not above preexercise levels until after 10 min from the time exercise ceased.

Prolactin and growth hormone levels in the current study provide an interesting comparison between these responses to stress. Growth hormone was greatly elevated in all but the one obese subject, but prolactin was not increased in any of the subjects after exercise. Boyden et al (22) have suggested on the basis of their studies that prolactin is increased in runners but not in untrained women. Our results confirm this, but Cummings and Rebar (5) did not find this difference. They found that prolactin was increased in eumenorrheic, but not amenorrheic runners after exercise. Prolactin obviously is more sensitive to differences in experimental conditions and experimental subjects than the other hormones measured, but the reasons for these differences are not clear from the available data. Certainly, prolactin and growth hormone are subject to different control mechanisms. Pituitary stalk section results in an abundant increase in prolactin secretion and a suppression or decrease in growth hormone secretion. A peptide, somatostatin, is the hypothalamic inhibitor of growth hormone secretion, whereas suppression of prolactin appears to be primarily achieved through secretion of dopamine into the portal vascular system. Thyrotropin releasing hormone stimulates release of prolactin and TSH, but not growth hormone. A separate releasing factor has been identified for stimulation of growth hormone release. Prolactin and growth hormone secretion are both stimulated by insulin-stimulated hypoglycemia (23) and both are secreted in response to certain stressful stimuli (24). Yet, immobilization of rats results in 10-fold increases in prolactin while growth hormone levels are decreased (25). Thus, it is not surprising to see disparate responses of growth hormone and prolactin to this stress.

Generally, the hormonal changes with exercise in the non-athletic women were similar to those observed by others in athletes. The primary difference is in the complete lack of a prolactin response in the non-athletes. The failure of the acute stress of the exercise program to affect ovulation may be related to the failure of exercise of this duration to affect prolactin secretion.

REFERENCES

1. Prior JC Luteal phase defects and anovulation: adaptive alterations occurring with conditioning exercise. Sem Reprod Endocrinol 3:27, 1985
2. Shangold MM Exercise and amenorrhea. Sem Reprod Endocrinol 3:35, 1985
3. Schwartz B, Cumming DC, Reordon E, Selye M, Yen SSC, Rebar RW Exercise-associated amenorrhea: a distinct entity? Am J Obstet Gynecol 141:662, 1981
4. Frisch RE Body fat, menarche, and reproductive ability. Sem Reprod Endocrinol 3:45, 1985
5. Cumming DC, Rebar RW Hormonal changes with acute exercise and with training in women. Sem Reprod Endocrinol 3:55, 1985
6. McArthur JW, Bullen BH, Beitins IZ, Pagano M, Badger TM, Klibanski A Hypothalamic amenorrhea in runners of normal body composition. Endorcin Res Commun 7:13, 1980

7. Fox SM, Naughton JP, Gorman PA Physical activity and cardiovascular health: the exercise prescription. Modern Concepts of Cardiovascular Disease 41:1, 1972
8. Winder WW, Hickson RC, Hagberg JM, Ehsani AA, McLane JA Training induced changes in hormonal and metabolic responses to submaximal exercise. J Appl Physiol: Respirat Environ Exercise Physiol 46:766, 1979
9. Brandenberger G, Follenius M, Heitter B Feedback from meal-related peaks determine diurnal changes in cortisol response to exercise. J Clin Endocrinol Metab 54:592, 1982
10. Chatterton, RT Jr., Haan JN, Jenco JM, Cheesman KL Radioimmunoassay of pregnanediol concentrations in early morning urine specimens for assessment of luteal function in women. Fertil Steril 37:361, 1982
11. Schalch DS, Parlow AF, Boon RC, Reichlin S Measurement of human luteinizing hormone in plasma by radioimmunoassay. J Clin Invest 47:665, 1968
12. Casper RC, Chatterton RT Jr., Davis JM Alterations in serum cortisol and its binding characteristics in anorexia nervosa. J Clin Endocrinol Metab 49:406, 1979
13. Shangold M, Freeman R, Thysen B, Gatz M The relationship between long-distance running, plasman progesterone, and luteal phase length. Fertil Steril 31:130, 1979
14. Prior JC, Cameron K, Ho Yuen B, Thomas J Menstrual cycle changes with marathon training: anovulation and short luteal phase. Can J Appl Sport Sci 7:173, 1982
15. Bonen A, Belcastro AN, Simpson AA Profiles of menstrual cycle hormones in teenage athletes. J Appl Physiol 50:545, 1981
16. Shangold MM, Gatz ML, Thysen B Acute effects of exercise on plasma concentrations of prolactin and testosterone in recreational women runners. Fertil Steril 35:699, 1981
17. del Pozo E, Wyss H, Tolis G, Alcaniz J, Campana A, Naftolin F Prolactin and deficient luteal function. Obstet Gynecol 53:282, 1979
18. Asch RH, Braunstein G, Abou-Samra M, Pauerstein CJ Luteal function in hypophysectomized rhesus monkeys: is the pituitary necessary for the maintenance of the corpus luteum? Fertil Steril 37:309A, 1982
19. Dale E, Gerlach D, Wilhite A Menstrual dysfunction in distance runners. Obstet Gynecol 54:47, 1979
20. Hale RW, Kosasa T, Krieger J, Pepper S A marathon: the immediate effect on female runners' luteinizing hormone, follicle stimulating hormone, prolactin, testosterone, and cortisol levels. Am J Obstet Gynecol 146:550, 1983
21. Baker ER, Mathar RS, Kirk RF, Williamson HO Female runners and secondary amenorrhea: correlation with age, parity, mileage, and plasma hormonal and sex-hormone-binding globulin concentrations. Fertil Steril 36:183, 1981

22. Boyden TW, Parmenter RW, Crosso D, Stanforth P, Rotkis T, Wilmore JH Prolactin responses, menstrual cycles and body composition of women runners. J Clin Endocrinol Metab 54:711, 1982
23. Nathan RS, Sachar EJ, Langer G, Tabrizi MA, Halpern FS Diurnal variation in the response of plasma prolactin, cortisol, and growth hormone to insulin-induced hypoglycemia in normal men. J Clin Endocrinol Metab 49:231, 1979
24. Rose, RM, Jenkins CD, Hurst M, Livingston L, Hall RP Endocrine activity in air traffic controllers at work. I. Characterization of cortisol and growth hormone levels during the day. Psychoneuroendocrinology 7:101, 1982
25. Lenox RH, Kant GJ, Sessions GR, Pennington LL, Mougey EH, Meyerhoff JL Specific hormonal and neurochemical responses to different stresses. Neuroendocrinology 30:300, 1980

Acknowledgement: Studies described in this report were supported by a contract with the U.S. Army Human Engineering Laboratory, Aberdeen Proving Ground, Maryland.

NEUROENDOCRINE CONTROL IN THE THERMAL STRESS

Vojislav M. Petrović

Department of Endocrinology and Metabolism
Institutes for Biological Research,
Physiology and Biochemistry
Faculty of Science, University of Belgrade
29 Novembra 142, Belgrade, Yugoslavia

INTRODUCTION

Stress may be defined in terms of any adjustment directed towards a reestablishment of internal homeostasis (Ganong, 1980). Starting from Selye's terminology, stress might be defined as such a type of response in which an increased ACTH secretion occurs (see Axelrod, 1980). However, the increased ACTH secretion and consequently an increased adrenocortical activity was also found in intensive muscular activity and swimming. In such a kind of activity if muscular work is not very intensive, the typical stress reaction of pituitary-adrenocortical system does not occur. Thus, it was suggested that at the present time a quantitative criteria for stress rather than a qualitative, should be used (Kozlowsski, 1980). Having in mind all available data about stress it seems necessary that the kind of stressor, used by different authors in order to provoke stress in laboratory animals, should be well defined. So the character and magnitude of the response to stress should be better understood.

The response of the organism to the given stressor was indicated as specific (Koslowski, 1980; Ganong, 1980), but some data suggesting unspecificity were also shown (Vigas, 1980). In the case of cold it was evidenced that this kind of stress produces many responses which may be defined to be specific and non specific (Le Blanc et al., 1971). Study on neuroendocrine control of the cold and heat stress have shown many similarities between thermal and physical or emotional stress. Results obtained in our study seem to confirm the concept of both, specific and non specific response of the organism exposed to thermal stress. These results together with the results obtained by other authors, will be presented and discussed in the present article.

Type of Stress and Site of Action

Stressful stimuli affect the function of biogenic amines in the central nervous system (CNS). It was shown that changes of amine levels depend on the type of stressor and the site of action (Palkovits et al., 1980). Serotonin shows an acute decrease in almost all brain area but in the case of adrenaline, noradrenaline and dopamine the effect seems initially to be selective for the hypothalamus and in particular for the arcuate and ventromedial nuclei (Palkovits et al., 1975; Kvetnansky et al., 1977).

According to the conceptual model proposed by Henry and Stephens (1977), a dual stress pathways exist. Some stressors, particularly psycho-social ones, activate either the pituitary-adrenocortical system or the sympathetic-adrenomedullary system. According to these authors the pituitary-adrenocortical system becomes activated when there is a loss of control by the organism, a state leading to depression. This type of stress is characterized by augmented ACTH and corticosterone secretion along with unaltered catecholamines, whereas testosterone level decreases. The hippocampus and septum are involved in the mechanism of this reaction. The sympathetic-adrenomedullary system is activated at the fight-flight reaction, when the organism is challenged in its control of the environment. In this type of stress, according to the same authors, noradrenaline and adrenaline as well as testosterone are increased, but corticosterone remains unchanged. The amygdala is primarily involved in the mechanism of this reaction. The sympathetic-adrenomedullary system is activated in the cold ambient as well. We have shown (Fig 1), that TH activity, regulated mainly by neuronal transsynaptic stimulation, under this condition was increased (Petrović et al., 1978).

In the last decade, forced immobilization was one of the most explored models of stress in the rat. This model seems to combine emotional stress and physical stress, resulting in both restricted mobility and aggression. During immobilization the sympathetic-adrenomedullary and pituitary-adrenocortical systems were highly

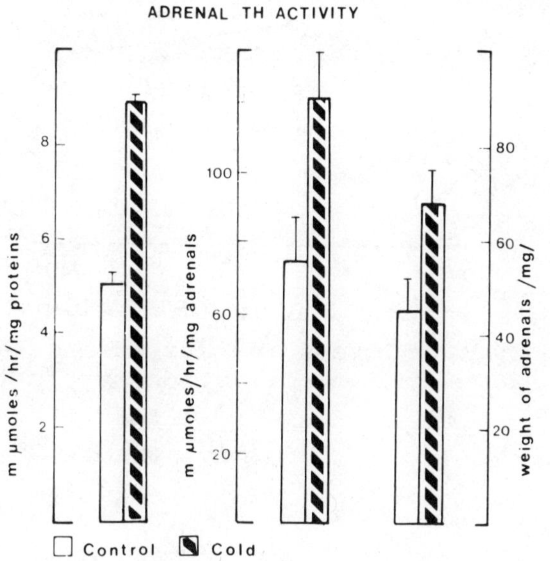

Fig. 1. Tyrosine hydroxylase (TH) activity in the adrenals of the ground squirrel exposed to cold in summer (Petrović et al., 1978).

activated (Kvetnansky et al., 1978; Kvetnansky and Mikulaj, 1970; Mikulaj et al., 1976; Kvetnansky, 1980). Adrenals adrenaline shows gradual decrease but plasma and urinary adrenaline were elevated at the beginning of immobilization. Plasma adrenaline later falls but urinary adrenaline kepps increassing during the six hours of immobilization (Fig. 2). The activity of catecholamine-synthesizing enzyme in the adrenals of immobilized rats was also increased.

It was shown that under stress, catecholamines synthesizing enzymes are regulated both via neuronal and endocrine pathways (Fig. 3). Tyrosine hydroxylase (TH) and dopamine-β - hydroxylase (DBH) are regulated mainly by neuronal transsynaptic stimulation and phenylethanolamine-N-methyltransferase (PNMT) is primarily under endocrine control (Kvetnansky, 1973; Petrović and Janić-Šibalić, 1976) (Fig. 4,5). However, both regulatory systems have been found to be involved in each induction.

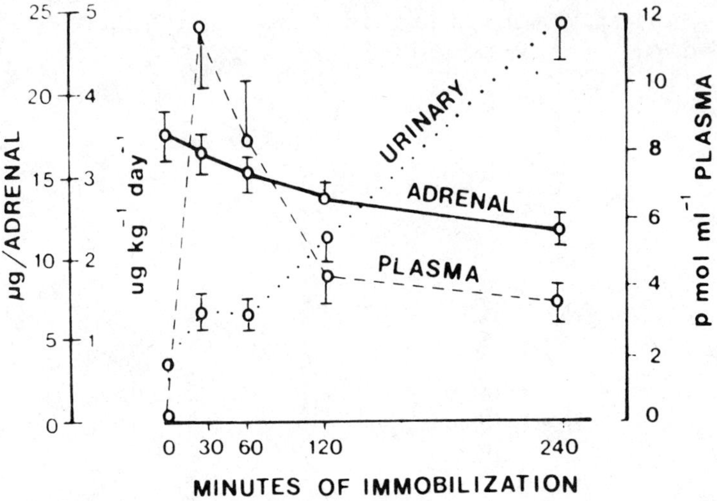

Fig. 2. Adrenaline levels in rats during the first exposure to immobilization stress (Kvetnansky, 1980).

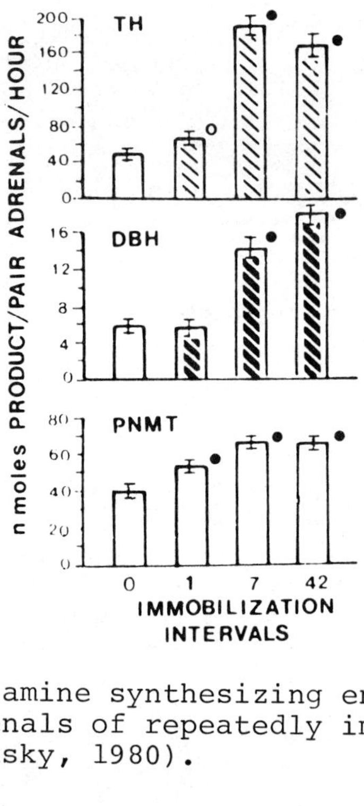

Fig. 3. Catecholamine synthesizing enzyme activity in the adrenals of repeatedly immobilized rats (Kvetnansky, 1980).

Although the physiological needs of organism, as regards the environment, are different in respect to physical trauma or social stress, the immediate response to stres-

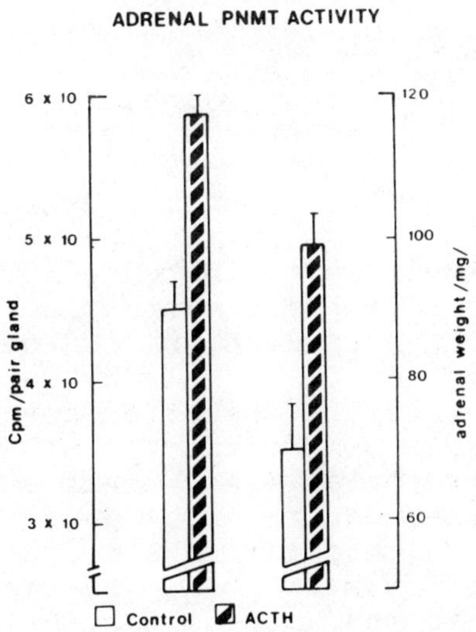

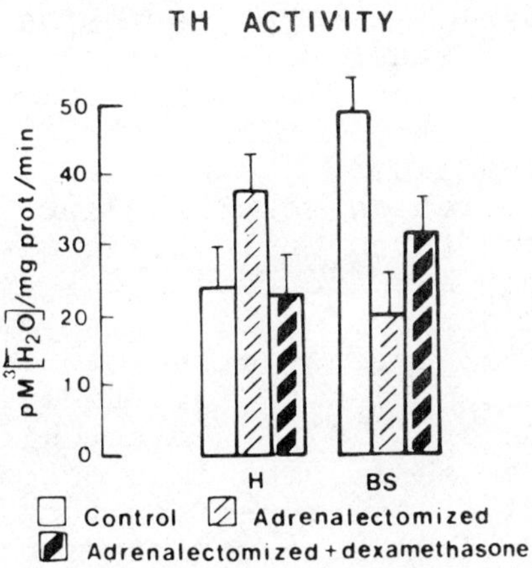

Fig. 4. Phenylethanolamine-N-methyl transferase activity and adrenals weight in ACTH treated ground squirrel in summer (Petrović and Janić-Šibalić, 1976).

Fig. 5. Effect of dexamethasone on TH activity in the hypothalamus and brain stem of the rat (Petrović et al., 1984).

sor shows many similarities (Kvetnansky et al., 1971; Petrović and Janić-Šibalić, 1977; 1980).

Brain Monoamines Regulating Pituitary-Adrenocortical Activity under Stress

The increase in ACTH secretion produced by stressful stimuli is mediated via neural pathways and corticotropine relesasing hormone (CRH) from the hypothalamus. This hormone was found in portal-hypophyseal blood and the consequence of its increase can be drawn on the basis of measurements of ACTH or glucocorticoids in the peripheral circulation, or on the basis of the output of glucocorticoids from the adrenal cortex (Ganong, 1974,

1980). It seems that CRH, like TRH, LHRH, somatostatin and dopamine, is secreted by the endings of nerve fibers that terminate in the median eminence of the hypothalamus. The largest amount of CRH is found in the ventral hypothalamus (Krieger er al., 1977). L-dopa and other compounds that increase the release of catecholamines in the brain inhibit stress-induced ACTH secretion. Epinephrine and norepinephrine both produce the inhibition of ACTH secretion in the stress, acting by the way of α-adrenergic receptors in the brain (Ganong, 1980). The α-adrenergic agonist clonidine, which crosses blood-brain barrier, inhibits stress-induced ACTH secretion (Weiner and Ganong, 1978). Stressful stimuli which increase ACTH secretion generally increase norepinephrine synthesis and turnover in the brain as well, but the significance of this increase and its relation to ACTH remain obscure. Contrary to the brain catecholamines the effect of central release of serotonine seems to be excitatory but some opposite results were also reported (see Weiner and Ganong, 1978). On the basis of many experimental data it may be assumed that monoamines, which act on CRH secretion, exert their effects inside the blood-brain barrier. Various observations indicate that monoamines, particularly adrenaline, which does not pass the blood-brain barrier, stimulate ACTH secretion by a direct action on the pituitary or stimulate corticotropin release in the intermediate lobe (see Kraicer et al., 1978, 1980).

Hypothalamo-Pituitary System in the Cold Stress

Cold stress induces a considerable burden on homeotherm and the meaning of the response is to maintain constant internal body temperature. This specific response consists of shivering, which increases heat production. As was evidenced many years ago, exposure to cold activates the sympathetic nervous system and hypothalamo-pituitary-adrenocortical system. In cold exposed animals a marked increase in the excretion of noradrenaline and adrenaline was found (Le Blanc, 1976; Le Blanc et al., 1971). There is much evidence that the activity of adrenal cortex of rats, guinea pigs and ground squirrels considerably increase during the initial phase of cold exposure (Boulouard, 1966; Schoenbaum, 1960; Petrović, 1976; Petrović et al., 1981) (Fig. 6). Bothe the sympathetic nervous system and the adrenal medulla are activated during exposure of animals to cold. It was evidenced that noradrenaline participates in central regulatory processes and together with other amines is important for the regulation of body temperature.

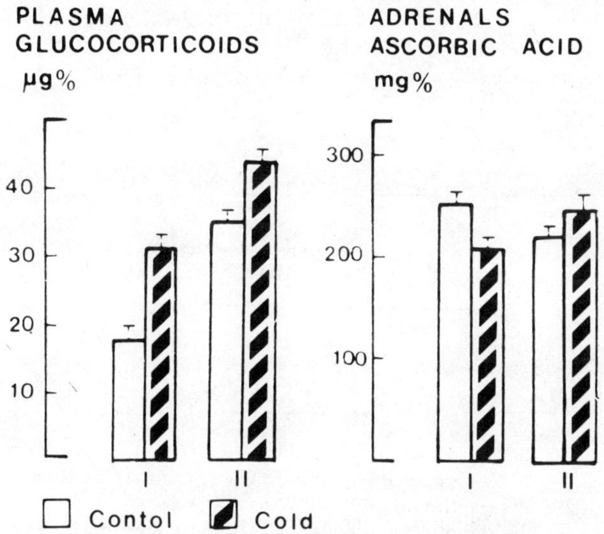

Fig. 6. Glucocorticoid plasma level and adrenals ascorbic acid content in the ground squirrel exposed to cold: I in captivity 1 year; II several days (1-7) after captivity (Petrović et al., 1981).

The reflex responses activated by cold ambient are controlled from the posterior hypothalamus. However, responses activated by warmth are controlled from the anterior hypothalamus. Stimulation of posterior hypothalamus causes shivering and the body temperature of animals wiht posterior hypothalamic lesions falls toward that of the environment. Stimulation of anterior hypothalamus causes cutaneous vasodilatation and sweating. The lesion of this region causes hyperthermia. It was evidenced that serotonin is a synaptic mediator in the centers controlling the mechanism activated by cold and norepinephrine may play a similar role in the centers activated by heat. This model was postulated for the monkey by Myers and Yaksh (1969). However it seems that this model is not applicable for other species such as ox, sheep, goat, rabbit and rat. Another model was suggested by Bligh et al. (1971) according to which serotonin acts to increased heat loss and to reduced heat production whereas norepinephrine pathways cause the inhibition of heat loss and activate heat production. According to this model norepinephrine pathways would be stimulated during the exposure of animals to cold (cold stress) and the serotonergic pathways would be activated during the exposure to heat. This concept has been supported by biochemical studies which showed that the serotonin turnover increases during the exposure to heat while the noradrenaline turnover increases during cold exposure (Simmonds, 1969, 1970; Beley et al., 1977);

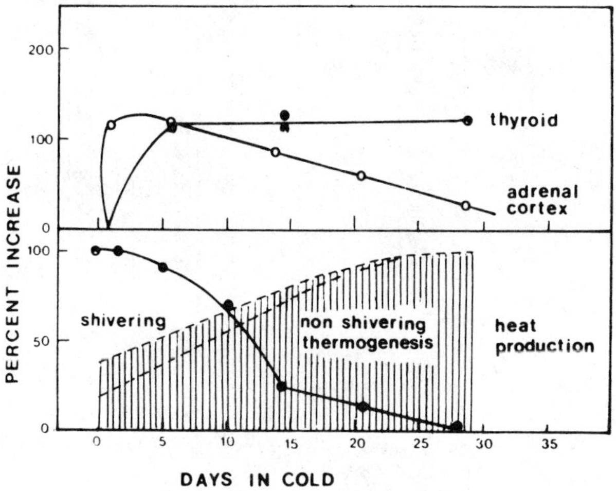

Fig. 7. Summary of endocrinological changes and thermogenesis during acclimation to cold (Hart, 1963).

The first reaction in the cold is a shivering heat production but in cold adapted homeotherm which possesses non-shivering thermogenesis the central aminergic transmission plays an important role (Fig. 7). Zeisberger and Brück (1973) suggested that the activation of noradrenaline structures in the brain of cold adapted guines pigs may stimulate some thermosensitive structures in the caudal hypothalamus which are supposed to generate the reference signal for impulses coming from primary thermosensors in the anterior hypothalamus. In such a mechanism, the setpoint for shivering could be lowered and NŠT could be induced predominantly.

In the hypothalamus disconnected rats, contrary to the controls (except those with anterior hypothalamic disconnection) a significant inhibition of corticosterone release upon exposure to cold was found (Chowers et al., 1972). Dupont et al., 1972) have demonstrated that hippocampal stimulation in the rat inhibits the pituitary adrenocortical response to stress. The similar effect has been previously found in the cat (Endröczi and Lissak,

1962) and rabbit (Kowakami et al., 1968). These results suggest that the role of the hippocampus and other components of the limbic system in the control of ACTH and also TSH secretion should be also taken into consideration for further systematic studies on neurohumoral mechanism involved in short-term exposure to cold (cold stress) as well as on adaptation to cold.

Adrenal Cortex and Thyroid

The increased activity of the adrenal cortex during the first few hours of cold exposure (Fig. 8) is due to the effect of ACTH stimulation, the concentration of which in the pituitary augmented considerably. Later phase of adrenocortical activity under cold conditions is probably

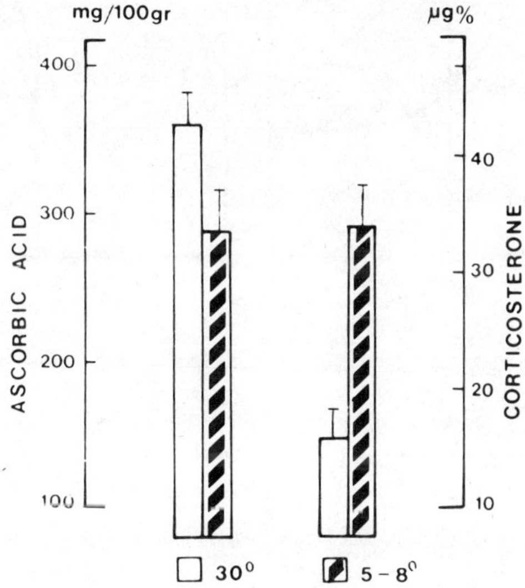

Fig. 8. Corticosterone plasma level and ascorbic acid content in the rat exposed to cold (Petrović and Janić, 1964).

related to the increased thyroid function (Fortier, 1966; Chaffee and Roberts, 1971). Because of the fact that in laboratory animals hypothalamo-pituitary adrenocortical system reacts immediately after cold exposure it is probable that feed back mechanism of activation in this case does not play a significant role, at least under the conditions of acute exposure. It is possible to conclude that under these conditions blood-corticoid levels do not appear to play a central role in the initiation or control of ACTH secretion. The neural drive seems to be capable of inducing and maintaining a sustained increase in blood-corticoid levels (Fortier, 1966; Petrović and Janić, 1964). It was found that could exposure resulted in the depletion of adrenal assorbic acid and cholesterol and in the decrease of eosinophilis.

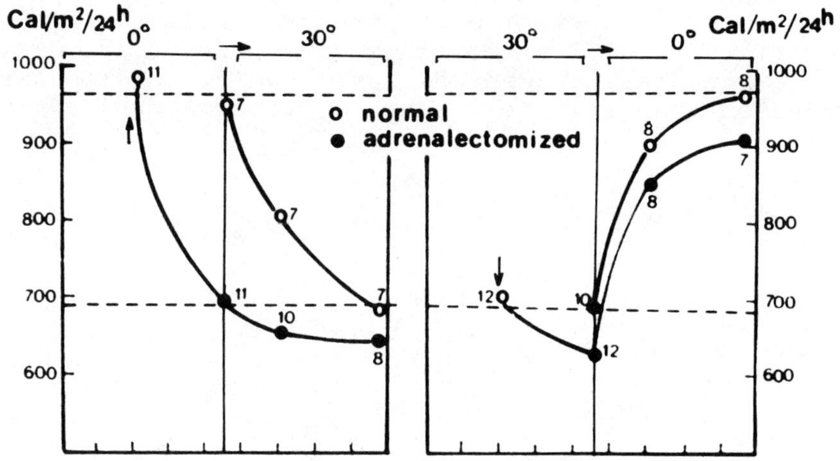

Fig. 9. Resting metabolism of control and adrenalectomized rats before and after changes of ambient temperature. Broken lines: the mean values of resting metabolism of control adapted to 0°C or to 30°C; horizontal arrows - the direction of changes of thermal environment; vertical arrows - the time of adrenalectomy (Petrović et al., 1961).

Not only in the rat but also in the normothermic ground squirrel or golden hamster an increase of circulating glucocorticoids during cold exposure was found (Boulouard, 1966; Schoenbaum, 1960; Petrović and Janić, 1964; Petrović et al., 1964). Furthermore a high level of circulating glucocorticoids, found in the active ground squirrel coming from a natural habitat, dit not prevent an additional increase under the conditions of cold exposure (Petrović and Janić, 1964). Cold exposure of the rat resulted in an increase of the adrenal weight, protein and RNA but not in DNA content and also an initial increase in the incorporation of labelled amino acids into the total and soluble proteins (Petrović et al., 1966; Petrović and Rajčić, 1969)

It seems that adrenal cortex is very important for the first reaction to cold but not indispensable for cold adaptation. A considerable amount of cold adaptation in the rat is possible without adrenals (Petrović and Andjus, 1960; Petrović et al., 1961), (Fig. 9).

The increased thyroid activity in cold exposed animals is brought about by an increased secretion of thyroid-stimulating hormone of the adenohypophysis (Hefco et al., 1975). In rats adapted to cold, basophil cells, which are responsible for TSH production, are more numerous than in the nonadapted controls and serum TSH is higher. In laboratory animals such as the rat, guinea pig and hamster, ventral hypothalamic lesions, which produce persistent oestrus, the basal pituitary-thyroid function appears normal, but thyroid

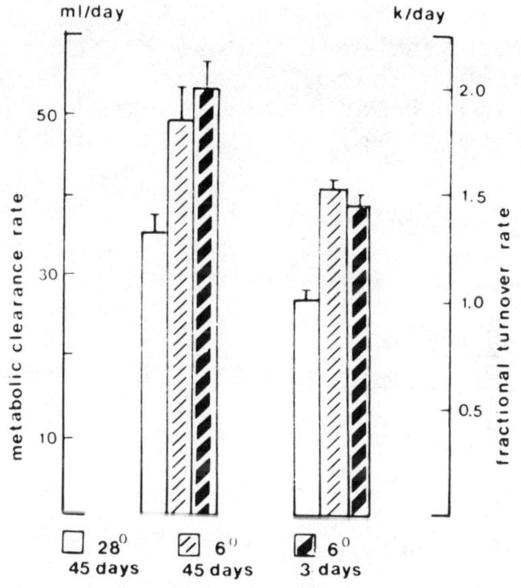

Fig. 10. Thyroxine turnover rate in rats exposed to cold (Héroux and Petrović, 1969).

activation does not occur when the animals are placed at 5°C (Knigge, 1960; D'Angelo, 1960). Cold exposure seems to activate neural mechanisms activating TSH discharge within increase in short time, being 0.5 and 3 hrs for the rabbit, rat, hamster and ground squirrel (Itoh, S. et al., 1969; Lachiver and Petrović, 1960; Héroux and Petrović, 1969). (Fig. 10).

Activation of Aminergic Structures in the Cold

As a consequence of the activation of the sympathetic nervous system and adrenal medulla during the exposure to cold, the amount of noradrenaline in the urine of these animals was about four times incresed (Jansky et al., 1976). The increased production of noradrenaline can be traced during the long-term stay in the cold. It was shown that relative increase in adrenaline production in the cold was greater than that of noradrenaline, but the release of this hormone was somewhat delayed and it returned towards the initial control level within the days of cold exposure (Leduce, 1961). The increase in adrenaline and noradrenaline production is reflected in the activity of catecholamine synthesizing enzymes in adrenals (Petrović et al., 1981) (Fig 11). In the case of noradrenaline, a dissociation between its synthesis and secretion was observed by Sellers et al. (1971). In spite of the fact that the relation between the rate of synthesis and secretion of noradrenaline during the exposure to cold changes it was registered that the absolute rate of NA synthesis always greatly exceeds the absolute rate of secretion (see Jansky et al., 1976).

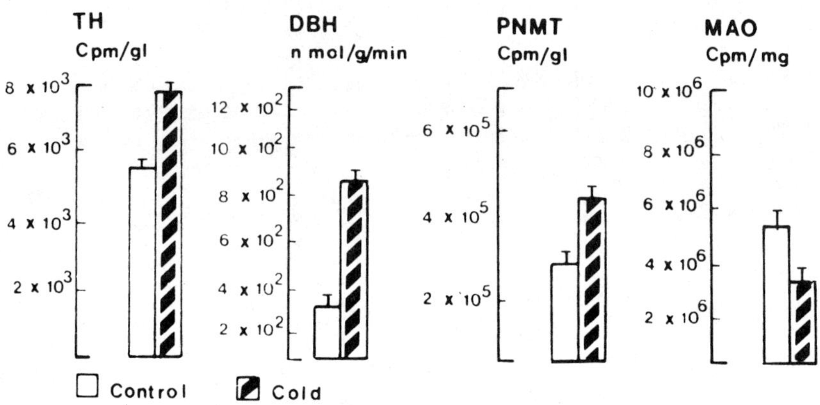

Fig. 11. Catecholamine synthesizing and degrading enzymes in the control ground squirrel and in that after 6 hrs of exposure to cold (Petrović et al., 1981).

Calorigenic action of NA release from the sympathetic nervous system is mainly responsible for the increased resistance to cold. Thus, to the certain extent the increased metabolism, due to exogenous NA, can be used as an indicator of the degree of adaptation of rats to cold (Mejsner and Jansky, 1971; Petrović and Marković-Djaja, 1973; Petrović and Maksimović, 1979). (Fig. 12). The physiological role of adrenaline during cold stress and cold adaptation is less than that of noradrenaline.

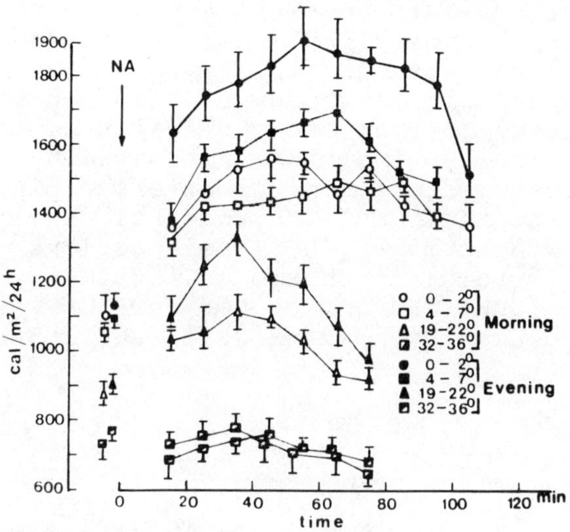

Fig. 12. The effect of noradrenaline on the heat production in the rat adapted to different environmental temperatures, measured at 30°C (Petrović and Maksimović, 1979).

Judging by the experiments of Himms-Hagen (1969), the effect of adrenaline (A) was evidenced also in the warm but it can be potentiated by cold adaptation. It seems that A is of secondary significance for the induction of NST in cold. Data of LeBlanc et al. (1971) indicate that A thermogenesis participates rather in animals exposed to an acute cold stress.

The biochemical effect of NA in cold stressed animals consists mainly of its lipolytic action in adipose tissues. In the brown adipose tissue (BAT) the free fatty acids (FFA), liberated by lipolytic action on NA, first induce a loosening of coupling between oxydation and phosphorylation, stimulate the respiration and are as a substrate (see Himms-Hagen, 1970). The heat released during the increased catabolism of FFA is utilized for maintaining the normothermic state.

Hypothalamo-Pituitary System in the Heat Stress

Environmental heat, like the cold, may affect the hypothalamus by skin neural receptors, spinal CNS and hypothalamic neural processes and functions responsive to this peripheral neural stimulation. Rises in body temperature in the heat ambient may directly affect hypothalamic neuroendocrine functions as well (Chap et al., 1977). Neural projections into cortical areas presumably mediate conscious thermal sensations and ascending noradrenergic tracts which connect the brain stem with the hypothalamus (see Gale, 1973). In the hypothalamic-pituitary neuroendocrine system, thermal and chemical receptors in the preoptic anterior hypothalamus, activated by the heat, influence the secretion from the anterior pituitary of adrenocorticotropin (ACTH), thyroid stimulating hormone (TSH) and growth hormone (GH). These actions are mediated by hypothalamic releasing hormones for thyrotropin (TRH) corticotropin (CRH) and growth hormone (GH). Vasopresin (ADH) is influenced by heat as well (see Johnson, 1976).

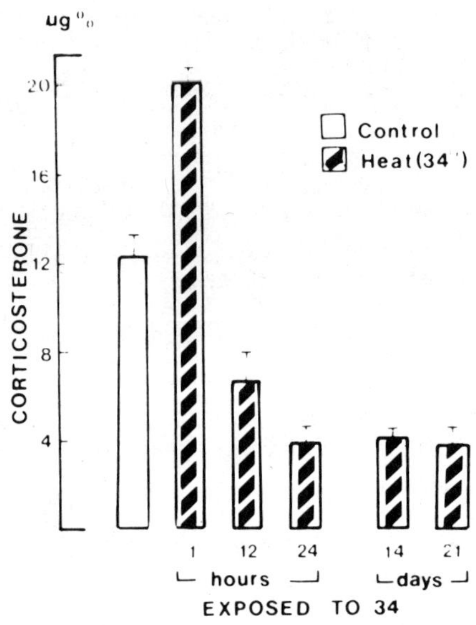

Fig. 13. Corticosterone plasma level in rats previously adapted to 20-22°C and exposed to 34°C as indicated (Petrović and Janić-Šibalić, 1980).

Acute heat exposure increases the plasma level of growth hormone but long term exposure causes a decline in the level of this hormone (Mitra and Johnson, 1972). Judging by an immediate increase of plasma corticosterone and cortisol level in animals upon acite exposure to heat (Christison et al., 1970, 1972) it may be concluded that hypothalamic-pituitary-adrenocortical system under this condition reacts similarly as in the cold (Fig. 13). The difference was evidenced a few hours later, when adrenocortical activity in the heat was significantly lower than in controls (Petrović and Janić-Šibalić, 1980).

Adrenal Cortex and Thyroid in the Heat Stress

Exposure of rats to heat (34°C) is characterized by an initial increase in the metabolic rate (MR), followed by a decline toward the level equal to that of the controls. It was suggested that this increase in MR may be due to increased adrenocortical activity in the first few hours of exposure to heat (Katby and Johnson, 1967). Later the same authors showed in the rat that a sudden exposure to heat (34°C) causes an increase in plasma corticosterone level with a maximum after 24 hrs. After this period the level of corticosterone in plasma was decreased below the control value. Contrary to this Bertin (1969) found that in the rat exposed to 30°C both adrenal and plasma cortitosterone levels are decreased in respect to the control and remain low for about one month. We have found an increase in corticosterone plasma level one and three hours after the exposure of animals to heat (34°C) but later the level of this hormone was decreased (Petrović et al., 1978).

Storm et al. (1981) reported that T_3/T_4 ratio was significantly different in animals expposed to room temperature (23 $\pm$ 1°C) than in those exposed to cold (4°C). Fractional disappearance rate (K) of T_4 and T_3 was lower at 35°C in comparison with 10°C and energy intake had no significant effect on K value (Macari et al., 1983). The same author concluded from experiment that the metabolism of thyroid hormones is influenced independently by both, ambient temperature and energy intake.

Catecholamines in the Heat Stress

Exposure to heat represents a special kind of stress under which not only the temperature but also the humidity is very important for the survival and the adaptation process (Suttanov, 1976). Our results have shown that gradual exposure to moderate heat (32 or 34°C) did not produce such a dramatic change in the parameters studied as did a sudden exposure to extreme heat of 36 or 38°C. Besides, a gradual exposure to heat eliminated the mortality of rats (Petrović et al., 1976). As shown in the figure 14, in rats exposed to heat of 36°C for one hour, a significant decrease in adrenal adrenaline was found, but noradrenaline content remained unchanged as compared with nonexpo-

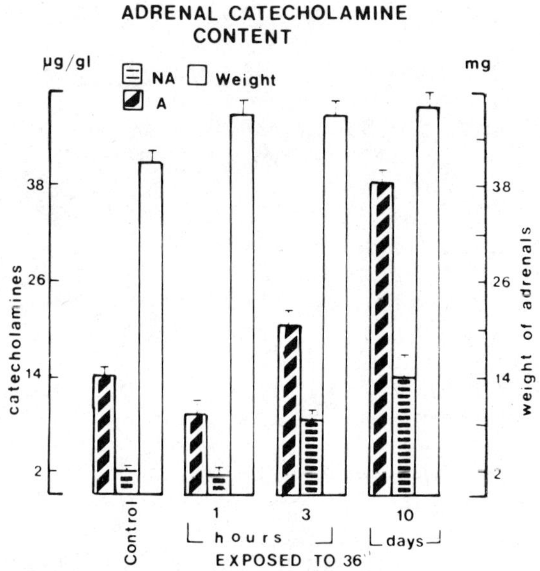

Fig. 14. Adrenal catecholamines content in rat exposed to 36°C (Petrović et al., 1976).

sed controls. Body temperature in animals exposed to heat for many hours rose to 38-39°C. In animals exposed to heat for 24 hours or 10 days adrenal adrenaline contents were significantly higher than in non exposed controls. The amount of adrenaline in urine was found to be significantly higher, whereas that of noradrenaline was lower as compared with the control (Fig. 15). It was suggested that in rats exposed to 36°C for 24 hrs or 10 days an increased biosynthesis of adrenaline occurred (Petrović et al., 1976).

In rats exposed to heat for one hour we did not get enough urine for catecholamine determination. The fact that in rats exposed to 36°C for 24 hrs or 10 days the noradrenaline content in urine was lower whereas in adrenals it was higher in comparison with controls, suggests low activity of sympathetic nervous system under these conditions.

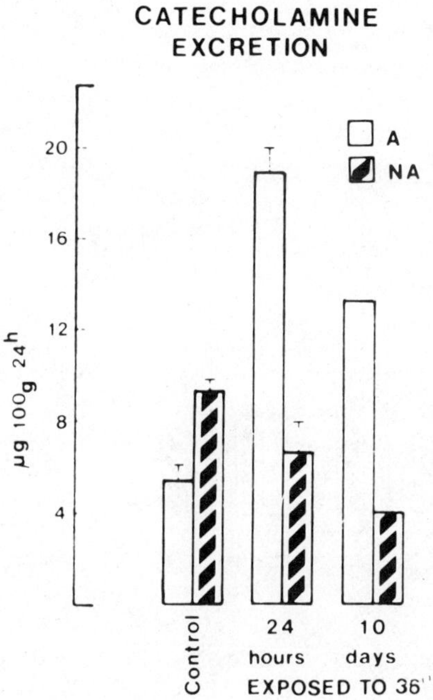

Fig. 15. Adrenaline and noradrenaline excretion in rats exposed to heat (Petrović et al., 1976).

It seems that during the first few hours of exposure to extreme heat the activity of hypothalamo-pituitary-adrenocortical system was increased. This was concluded on the basis of an increased corticosterone level in the plasma. Adrenaline synthesis and excretion were also incressed.

The exposure of rats to 36°C produced the mortality of about 20%. In order to avoid or minimize the mortality of rats exposed to heat and to enable them to adapt to heat we decided in the second experiment to expose animals to 34°C, Under this condition we found, as we did before, an increase in corticosterone plasma level in animals exposed to 36°C for 1 and 3 hrs, followed by a significant decrease, phenomenon already observed in rats exposed to 36°C (Petrović et al., 1976; Petrović and Janić-Šibalić, 1980). In the same animals, exposed to heat for 3 hrs a higher PNMT activity in the adrenals was found, as compared with control adapted to 20-24°C. However, in 1, 6 and 24 hours exposed rats, PNMT activity was at about the same level as in non exposed controls. TH activity in the adrenals of the same animals was somewhat lower in rats exposed to 34°C but as compared to non exposed controls the difference was not significant (Fig. 16).

Monoamine oxidase (MAO) activity in the liver, heart heart, kidney, lung, brown fat and hypothalamus in rats

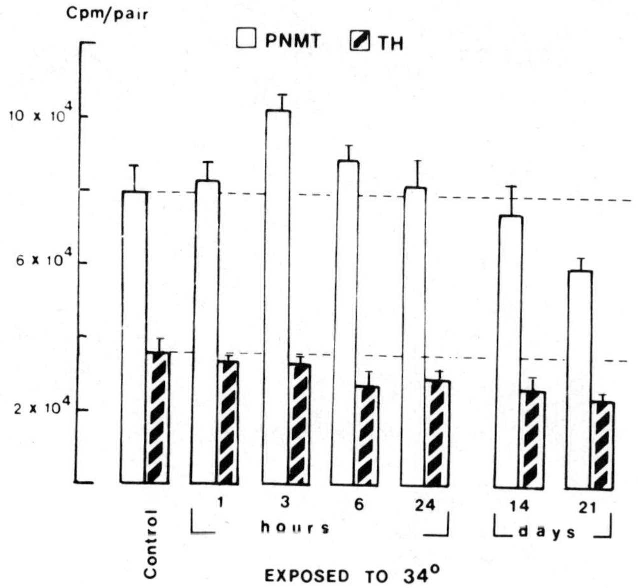

Fig. 16. Phenylethanol-N-methyltransferase (PNMT) and tyrosine hydroxylase (TH) activity in the adrenals of rats exposed to heat (34°C) (Petrović and Janić-Šibalić, 1980).

exposed to heat for 1, 3, 6 and 24 houurs was at about the same level as in the non exposed controls except for the hypothalamus of 6 hour exposed rats (Fig. 17,18).

The increase in PNMT activity found in our experiments in the adrenals of rats exposed to 34°C for 3 hrs indicates an increase in the methylation of nor-adrenaline into adrenaline. We have previously observed that shortly after being exposed to heat rats excreted more adrenaline per 100 g/24 h than controls. In addition, adrenaline content of adrenals in these animals was decreased (Petrović et al., 1976).

Taking into consideration all these data together with the fact that corticosterone level in plasma of our animals exposed to 34°C for 1 and 3 hrs was also elevated we suggest that the first reaction to heat has similarity to the pattern of the "alarm reaction".

As it has been shown that glycocorticoids play a significant role in the activation of PNMT in the adrenals, we may suggest that the transient increase in the activity of this enzyme in the heat, as found in our second experiment, might be due to an increase in adrenocortical

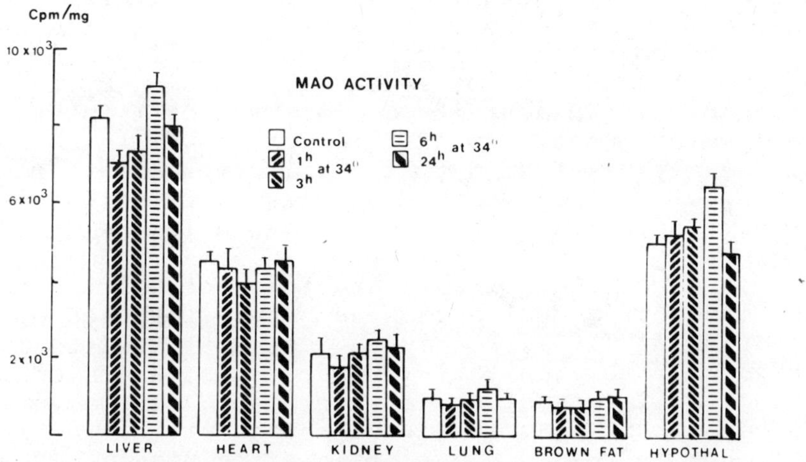

Fig. 17. Monoamine oxidase (MAO) activity in the rat tissues after the exposure to heat (Petrović and Janić-Šibalić, 1980).

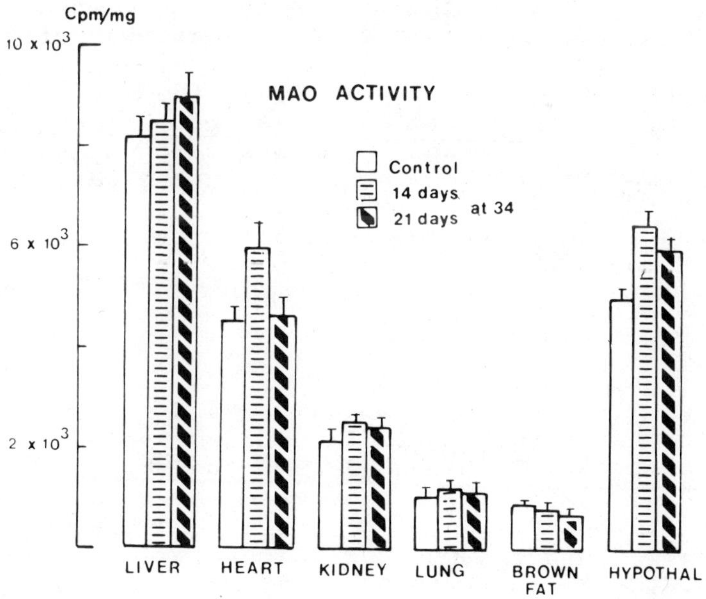

Fig. 18. Monoamine axigase (MAO) activity in the tissues of rats adapted to Reat. (Petrović and Janić-Šibalić, 1980).

activity. Thus, our experiment shows that the transient reaction to heat is not associated with a significant increase in catecholamine synthesis in general but probably only with a short stimulative effect of elevated glycocorticoids on the transferase activity and consequently on the adrenaline synthesis. Judging by the fact that PNMT and TH activity as well as corticosterone plasma level in heat adapted rats were lower than in controls it may be assumed that a hot environment produces in long exposed animals a suppression in adrenocortical activity as well as in adrenal catecholamine synthesis.

In conclusion, if we take into account the conceptual model of a dual stress pathways prorposed by Henry and Stephans (1977) we may suggest that the thermal stress activates both pituitary-adrenocortical and sympathetic-adrenomedullary system. The increased ACTH secretion and consequently an increased adrenocortical activity was found in the cold but also in the first few hours of the heat stress. Sympathetic-adrenomedullary system was activated by the cold but this activation was also observed at the beginning of heat exposure. The increased PNMT activity and consequently the augmented adrenaline synthesis and excretion were found in cold exposed animals. This increase was also observed in heat exposed animals but only at the beginning of the exposure. It seems that hormonal rather than neural way of the activation of the adrenal medulla occurs in the first period of the heat exposure. Later on, in the heat ambient, contrary to cold, the activity of sympathetic-adrenomedullary system was low and hypokinesis, hypophagia and a sexual abstination were observed in the rat. From the results reported and discussed here it way be concluded that the response in the cold and heat stress may be defined to be specific as well as non specific.

REFERENCE

Axelrod, I., 1980, Catecholamines and stress: A brief informal history, in: "Catecholamines and Stress-Recent Advances", E. Usdin, R. Kventnansky and I.J. Kopin eds., Elxevier/North-Holland, Amsterdam, pp. 3-5.

Beley, A., Beley, P., Rochette, L. and Bralet, J., 1977, Time dependent changes in the rat of noradrenaline synthesis in various rat brain areas during cold exposure, Pflügers Arch., 368: 225-229.

Bertin, R., 1969, Pharmacodinamie - Teneurs surrennaliéne et plasmatique en corticostérone chez le rat adapté a diverse temperatures, C.R.Soc.Biol., 1963: 2108-2112.

Bligh, J., Cottle W.H. and Maskrey, M., 1971, Influence of ambient temperature on the thermoregulatory response to 5-hydroxytryptamine, noradrenaline and acetylcholine injected into the lateral cerebral ventricles of sheep, goats and rabbits, J.Physiol., 212: 377-392.

Boulouard, R., 1966, Adrenocortical activity during adaption to cold in the rat: role of Porter-Silber chromogens, Fed. Proc., 25: 1195-1199.

Chaffee, R.R. and Roberts, J.C., 1971, Temperature acclimation in birds and mammals, Ann.Rev.Physiol., 33: 155-203.

Chap, Z., Bedrak, E. and Sod-Moriah, A., 1977, Effect of heat acclimation on testicular enzymes involved in androgen biosynthesis via the 5-ene pathway, Austr. J.Biol.Sci., 30: 85-95.

Chowers, J., Conforti, N. and Feldman, S., 1972, Body temperature and adrenal function in cold-exposed hypothalamic disconnected rats. Am.J.Physiol., 223: 341-345.

Christison, G.I. and Johnson, H.D., 1972, Cortisol turnover in heat-stressed cows, J.Animal Sci., 35: 1005-1010.

Christison, G.I., Mitra, R. and Johnson, H.D., 1970, Glucocorticoids in acutely heat stressed steers, J.Animal Sci., 31: 219-220.

D'Angelo, S.A., 1960, Hypothalamus and endocrine function in persistent oestrus rats at low environmental temperature, Am. J.Physiol., 199: 701-706.

Dupont, A., Bastarache, E., Endröczi, E. and Fortier, C., 1972, Effect of hippocampal stimulation on plasma thyrotropin (TSH) and corticosterone responses to acute cold exposure in the rat, Can.J.Physiol. Pharmacol., 50: 364-367.

Endröczi, E. and Lissak, K., 1962, Interrelations between palaco-cortical activity and pituitary-adrenocortical function, Acta Physiol. Acad. Sci. Hung., 21: 257-263.

Fortier, C., 1966, Nervous control of adrenocorticotrophic hormone secretion, in: "The Pituitary Gland", G.W. Harris and B.T.Donovan, eds., Butterworth, London, pp. 195-234.

Gale, C.C., 1973, Neuroendocrine aspects of thermoregulation, Ann. Rev. Physiol., 35: 391-430.

Ganong, W.F., 1974, The role of catecholamines and acetylcholine in the regulation of endocrine function, Life Sci., 15: 1401-1414.

Ganong, W.F., 1980, Participation of brain monoamines in the regulation of neuroendocrine activity under stress, in: "Catecholamines and Stress; Recent Advances", E. Usdin, R.Kventnansky and I.J.Koppin, eds., Elsevier/

North-Holland, Amsterdam, pp. 115-124.

Hefco, E., Krulich, L., Illner, P. and Larsen, P.R., 1975, Effect of acute exposure to cold on the activity of the hypothalamic-pituitary-thyroid system, Endocrinology, 95: 1185-1195.

Henry, H.P. and Stephens, P.M., 1977, "Stress, Health and the Social Environment", Springer Verlag, New York, pp. 1-282.

Heroux, O. and Petrović, V.M., 1969, Effect of hight and low bulk diets on the thyroxine turnover rate in rats acute and chronic exposure to different temperatures, Can.J.Physiol.Pharmacol., 47: 963-968.

Himms-Hagen, J., 1969, The role of brown adipose tissue in the calorigenic effect of adrenaline and noradrenaline in cold acclimated rats, J.Physiol., 205: 393-404.

Himms-Hagen, J., 1970, Regulation of metabolic processes in brown adipose tissue in relation to nonshivering thermogenesis, Adv.Enzyme Regulation, 8: 131-142.

Itoh, S., Hiroshige, T., Koseki, T. and Nakotsugawa, T., 1969, Release of thyrotropin in relation to cold exposire, Fed. Proc., 25: 1187-1192.

Jansky, L., Mejsnar, J. and Moravec, J., 1976, Catecholamines and cold stress, in: "Catecholamines and Stress, - Recent Progress", E, Usdin, R, Kvetnasky and I. J. Kopin, eds., Pergamon Press, Oxford, 419-434.

Johnson, H.D., 1976, Effect of heat on endocrine responses of domestic and laboratory animals, in: "Progress in Biometeorology", S.W.Tromp ed., Swets and Zeitlinger, B.V., Amsterdam, pp. 27-32.

Katby, S. and Johnson, H.D., 1967, Rat adrenal cortical activity during exposure to a high (34°C) ambient temperature Life Sci., 6: 1121.

Kawakami, M., Seto, R., Terasawa, E., Yoshida, K., Miyamoto, T. and Hattatori, Y., 1968, Influence of electiral stimulation and lesion in limbic structure upon biosynthesis of adrenocorticoids in the rabbit, Neuroendocrinology, 3: 337-348.

Knigge, K.M., 1960, Neuroendocrine mechanisms influencing ACTH and TSH secretion and their role in acclimation, Fed.Proc., 19: 45-51.

Kozlowski, S., 1980, Panel discussion on stress theory, in: "Catecholamines and Stress; Recent Advances", E. Usdin, R.Kvetnansky and I.J.Kopin eds, Elsevier/ North-Holland, Amsterdam, pp. 583-584.

Kraicer, J., Elliot, N.L. and Zimmerman, A.E., 1978, In vitro release of ACTH from dispersed rat Parts intermedia cells. III. Multiple forms of ACTH biological activity, Neuroendocrinology, 27; 86-96.

Kraicer, J., Zimmerman, A.E., and Moor, B.C., 1980, Role

of biogenic amines in the control of secretion of pars intermedia ACTH and related peptides, in: "Catecholamines and Stress - Recent Advances", E.Usdin, R.Kvetnansky, and I.J. Kopin, eds, Elsevier/North Holland/Amsterdam, pp. 131-136.

Krieger, D.T., Liotta, A., and Brownstein, M.J., 1977, Corticotropin releasing factor. Distribution in normal and brattleboro rat brain and effect of differentiation hypophysectomy and steroid treatment in normal animals, Endocrinology, 100: 227-237.

Kvetnansky, R., 1973, Frontiers in Catecholamine Research, E. Usdin and Snyder, S. eds., Pergamon Press, Oxford, pp. 223-229.

Kvetnansky, R., 1980, Recent progress in catecholaminess under stress, in: Catecholamines and Stress: Recent Advances, E. Usdin, R.Kvetnansky and I.J. Kopin, eds., Elsevier/North-Holland, Amsterdam, pp. 7-18.

Kvetnsky, R., Gewirtz, G.P., Weise, V.K. and Kopin, I.J., 1971, Catecholamine-synthesizing enzymes in the rat adrenal gland during exposure to cold. Am. J.Physiol., 220: 928-931.

Kvetnansky, R. and Mikulaj, L., 1970, Adrenal and urinary catecholamines in rats during adaptation to repeated immobilization stress, Endocrinology, 87: 738-743.

Kventnansky, R., Palkovits, M., Mitro, A., Torda, T. and Mikulaj, L., 1977, Catecholamines in individual hypothalamic nuclei of acutely and repeatedly stressed rats, Neuroendocrinology, 23: 257-267.

Kvetnansky, R., Sun, C.L., Lake, C.R., Thoa, N., Torda, T. and Kopin, I.J., 1978, Effect of handling and forced levels of epinenphrine, norepinephrine and dopamine β hydroxalase, Endocrinology, 103: 1868-1874.

Lechiver, F. and Petrović, V.M., 1960, Activité thyroidienne comparée de deux hibernants: le lerot (Elliomys quercinus) et le Spermophile (Citellus citellus) et d'un homeotherme, le rat au cours de l'exposition au froid pendant l'été, C.R.Acad.Sci. (Paris), 250: 3883-3885.

LeBlanc, J., 1976, The role of catecholamines in adaptation to chronic and acute stress, in: "Catecholamines and Stress", E. Usdin, R.Kvetnansky and I.J.Kopin, eds., Pergamon Press, Oxford, pp. 409-418.

LeBlanc, J., Roberge, C., Vallières, J. and Oakson, G., 1971, The sympathetic nervous system in short term adaptation to cold, Can,J.Physiol.Pharmacol., 49: 96-101.

Leduc, J., 1961, Excretion of catecholamines in rats exposed to cold, Acta Physiol.Scand., 51: 94-101.

Macari, M., Dauncey, M.J., Ramsden, D.B. and Ingram, D. L., 1983, Thyroid hormone metabolism after acclimatization to a warm or cold temperature under conditions of high or low energy intake, Quart. J. Exp. Physiol., 68: 709-718.

Mejsnar, J., and Jansky, L., 1971, Methods for estimating of nonshivering thermogenesis, in: "Nonshivering thermogenesis, "L.Jansky, ed., Academia, Prague, pp. 27-36.

Mikulaj, L., Kvetnansky, R., Murgas, R., Parizkova, J. and Vancel, P., 1976, in: "Catecholamines and Stress" E.Usdin, R.Kvetnansky and I.J.Kopin, eds., Pergamon Press, Oxford, pp. 445-455.

Mitra,R. and Johnson, H.D., 1972, Growth hormone rasponse to cute thermal exposure in cattle, Proc.Soc.exp. Biol., 139: 1086-1089.

Myers, R.D. and Yaksh, T.L., 1969, Control of body temperature in the unanasthetized monkey by cholinergic and aminergic systems in the hypothalamus, J.Physiol., 202: 483-500.

Palkovits, M., Kabayashi, R.M., Kizer, J.S., Jacobowitz, D.M. and Kopin, I.J., 1975, Effects of stress on catecholamines and tyrosine hydroxylase activity of individual hypothalamic nuclei, Neuroendocrinology, 18: 144-153.

Palkovits, M., Mezey, E. and Feminger, A., 1980, Neuroanatomical basis for the activation of brain monoergic system under stress. in: "Catecholamines and Stress; Recent Advances", E.Usdin, R.Kvetnansky and I.J.Kopin, eds, Elsevier/North-Holland, Amsterdam, pp. 21-29.

Petrović, V.M., 1976, Effects of acute and chronic exposure to cold on the endocrine system of laboratory animals, in: "Progress in Biometeorology, S.W.Tromp, ed., Swets and Zeitlinger, B.V., pp. 42-48.

Petrović, V.M. and Andjus, R.K., 1960, Métabolisme de base et adaptation therqmique du rat; role de la thyroide et des surrénales, J.Physiol., (Paris), 52: 191-192.

Petrović, V.M., Andjus, R.K. and Dukić, S., 1961, Role de la thyroid et des surrénales dans l'adaptation thermique du rat, Arch.Biol.Sci. (Beograd), 13: 7-20.

Petrović, V.M., Davidović, V. and Janić-Šibalić, V., 1976, Catecholamine synthesis, release and excretion and adrenocortical activity in the heat-stressed rat, in: "Catecholamines and Stress", E.Usdin, R. Kvetnansky and I.J. Kopin, eds., Pergamon Press, Oxford, pp. 437-433.

Petrović, V.M. and Janić, V., 1964, Comparative study of the effect of cold on 17, 21 hydroxi-20-ketosteroids and adrenal ascorbic acid in the rats and ground squirrels, Arch. Biol.Sci., 16: 145-153.

Petrović, V.M. and Janić-Šibalić, Vera, 1976, Adrenocortical control of phynylethanolamine-N-methyl transferase and monoamine oxidase activity in the ground squirrel (Citellus citellus) during the summer, Gen. Comp.Endocrinol. 29: 492-497.

Petrović, V.M. and Janić-Šibalić, V., 1977, Regulation of adrenal catecholamine synthesis in the ground squirrel (Citellus citellus), Bull. Acad.Serbe Sci., 60: 83-89.

Petrović, V.M. and Janić-Šibalić, V., 1978, Effect of corticotropin and dexamethasone on monoamine oxidase activity in the rat brain, Bull.Acad.Serbe Sci., 61: 1-4.

Petrović, V.M. and Janić-Šibalić, V., 1980, Catecholamine synthesizing and degrading enzymes in the heat stressed or adapted rats, in: "Catecholamines and Stress", E.Usdin, R.Kvetnansky and I.J. Kopin, eds., Elsevier/North Holland, Amsterdam, pp. 365-370.

Petrović, V.M., Janić-Šibalić, V., Aminot, A. and Roffi, J., 1978, Adrenal thyrozine hydroxilase activity in the ground squirrel-effect of cold and arousal from hibernation, Comp.Biochem.Physiol., 61C: 99-101.

Petrović, V.M., Janić-Šibalić, V. and Cvijić, G., 1981, Adrenocortical activity and catecholamines synthesizing and degrading enzymes in the ground squirrel exposed to cold or aroused from hibernation, Acta Universitas Caroline-Biologica (Prague), 245-248.

Petrović, V.M., Janić-Šibalić, V. and Cvijić, G., 1984, Effect of dexamethasone on catecholamines biosynthesis in the brain regions of the rat, Proc. Meeting Yugoslav End. Soc. (in press).

Petrović, V.M., Janić, V. and Dukić, S., 1964, L'action du froid sur l'activité corticosurrénalienne chez le spermophile, J.Physiol., 56: 631-632.

Petrović, V.M., Maksimović, K., 1979, Adaptation to cold and diurnal fluctuation of the sensitivity to noradrenaline in the rat, Bull.Acad.Serbe Sci. (Belgrade), 66: 81-86.

Petrović, V.M. and Marković-Djaja, L., 1973, A comparative study of the calorigenic action of noradrenaline in the rat and ground squirrel adapted to different temperatures, Experientia, 29: 1295-1296.

Petrović, V.M. and Rajčić, O., 1969, Effect of prolonged cold exposure and ACTH administration on RNA, DNA and protein content in adrenals and liver of rat and ground squirrel, Fed.Proc., 28: 1247-1250.

Petrović, V.M., Rajčić, O., Hudnik-Plevnik, T., 1966, Étude comparée de l'action du froid et de l'ACTH, sur le taux des acides nucléiques et de protéins dans la surrénale et dans le foie chez le rat et le spermophile, J.Physiol. (Paris), 58 —590-591.

Schoenbaum, E., 1960, Adrenocortical function in rats exposed to low environmental temperatures, Fed.Proc., 19: 85-88.

Sellers, E.A., Steiner, G., Flattery, R.V., Shum, A., Johnson, G.E. and Schönbaum, E., 1971, Activity of the sympathetic nervous system during cold exposure, in: "Nonshivering Thermogenesis", L.Jansky, ed., Academia, Prague, pp. 271-279.

Simmonds, M.A., 1969, Effect of environmental temperature on the turnover of noradrenaline in hypothalamus and other areas of rat brain, J.Physiol., 203, 199-210.

Simmonds, M.A., 1970, Effect of environmental temperature on the turnover of 5-hydroxytryptamine in various areas of rat brain, J.Physiol., 211: 93-108.

Storm, H., Hardelveld E. and, Kassenaar, A.A.H., 1981, Thyroid hormone-catecholamine interrelationship during exposure to cold, Acta Endocrinologica,97: 91-97.

Suttanov, F.F., 1976, Catecholamines and heat stress, in: "Catecholamines and Stress", E.Usdin, R.Kvetnansky and I.J.Kopin, eds, Pergamon Press, Oxford, pp. 435.

Vigaš, M., 1980, Contribution to the understanding of the stress concept, in: "Catecholamines and Stress; Recent Advances", E.Usdin, R.Kvetnansky and I.J. Kopin, eds., Elsevier/North-Holland, Amsterdam pp. 573-578.

Weiner, R.I. and Ganong, W.F., 1978, Role of brain monoamines and histamine in regulation of anterior pituitary secretion, Physiol.Rev., 58: 905-959.

Zeisberger, E. and Brück, R., 1973, Effect of intrahypothalamically injected noradrenergic and cholinergic agents on thermoregulatory responses, in: "The Pharmacology of Thermoregulation", E.Schönbaum, E. and P.Lomax, eds., Karger, Basel, pp. 232-246.

THE SIGNIFICANCE OF THE CHOLINERGIC-ADRENERGIC INTERACTIONS IN THE RESPONSE OF THE RAT TO IMMOBILIZATION STRESS

S. Stepanović, V.M. Varagić, J. Nikolić, and R. Kvetnansky*

Institute "Boris Kidrič", Vinča, Department of Pharmacology Faculty of Medicine, Belgrade, Yugoslavia and *Institute of experimental endocrinology, Bratislava, Szhechoslovakia

INTRODUCTION

A conceptual model of dual stress pathways has been postulated by Henry and Stephens (1977). Some stressors, particularly the psychosocial ones activate the pituitary-adrenocortical system, or the sympatho-adrenomedullary system. The first system is activated particularly when there is a loss of control by the organism, a state known to lead to depression. This type of stress is characterized by an increased secretion of corticosterone and corticotropine, whereas the secretion of catecholamines is unaltered. On the other hand, the sympatho-adrenomedullary system is particularly activated during the "fight and flight" reaction, in which the organism is chalanged in its control of the environment. In this type of stress the release of catecholamines is significantly increased, whereas the plasma corticosterone level remains unchanged. In the central nervous system, amygdala is thought to the primarily involved in this type of stress reaction.

A central cholinergic mechanism is known to participate in the peripheral adrenergic activation, thus leading to an increase in blood pressure (Varagić, 1955). For this reason, all the anticholinesterases which penetrate the blood-brain barrier produce an increase in blood pressure, both in conscious and anaesthetized animal. The pressor response to physostigmine and other anticholinesterases is the result of a complex interaction between cholinergic and adrenergic mechanisms, and this interaction might have functional implications under certain physiological and pathological conditions.

Kvetnansky (1980a) has put forward a hypothesis that adaptation on repeated stress involves an enchanced activity of the sympatho-adrenomedullary system and its availability for an intensified response to a different stressogenic stimulus. It was therefore of interest to investigate the effect of physostigmine on the response to immobilization stress, as judged by plasma catecholamine levels.

MATERIALS AND METHODS

Male rats of the Wistar strain, bred under standard conditions and weighing 300-320 g, were used. First group of animals was treated with eserine (physostigmine) in the doses of 200,400 and 800 μg/kg intraperitoneally (ip.). In the second group immobilization stress lasted from 15 to 90 min. Immobilization was performed by forcibly fixing the animal to a board. All four limbs were fixed and the motion of the head was limited by one metal loop fixed over the neck area (Kvetnansky and Mikulaj, 1970; Kvetnansky et al., 1978). A separate series of animals was pretreated by eserine (200,400 and 800 μg/kg ip.), and 30 sec after injection of eserine the same animals were subjected to immobilization for 15, 40 and 90 min, respectively.

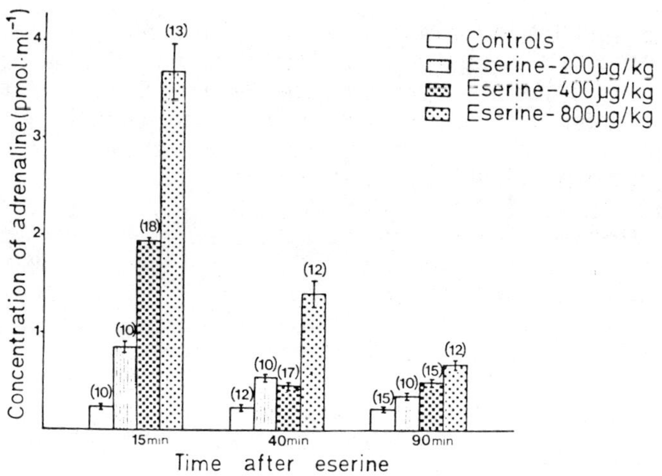

Fig. 1. The effect of increasing doses of eserine (200,400 and 800 μg/kg) on the plasma level of adrenaline (15,40 and 90 min after intraperitoneal injection of eserine). The number of experiments is shown in brackets.

In all groups of animals the permanent polyethylene catheter was introduced under general pentobarbiton anaesthesia into the tail artery, 24 hours before the experiment. In all three groups of animals blood samples (0.5 to 0.6 ml) were collected via the catheter at 15,40 and

90 min after treatment with eserine, or after pretreatment both by eserine and immobilization. This technique allowed the collection of blood without producing any disturbance to the animals.

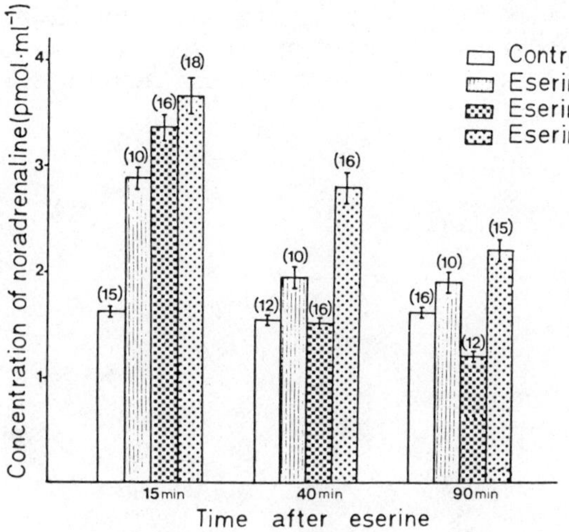

Fig. 2. The effect of increasing doses of eserine (200, 400 and 800 µg/kg, intraperitoneally) on the plasma level of noradrenaline (15,40 and 90 min after injection of eserine). The number of experiments is shown in brackets.

The estimation of catecholamines in plasma was done using a radioenzymatic method, slightly modified, as originally described by Weise and Kopin (1976). The blood samples were collected in iced heparin-treated tubes and centrifuged at 5000 g at - 2°C for 15 min. Aliquots of plasma were removed for determination of catecholamines (200 µl). Deproteination was done using 0.6 N perchloric acid containing 2% EGTA and 0.2 % $MgCl_2 \cdot H_2O$. The samples were vortexed and once again centrifuged at 5000 g at - 2°C for 15 min. Catecholamines in portions of 200 µl were converted to their ^{3}H-O-methylated derivatives by using S-^{3}H-adenosyl-methionine and catechol-O-methyltransferase (COMT). The O-methylated derivatives of catecholamines were extracted along with unlabelled carrier, as described by Da Prada and Zürcher (1976). Finally, the O-methylated derivatives were oxidized with periodate (Peuler and Johnson, 1977).

Results were expressed as the mean ±S.E.M. Statistical significance was calculated by Student's - t-test.

RESULTS

The effect of increasing doses of physostigmine (eserine) on the plasma catecholamine levels. - The increasing doses of eserine (200, 400 and 800 μg/kg b.w.) were found to produce a dose-dependent increase in the plasma concentration of adrenaline (Fig.1). Eserine was injected intraperitoneally and this was reason that the first blood samples were taken 15 min after injection of eserine. The highest increase in the plasma level of adrenaline was found 15 min injection of eserine, but this increase, although to a less degree, persisted even 90 min after injection of eserine, but with a clear tendency of restoring the normal level adrenaline.

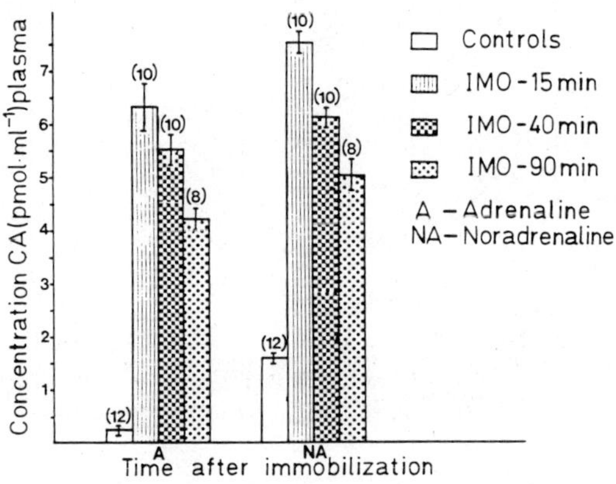

Fig. 3. The effect of forced immobilization for 15,40 and 90 min on the plasma catecholamine levels.

Similarly, the intraperitoneal injection of eserine produced a dose-dependent increase in the plasma concentration of noradrenaline (Fig.2.). Here again, the maximal response was found 15 min after injection of eserine, but 90 min after injection of eserine a tendency towards normalization of plasma level of noradrenaline was observed.

The effect of immobilization on the plasma catecholamines levels. - The immobilization of rats for 15, 40 and 90 min produced a highly significant increase in plasma levels both of adrenaline and noradrenaline (Fig.3.). The highest increase of both catecholamines was found after 15 min of immobilization, whereas the lower values were found after 40 and 90 min of immobilization. Still, the values of both adrenaline and noradrenaline after 90 min of immobilization were well above the control values.

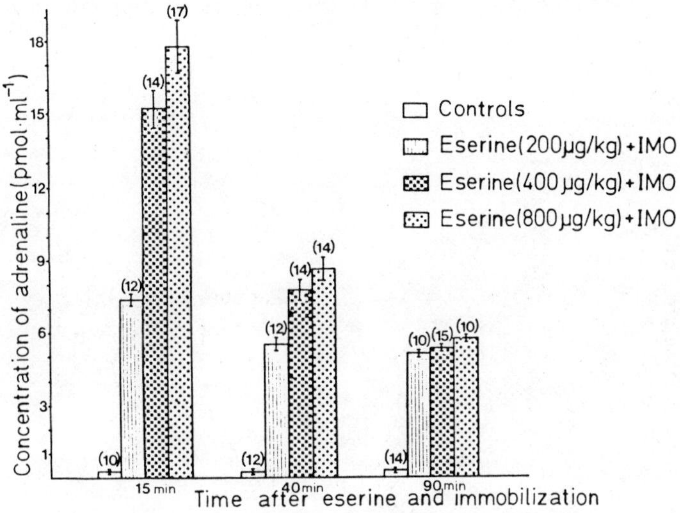

Fig. 4. The effect of forced immobilization for 15, 40 and 90 min on the plasma level of adrenaline in the eserine-pretreated rat (200, 400 and 800 µg/kg, intraperitoneally). The number of experiments is shown in brackets.

<u>The effect of immobilization in the eserine-pretreated animals on the plasma catecholamine levels.</u>- The plasma catecholamine levels after immobilization for 15, 40 and 90 min in the eserine-pretreated animals (200, 400 and 800 µg/kg) were significantly higher than in the animals treated either by increasing doses of eserine alone, or after immobilization alone.

The values for adrenaline are shown in Fig.4. and the values for noradrenaline in Fig.5. (Note the scale on the ordinate in both figures). Evidently, the increased response of catecholamine stores after immobilization of the animal was not more summation of the effect of eserine and of immobilization themselves, but a genuine potentiation produced by eserine. This potentiating effect of eserine was particularly pronounced 15 min after injection of eserine, but it was still present even 90 min after injection of eserine in lower degree.

Comparison of the effects of eserine, immobilization and a combined action of eserine and immobilization, on the plasma catecholamine levels. - All the data obtained with various types of treatment are shown in Fig.6. and 7. For comparison, all the data in these figures are shown againist the same scale on the ordinate. It is evident that both adrenaline and noradrenaline are significantly higher in both eserine-pretreated and immobilized animals than after any these treatments alone. Still, the combined action of eserine and immobilization was more apparent on the levels of noradrenaline than on adrenaline.

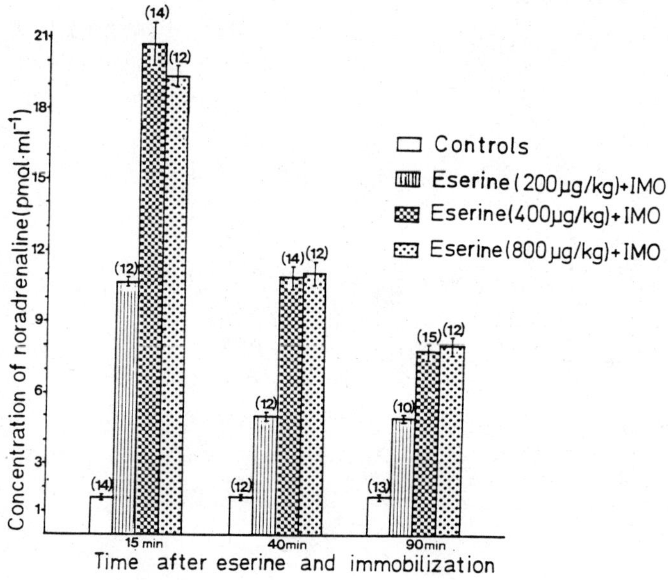

Fig. 5. The effect of forced immobilization for 15,40 and 90 min the plasma level of noradrenaline in the eserine-pretreated rat (200,400 and 800 µg/kg, intraperitoneally). The number of experiments is shown in brackets.

DISCUSSION

It was found in the present experiments that the increasing doses of eserine regularly produced a dose-dependent increase in the plasma concentration of both adrenaline and noradrenaline. It has been already reported that eserine produces a blood pressure rise both in urethane-anaesthetized and conscious rats (Varagić, 1955; Varagić and Krstić, 1966; Brezenoff and Giuliano, 1982). The time course and the peak of the increase in the plasma catecholamine levels roughly corresponds to the time course and the peak of the hypertensive response to eserine and to the time course and the peak of the increased neuronal activity in the peripheral sympathetic after injection of eserine (Stamenović and Varagić, 1970).

The doses used to produce a dose-dependent blood pressure rise in the anaesthetized rat ranged from 25 to 100 ug/kg, and only occasionally up to 200 ug/kg (Varagić, 1955). These doses presumably act by increasing the peripheral noradrenergic influences and in increase in the peripheral vascular resistence (Varagić, et al., 1969). The hypertensive effect of eserine is also present in the adrenalctomized animal, indicating that the liberation of adrenaline from the adrenals does not contribute to the blood pressure rise after injection of eserine. In the present experiments the doses of eserine ranged from 200 to 800 ug/kg. All the doses used in the present experiments produced an increase of both adrenaline and noradrenaline in the plasma. Most probably, the higher dose range and the somatic changes produced by higher doses of eserine in the conscious animals (e.g. fasciculation of the skeletal muscles) have contributed to an increased liberation of adrenaline from the adrenals.

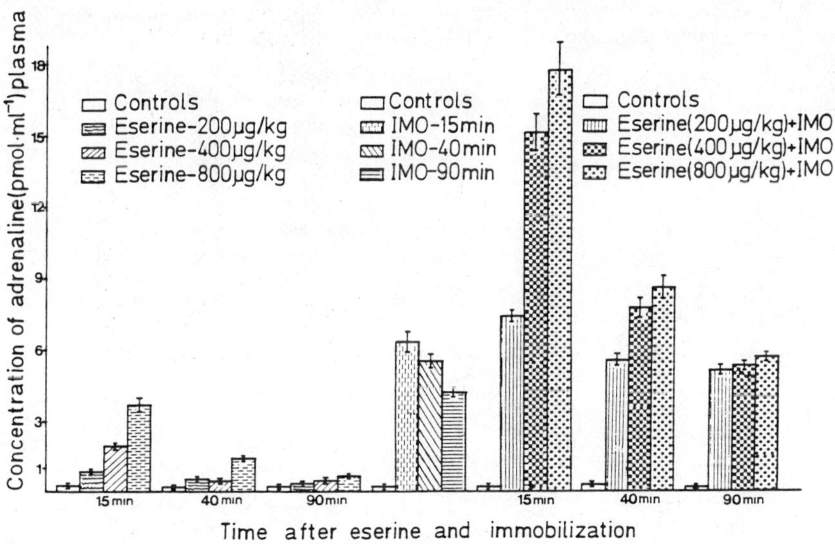

Fig. 6. Comparative effects of eserine (200, 400 and 800 ug/kg intraperitoneally) and of immobilization (15, 40 and 90 min), as well as of a combination of eserine and immobilization, on the plasma levels of adrenaline.

The method used in this work for collection of blood samples has made it possible to study the effects of minor psychosocial stressors (handling, opening the cage etc.) on the plasma catecholamine levels (Kvetnansky, 1980). The same method has been previously used for studyng the effect of forced immobilization on the plasma catecholamine levels (Kvetnansky, 1980a) This model of stress combines the emotional stress (escape reaction) and physical stress (muscle work), thus resulting in both restricted mobility and aggression. It has been shown that the initial response to immobilization involves primarily stimulation of the adreno-medullary system, leading to an increase in the plasma adrenaline level. With the prolongation of the immobilization stress, the peripheral adrenergic system becomes increasingly activated, leading to an increase in the plasma noradrenaline level (Kvetnansky et al., 1978).

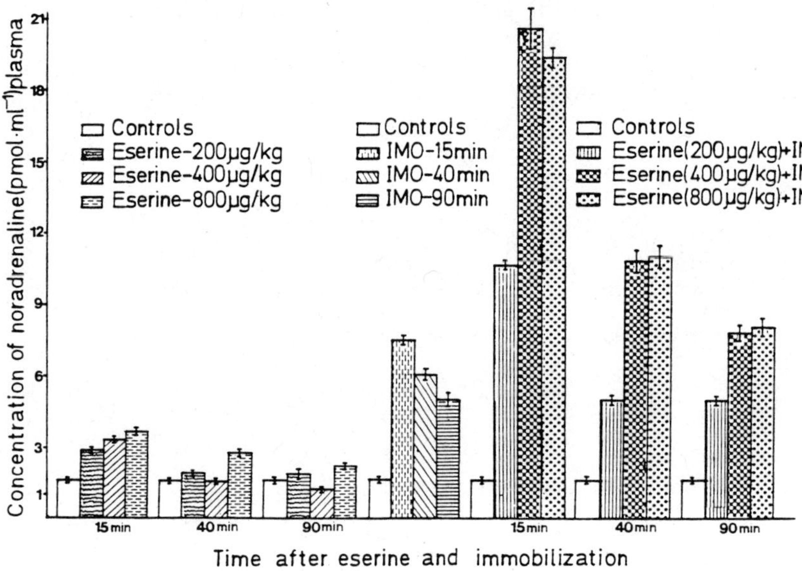

Fig. 7. Comparative effects of eserine (200, 400 and 800 µg/kg, intraperitoneally) and of immobilization, as well as of a combination of eserine and immobilization, on the plasma level of noradrenaline.

In the present experiments the animals were immobilized for 15, 40 and 90 min. By the time when the first blood samples were taken (15 min), the plasma levels of both adrenaline and noradrenaline were increased to almost equal levels. After 40 min of immobilization the plasma catecholamine levels were lower, and after 90 min of immobilization they were significantly lower than after 15 min of immobilization. Still, even these levels of catecholamine were high above the control values for both catecholamines. These findings are in accordance with those of Kvetnansky et al., (1978).

In the eserine-pretreated animals immobilization produced significantly higher levels in the plasma catecholamines than in the control untreated immobilized animals. The values obtained in the eserine-pretreated animals were not a simple summation of the effects of eserine and of immobilization by themselves. This effect might be characterized as a potentiating response to immobilization produced or coupled with the eserine pretreatment.

Both the effects of eserine and immobilization can be classified as stressors and therefore the action of immobilization in the eserine-pretreated animals can be estimated as the action of double stressors on the animals. In rats repeatedly stressed by forced immobilization, an increased catecholamine synthesis was observed (Kvetnansky et al., 1971). Kvetnansky (1980) has even put forward a hypothesis that adaptation to repeated stress involves an enhanced activity of the sympatho-adrenomedullary system and the availability for an intensified response to a different stressogenic stimulus. The pretreatment with eserine presumably creates the physiological circumstances similar to those after repeated stressogenic stimuli, as judged by an increased plasma catecholamine levels. It is therefore possible that a central cholinergically mediated activation of the peripheral adrenergic system by eserine produces a state of an increased readyness and availability for an intensified response to stressogenic stimuli.

SUMMARY

The increasing doses of eserine (200, 400 and 800 µg/kg, intraperitoneally) regularly produced a dose-dependent increase in the plasma concentrations of both adrenaline and noradrenaline. This increase in the plasma catecholamines roughly corresponds to the time course an the peak of the hypertensive response to eserine in the rat . The increase in the plasma catecholamine levels after injection of eserine is due to a central cholinergically mediated activation of the peripheral adrenergic system, as well as to the somatic effects of eserine.

Forced immobilization of the rat for 15, 40 and 90 min produced an increase in plasma levels of both adrenaline and noradrenaline. The highest increase was obtained after 15 min of immobilization. After 40 and 90 min of immobilization the plasma catecholamine levels were lower in comparison with the 15 min period, but still well above the control values, before the animals were subjected to immobilization.

In the eserine-pretreated animals immobilization produced significantly higher levels of catecholamines than in the control untreated animals. The potentiated response is due to the action of double stressors. The pretreatment with eserine presumably acts by creating the physiological circumstances similar to those after repeated stressogenic stimuli. It is therefore possible that a central cholinergically mediated activation of the peripheral adrenergic system by eserine produces a state of an increased readyness an availability for an intensified response to stressogenic stimuli.

ACKNOWLEDGEMENT: The authors are indebted to Miss Gordana Milenković for technical assistance in carrying out the experiments and in the preparation of the manuscript.

REFERENCES

Brezenoff,H.E.Giuliano,R.,1982, Cardiovascular control by cholinergic mechanisms in the central nervous system, Ann.Rev. Pharmacol. Toxicol., 22,341.

Da Prada, M., Zürcher,G., 1976, Simultaneous radioenzymatic determination of plasma and tissue adrenaline, noradrenaline and dopamine within the femtomole range, Life Sci., 19. 1161.

Henry,H.P., Stephens, P.M., 1977, Stress, health and the social environment, Springer Verlag, New York, 1, 282.

Kvetnansky, R., Mikulaj, L., 1970, Adrenal and urinary catecholamines in rats during adaptation to repeated immobilization stress, Endocrinol., 87, 738.

Kvetnansky, R., Weise, V.K., Gerwitz, G.P.Kopin, I.J., 1971, Enhanced synthesis of adrenal dopamine-β - hydroxylase induced by repeated immobilization in rats. Mol.Pharmacol., 7, 81.

Kvetnansky, R., Sun,C.L.,Lake,C.R.,Thoa,N.,Torda,T., Kopin, I.J.,1978, Effect of handling and forced immobilization on rat plasma levels of epinephrine,norepinephrine and dopamine-beta-hydroxylase. Endocrinol., 103, 1868.

Kvetnansky, R., 1980, Plasma catecholamines in emergency situations. In Homeostsis in injury and shock, Adv.Physiol. Sci. Eds. Z.Biro, A.G.Kovach, J.J., Spitzer and H.B. Stoner, Pergamon Press. Akademiai Kiado 26, 121.

Kvetnansky, R., 1980a, Recent progress in catecholamines under stress. In catecholamines and stress-recent advances. Eds. E. Usdin, R.Kvetnansky, I.Kopin, Elsevier North-Holland Inc., 7, 18.

Peuler,Y., Johnson,G., 1977, Simultaneous single isotope radioenzymatic assay of plasma norepinephrine, epineprhrine and dopamine, Life Sci., 21, 625.

Stamenović, B., Varagić,V.M., 1970, The effect of eserine on the efferent neuronal activity in the cervical sympathetic of the rat, Neuropharmacol., 9, 561.

Varagić,V.M., 1955, The action of eserine on the blood pressure of the rat, *Br. J.Pharmacol.*, 10, 349.

11

Varagić,V.M., Krstić, K., 1966, Adrenergic activation by anticholinesterases, Pharmacol. Rev., 18, 799.

Varagić, V.M., Žugić,M., Kentera, D., 1969, The effect of eserine on some circulatory parameters in the rat. *Iugoslav. Physiol. Pharmacol.* Acta, 5, 59.

Weise, V., Kopin, I., 1976, Assay of catecholamines in human plasma: Studies of a single isotope radioenzymatic technique, *Life, Sci.*, 19, 1673.

ENDOGENOUS PEPTIDES IN CIRCULATORY SHOCK

Winfried Krause, Karen Nieber
and Peter Oehme

Institute of Drug Research
Academy of Sciences of the GDR
DDR-1136 Berlin-Friedrichsfelde

INTRODUCTION

Circulatory shock may be considered as a special and severe form of stress. It is a complex syndrome and is characterized by a severely disturbed hemostasis of the entire organism.

Circulatory shock states are caused by different conditions such as hemorrhage, endotoxins, neurogenic dysregulations, acute heart failure, or others. Despite the differences in pathogenesis the result is quite similar in all of these cases. There is a disproportion between the volume of the circulating blood and the capacity of the blood vessels and it results in a so-called low flow syndrome. The low blood flow leads to an insufficient supply of the organism with oxygen and other essential nutrients.

Acute loss of blood or plasma, often in combination with tissue trauma, initiates a strong activation of the neurohumoral system. This defense reaction of the organism is quite similar to other typical stress reactions: The sympathetic nervous system is extremly activated, catecholamines are released from the adrenals. Enkephalins and larger enkephalin-like peptides, which are synthesized and stored along with the catecholamines in the chromaffin granules of the adrenal medulla, are also released into the blood by sympathetic activation. Possibly, they serve in the adaptive response to stress, including circulatory shock. Some other typical alterations in circulatory shock are enhanced plasmatic concentrations of ß-endorphin, released together with ACTH, of vasopressin and of angiotensin.

In a mild shock state these reactions will be sufficient to normalize circulation and the sufficient perfusion of all the organs and tissues of the body. However, in more severe shock states the extreme blood levels of the catecholamines and the other vasoactive substances cause strong changes in the distribution of blood between the different tissues and organs. This redistribution of flow favours mainly the heart, brain, liver and the kidneys, which are relatively highly perfused even during shock. On the other side, the blood flow to the abdominal organs and to the striated muscles is highly reduced (Bond et al., 1967; Rutherford et al. 1968). Therefore, the first hypoxic damages occur in these slowly perfused tissues. Some of such damages are

- increased permeabilities of cell membranes,
- occurence of proteolytic enzymes in the circulating blood,
- activation of enzymes that initiates blood coagulation.

All of these reactions, starting in the periphery and not in the CNS, will disturb the cell function and release biologically active compounds which will overcompensate the vasoconstriction induced by central regulation via sympathetic nerves and other mechanisms. This way circulation will progressively become dysregulated and an irreversible shock state will be reached within a short period of time. But, not all of the factors contributing to the progress of shock toward irreversibility have been elucidated yet.

Until today the effective treatment of severe circulatory shock states is an unsolved problem also in human medicine. All therapeutic effort is often unsuccessful if the shock state has already lasted for more than 2 hours only. This explains that at present many groups of scientists are looking for further unknown pathophysiological mechanisms which may offer new possibilities of more effective treatment of circulatory shock.

In 1978 Holaday and Faden suggested that the endogenous opiates released from the pituitary or from other tissues after stress could possibly play and important role in the pathophysiology of circulatory shock. They observed that the opioid receptor blocker naloxone significantly improves arterial pressure and enhances the survival rate of animals subjected to different forms of circulatory shock.

A great number of experiments to evaluate the mechanisms responsible for the shock-protective activity of naloxone has been published by this group. But the mechanisms seem to be quite complex. For instance, further more specific blockers of the μ- and δ-opioid receptors showed no clear results regarding their shock-protective activity. Some experiments indicate that the cardiovascular disturbances in shock are mediated by low affinity opioid (δ-) receptors. In fact, the selective δ-receptor antagonist M 154,129 reverses the endotoxic shock in the rat (Holaday et al., 1982). On the other hand, naloxazone, the hydrazone derivative of naloxone, is a selective and irreversible blocker of the high affinity (μ-) opioid receptor binding site. This opioid antagonist, at doses which effectively block high affinity opiate binding, failed to either block or reverse the endotoxic shock produced by E. coli liposaccharide endotoxin in the conscious rat (Holaday et al., 1983). But, another finding was very surprising and is not fully explainable yet. Pretreatment of the animals with naloxazone effectively prevented the well established therapeutic effects of subsequent naloxone injections following endotoxic shock hypotension. This suggests a possible functional interaction between the different opioid receptor subtypes.

During the past years more attention was paid to the role of the adrenals with reference to their regulatory function against stress as well as circulatory shock. Endogenous opioids seem to be involved in both cases. Central application of opioid peptides like ß-endorphin may increase the sympathetic outflow. On the other hand, peripherally administered morphine or related compounds decrease the sympathetic tone (Van Loom et al., 1981; Holaday, 1983a). Because the concentrations of endogenous opioids have been found enhanced in circulatory shock, opiate antagonists may be expected to restore the cardiovascular dysfunction by reversing the sympathetic changes via influencing the adrenal medullae.

Analogous mechanisms may be involved in other stress reactions. Naloxone-sensitive stress analgesia is not only reduced by lesion of central opioid-rich structures but also by removal of the adrenal medullae (Lewis et al., 1982). It has been postulated that not only enkephalin-like peptides (originated from the CNS) but also related peptides (originated from the adrenal medulla) are critically involved in mediating stress analgesia in the rat.

Furthermore, adrenal medullary integrity is required for naloxone to exert pressor effects in endotoxaemic rats (Holaday et al., 1983b). In a similar way removal of the adrenal medullae blocks the pressure response to naloxone in hemorrhagic shock (Patton et al., 1982). Adrenalectomized animals also react very more sensitive against inducers of circulatory shock, for example toxins.

Another peptide, which is involved in the regulation of stress susceptibility and the release of catecholamines from the adrenal medulla, is the undecapeptide substance P. It is an important modulator of many physiological and pathophysiological processes. Oehme and Hecht have found out that substance P also prevents stress-induced disorders (Oehme et al., 1980; Hecht et al., 1980). Substance P-like immunoreactivity has been found in fibers and cells of the adrenal medulla of rats (Görne et al., 1984). Substance P inhibits the release of catecholamines from chromaffin cells (Livett et al., 1979) as well as the raise of blood pressure in stressed rats (Roske et al., 1983). Furthermore, the level of substance P-like immunoreactivity is lower in the adrenal medullae and in blood plasma of chronically stressed animals than in the controls (Rathsack et al., 1983). Therefore we investigated the shock susceptibility of rats that were prophylactically treated with substance P for 4 days.

Many recent studies suggest that several other hypothalamic peptides, in addition to their endocrine activity, exert direct effects on the central nervous system. Some of these peptide factors interact with endogenous opiates administered either acutely or chronically. For example, TRH antagonizes the ß-endorphin-induced hypothermia and catalepsy (Holaday et al., 1978a) and also the ß-endorphin-induced depression of motor activity (Tache et al., 1977). Similarly TRH antagonizes the hypothermia and respiratory depression produced by morphine (Horita et al., 1976).

Multiple injections of TRH inhibit the development of physical dependence on morphine. Like other compounds that antagonize the effects of endogenous opioids TRH has also protective activity against circulatory shock (Holaday et al., 1981). On the other hand, some other effects induced by morphine or ß-endorphin are not blocked by TRH, for instance morphine-induced analgesia.

Another peptide released from the hypothalamus is the α-melanocyte-stimulating release-inhibiting factor (or MSH release-inhibiting factor), abbreviated as MIF, MIF-1 or PLG. The structure of this tripeptide is Pro-Leu-Gly-NH_2. The same sequence of these three amino acids is also contained in the nonapeptide oxytocin. Therefore oxytocin has been postulated as a precursor of MIF.

The tripeptide MIF does not only inhibit the release of the melanocyte-stimulating hormone, but also, like TRH, interacts with the development of tolerance to morphine (Bhargava et al., 1980; Bhargava and Kim, 1982). Treatment with MIF antagonizes the acute analgesic effects of enkephalins and morphine in the tail flick test on mice. Furthermore, MIF inhibits the effect of morphine on transmurally stimulated guinea pig ileum in vitro. The acute morphine-induced catalepsy is also antagonized by MIF. On the other hand, MIF stimulates the dopamine turnover in the striatum.

All these effects of MIF led us to study whether MIF - like naloxone or TRH - is able to cause some prolongation of survival times or to increase the survival rates of rats submitted to hemorrhagic shock.

MATERIALS AND METHODS

Male Wistar rats weighing 280 - 300 g were used. The animals were fasted overnight, except for water ad libitum. After producing anesthesia by intraperitoneal injection of 80 mg/kg of crotylbarbital, the left carotid artery was dissected and cannulated for bleeding the animal and for registration the blood pressure. The left femoral vein was cannulated for drug infusion and for application of 250 U/kg of heparin.

In order to induce hemorrhagic shock the animals were bled through the carotid catheter into a reservoir in which a constant pressure of 70 mm Hg was maintained. 12 minutes later the pressure was lowered to 60 mm Hg, after another 12 minutes the pressure was maintained for 12 minutes at 50 mm Hg and finally lowered to 40 mm Hg. At this level the animals were maintained for 45 minutes. During this period the animals released their blood into the reservoir until the blood pressure had dropped to the level inside the reservoir. On the other hand, animals underwent a reinfusion, if their blood pressure reached values lower than the pressure inside the reservoir. Such spontaneous reinfusion indicates that the shock has already become irreversible.

After maintaining the blood pressure at 40 mm Hg for 45 minutes the bleeding was stopped by clamping the reservoir. The shed blood remained for additional 45 minutes in the reservoir, before it was returned to the animals. All animals were monitored up to 5 hours. Animals having survived the hemorrhage for 5 hours were considered as survivors.

For investigating drugs in the model of the so-called "gut dependence" we used the isolated ileum of rats pretreated chronically in vivo with 25 mg/kg of morphine daily for 5 days. In vitro the gut of these animals developed a typical contraction after administration of naloxone. The details of the method have been described elsewhere (Nieber and Oehme, 1981). The contraction induced by naloxone was fully antagonized by morphine. The ileum of the animals being not dependent on morphine did not react to naloxone.

Statistical analysis was carried out by using the parameter free U test (Mann and Whitney, 1947) to compare the survival times between the groups treated with drugs and treated with saline. Only for p values less than 5 % the differences were considered statistically significant.

The peptides, MIF and substance P, were synthetized in our institute by Bienert and Ehrlich.

RESULTS

Figure 1 shows the changes in survival rate and survival time following treatment with MIF, tested in rats submitted to hemorrhagic shock. MIF solved in 1.8 ml of saline was infused intravenously for 3 hours. The infusion was started 60 minutes after the beginning of bleeding. The animals of the simultaneously investigated control group received the same volume of saline.

A dose of 2 mg/kg MIF significantly increased survival times relative to controls. In figure 1 the ordinate indicates how many of the 14 rats treated either with MIF or with saline were still alive after a certain periods of time. The differences between both groups are statistically significant at a p value less than 0.01. 5 hours after starting the shock induction the survival rate was 36 % in the group treated with MIF and only 7 % in the control group. A smaller dose of MIF (0.5 mg/kg for 3 hours) produced smaller effects. Although the differences in survival time were no longer significant at this lower dose the effects had the same tendency. Also, the survival rate was higher: 30 % in animals treated with this lower dose of MIF versus 5 % in control animals.

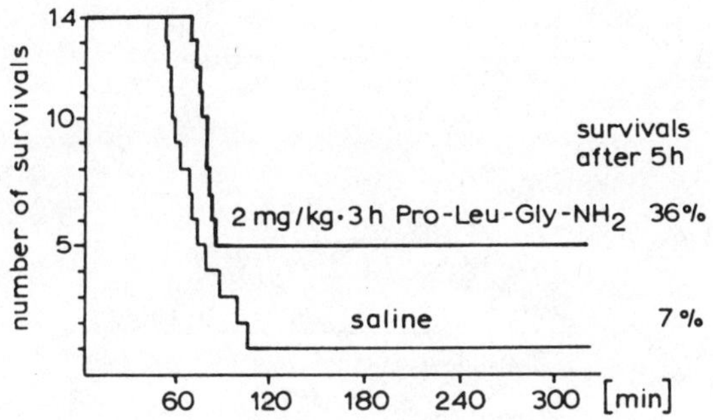

Fig. 1. Hemorrhagic shock in rats. Animals treated with MIF survive longer than controls ($p < 0.01$)

For comparing the effects of MIF with those of naloxone we repeated the experiments carried out by Faden and Holaday (1979) in conscious rats on our model. A dose of 4 mg/kg naloxone (about one half of the dose used by Faden and Holaday) increased the survival rate after 5 hours from 10 % to 45 %. This means that the activities of MIF and naloxone at the doses used were in the same range.

For investigating the mechanism of the protective action of MIF against hemorrhagic shock we tested MIF in the model of the so-called "gut dependence". The results are shown in figure 2.

Figure 2 A demonstrates that MIF, like the opiate antagonist naloxone, was able to contract the ileum of morphine-dependent rats. But the amplitude of the MIF-induced contraction was lower than that of naloxone. Naloxone, given after MIF, produced an additional contraction. Both contractions were completely antagonized by morphine (figure 2 C). The ileum of not morphine-dependent, saline-treated animals did not react on MIF as it didn't on naloxone.

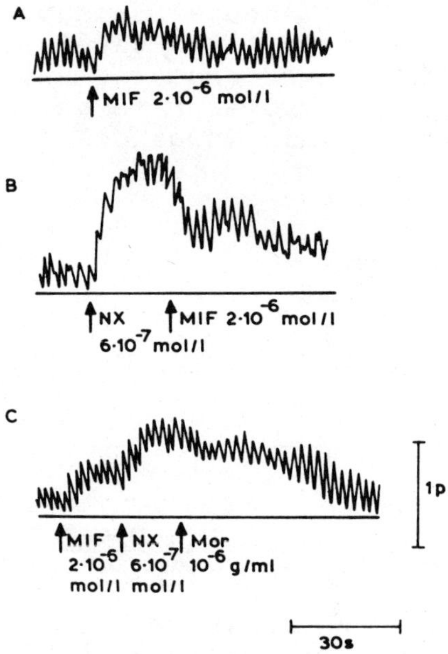

Fig. 2. Isolated ileum of morphine-dependent rats. Contractions ("gut dependence") are induced by MIF or Naloxone (NX). Mor = morphine. See text for further explanations

Figure 2 B shows that MIF was able to antagonize the naloxone-induced contraction partially, whereas morphine completely antagonized the contraction.

For investigating the shock susceptibility of rats, pretreated with substance P, the experimental protocol was very similar to that described for testing MIF. The only difference was that the substance P was not administered by infusion, but was given intraperitoneally, at a daily dose of 250 µg/kg for 4 days. For injection the drug was solved in 0.2 ml of saline which additionally contained acetic acid in a very low concentration (0.01 vol %). The control animals were given the solution of saline and acetic acid only. 20 - 24 hours after the last administration of substance P the shock induction was started.

The results of this experiments showed that substance P, even if administered subchronically, had no influence on the shock susceptibility of rats, although it prevents very effectively other stress induced disorders when using the same doses and the same time spacing. In the group pretreated with substance P only 20 % of the 10 investigated rats survived the hemorrhagic shock for 5 hours. In the control group one of 10 animals survived. Regarding the survival times there was also no detectable difference to the control group.

DISCUSSION

The obtained results indicate that the tripeptide MIF, like naloxone and TRH, is therapeutically active against lethal consequences of hemorrhagic shock. Which mechanisms can be supposed at present for this protective activity of MIF? There are some results which implicate an interaction with opioid and dopaminergic pathways in the central nervous system. Possibly related mechanisms, which occur additionally in the peripheral nervous system, may also contribute to the therapeutic effects of MIF against circulatory shock.

Both morphine and ß-endorphin release the α-melanocyte-stimulating hormone (α-MSH) from the pituitary gland (Celius, 1980). Inasmuch as the release of MSH is controlled by the hypothalamic MIF, an interaction between the opioids and the peptide hormone is likely to exist.

Treatment with MIF blocks the development of tolerance to the cataleptic action of morphine (Bhargava and Kim, 1982). Since the opiates may produce their cataleptic action by interacting with the dopaminergic systems in the brain the shock-protective effect of MIF may be caused not only by an interaction with opioid pathways but also indirectly via dopaminergic pathways. Dopamin is currently counted among the most useful drugs in treatment of patients and animals in circulatory shock.

Other studies suggest that the dopamine receptor supersensitivity develops as a consequence of chronic morphinization, because the dopaminergic transmission is chronically depressed by morphine. MIF has been shown to block morphine-induced receptor supersensitivity (Bhargava, 1980).

Some experiments support the view that MIF interacts more directly with the dopaminergic systems in the brain since MIF potentiates the effects of dopaminergic agonists, like L-DOPA or apomorphine, and stimulates the dopamine turnover in the striatum (Plottnikoff et al., 1971; Kostrezewa et al., 1978).

Our experiments on the "gut dependence" in vitro demonstrate that MIF antagonizes the action of morphine similar to naloxone. But this must be a functional antagonism. The site of action must be different from that of naloxone since MIF does not compete effectively with etorphine binding in the rat striatum (Czionkowski, 1978). On the other hand, specific MIF receptors in the central nervous system has been suggested that might facilitate nigrostriatal dopaminergic transmission (Chiu et al., 1983). Analogously the presence of specific binding sites for MIF may be supposed also in the peripheral nerves of the gut. Excitation of these receptors could possibly modulate the biological activity of endogenous opioids. Such an interaction may produce not only the contraction of morphine-dependent gut but also the therapeutic effects against hemorrhagic shock. But, at present we don't know exactly the mechanism of these effects of MIF, nor do we know exactly the pathophysiological basis of the therapeutic effects of dopamine or naloxone in treatment of circulatory shock.

Substance P even when given subchronically failed to exert some protective activity against circulatory shock under our experimental conditions. This result agrees well with those of the experiments carried out by Kovacs et al. (1977), who investigated substance P after acute administration and also didn't find any protective activity against hemorrhagic shock.

We gave substance P subchronically since under thes conditions it prevents other stress induced disorders very effectively and is inhibits the release of catechol amines from the adrenals. We expected analogous full effects with respect to shock protection since exogenic administration of catecholamines decreases the survival rate in circulatory shock and α-blockers have also shock protective activity. But this expection failed. Evidently, endogenous regulation is more complex in vivo.

SUMMARY

Endogenous peptides play a pathophysiological role in stress and circulatory shock, especially the endogenous opioids. Opioid receptor blocking agents, such as naloxone, are known to improve cardiovasculary function and survival in different shock states. The results of this paper indicate that the melanocyte-stimulating hormone release-inhibiting factor (MIF, Pro-Leu-Gly-NH_2) is also therapeutically active against hemorrhagic shock in rats. Furthermore, MIF, like naloxone, is able to contract the ileum of morphine-dependent rats. Since MIF does not block the opioid receptors we suggest that both effects are caused by an indirect anti-opioid action. Substance P, a protective agent against stress-induced disorders, shows no therapeutic activity in experimental shock.

REFERENCES

Bhargava, H. N., Walter, R., and Ritzmann, R. F., 1980, Development of narcotic tolerance and physical dependence. Effects of Pro-Leu-Gly-NH_2 and cyclo (Leu-Gly), Pharmacol. Biochem. Behav. 12:73.

Bhargava, H. N., 1980a, Cyclo(Leucylglycine) inhibits the development of morphine-induced analgesic tolerance and dopamine receptor supersensitivity in rats, Life Sci. 27:117.

Bhargava, H. N., and Kim, H. S., 1982, Structure activity relationship studies with hypothalamic peptide hormones. I. Effect of melanotropin release-inhibiting factor and analogs on tolerance to morphine in the rat, J. Pharmacol. Exp. Therap. 220:394.

Bond, R. F., Manley jr., E. S., and Green, H. D., 1967, Cutaneous and sceletal muscle vascular responses to hemorrhage and irreversible shock, Amer. J. Physiol. 212:488.

Celis, M. E., 1980, Effects of different opiate agonists on melanocyte-stimulating hormone release: In vivo and in vitro studies, Can. J. Physiol. Pharmacol. 58:326.

Chien, S., 1967, Role of the sympathetic nervous system in hemorrhage, Physiol. Rev. 47:214.

Chiu, S., Wong, Y.-W., Ferris, J. A., Johnson, R., and Mishra, R. K., 1983, Binding studies of L-prolyl-L-leucyl-glycinamide (PLG), a novel antiparkinsonian agent, in normal brain, Pharmacol. Res. Commun. 15:41.

Czionkowski, A., Hollt, V., and Herz, A., 1978, Binding of opiate and endogenous opioid peptides to neuroleptic receptor sites, Life Sci. 22:953.

Faden, A. I., and Holaday, J. W., 1979, Opiate antagonists: A role in the treatment of hypovolemic shock, Science 205:317.

Görne, R. C., Pfister, C., Rathsack, R., and Oehme, P., 1984, Zur zellulären Verteilung von Substanz P im Nebennierenmark der Ratte, Biomed. Biochim. Acta 43:135.

Hecht, K., Oehme, P., Kolometsewa, I. A., Ljowschina, I. P., Poppei, M., and Airapetjanz, M. G., 1980, Effect of substance P analogue on chronic deprivation of sleep of wistar rats under stress, in: "Neuropeptides and Neural Transmission", C. A. Marsan and W. Z. Traczyk, eds., IBRO Series, Vol. 7, Raven Press, New York, p. 159.

Holaday, J. W., and Faden, A. I., 1978, Naloxone reversa of endotoxin hypotension suggests role of endorphin in shock, Nature (London) 275:450.

Holaday, J. W., Tseng, L. H., Loh, H. H., and Li, C. H., 1978a, Thyrotropin-releasing hormone antagonizes ß-endorphin hypothermia and catalepsy, Life Sci. 22:1537.

Holaday, J. W., D'Amato, R. J., and Faden, A. I., 1981, Thyrotropin-releasing hormone improves cardiovascular function in experimental endotoxic and hemorrhagic shock, Science 213:216.

Holaday, J. W., Ruvio, L. E., Johnson, C. E., and D'Amato, R. J., 1982, M 154.129, a putative δ-antagonist, reverses endotoxic shock without altering morphine analgesia, Life Sci. 31:2359.

Holaday, J. W., Pasternak, G. W., D'Amato, R. J., Ruvio, B. A., and Faden, A. I., 1983, Naloxazone lacks therapeutic effects in endotoxic shock yet blocks the effects of naloxone, Europ. J. Pharmacol 89:293.

Holaday, J. W., 1983a, Cardiovascular effects of endogenous opiate systems, Ann. Rev. Pharmacol. Toxicol. 23:541.

Holaday, J. W., D'Amato, R. J., Ruvio, B. A., Feuerstein, G., and Faden, A. I., 1983b, Adrenalectomy blocks pressor responses to naloxone in endotoxic shock: Evidence for sympathomedullary involvement, Circ. Shock 11:201.

Horita, A., Carino, M. A., and Chestnut, R. M., 1976, Influence of thyrotropin-releasing hormone (TRH) on drug induced narcosis and hypothermia in rabbits Psychopharmacol. 49:57.

Kostrezewa, R. M., Kastin, A. J., and Sobrian, S. K., 1978, Potentiation of apomorphine action in rats by l-prolyl-l-leucyl-glycine-amide, Pharmacol. Biochem. Behav. 9:375.

Kovách, A. G. B., Rosell, S., Koltay, E., Sandor, P., Szabo, L., Ligeti, L., and Urbanics, R., 1977, Cardiovascular effects of substance P during hemorrhagic shock and hypotension, in: "Substance P", U. S. von Euler and B. Pernow, eds., Raven Press, New York, p. 321.

Lewis, J. W., Tordoff, M. G., Sherman, J. E., and Liebeskind, J. C., 1982, Adrenal medullary enkephaline-like peptides may mediate opioid stress analgesia, Science 217:557.

Livett, B. G., Kozousek, V., Mizobe, F., and Dean, D. M., 1979, Substance P inhibits nicotinic activation of chromaffin cells, Nature (London) 278:256.

Oehme, P., Hecht, K., Piesche, L., Hilse, H., Morgenstern, E., Poppei, M., 1980, Substance P as a modulator of physiological and pathological processes, in: "Neuropeptides and Neural Transmission", C. A. Marsan and W. Z. Traczyk, eds., IBRO Series, Vol. 7, Raven Press, New York, p. 73.

Mann, M. B., Whitney, D. R., 1947, On a test of whether one of two random variables is stochastically larger than the other, Ann. Math. Statist. 18:50.

Nieber, K., and Oehme, P., 1981, "Gut dependence" auf Opiate bei Ratten mit spontaner Hypertonie, Pharmazie 36:515.

Patton, M. L., Gurll, N. J., Reynolds, D. G., Vargish, T., and Ganes, E. M., 1982, Adrenalectomy abolishes the naloxone effect in hemorrhagic shock, Circ. Shock 9:173.

Plottnikoff, N. P., Kastin, A. J., Anderson, M. S., and Schally, A. V., 1971, Dopa potentiation by a hypothalamic factor MSH release-inhibiting hormone (MIF), Life Sci. 10:1279.

Rathsack, R., Oehme, P., Roske, I., and Hilse, H., 1983, Substance P-like immunoreactivity in plasma and adrenal medulla of rats with spontaneous hypertension and WKY rats under acute stress, Biomed. Biochim. Acta 42:955.

Roske, I., Rathsack, R., Hilse, H., and Oehme, P., 1983, Verhalten von Blutdruck und "Substance P-like immunoreactivity" (SPLIR) im Plasma von Ratten mit genetisch fixierter Hypertonie (SHR) unter chronisch intermittierender Immobilisation, Biomed. Biochim. Acta 42:731.

Rutherford, R. B., Kaihara, S., Schwentker, E. P., and Wagner jr., H. N., 1968, Regional blood flow in hemorrhagic shock by the distribution of labelled mocrospheres, Surg. Forum 19:14.

Tache, Y., Lis, M., and Collu, R., 1977, Effects of thyrotropin-releasing hormone on behavioral and hormonal changes induced by ß-endorphin, Life Sci 21:841.

Van Loom, G. R., Appel, N. M., and Ho, D., 1981, ß-Endorphin-induced stimulation of central sympathetic outflow: ß-Endorphin increases plasma concentrations of epinephrine, norepinephrine and dopamine in rats, Endocrinology 109:46.

PINEAL GLAND AND OPIOID PEPTIDES MIGHT BE INTERVENING VARIABLES IN INITIAL STRESS-INDUCED PROLACTIN SURGE

J. Milin[1], J. Martinović[3], M. Demajo[3], B. Banić[2] and R. Milin[4]

Dept. of Histol. and Embryol.[1], Dept. of Pharmacol.[2], Fac. of Med., Novi Sad; Inst. for Nuclear Scis.[3], Belgrade; Serbian Acad. of Scis. and Arts[4], Belgrade, Yugoslavia

INTRODUCTION

Several lines of studies have shown that the pineal gland (PG) and opioid peptide (OP) producing structures could be considered to be the first mediators between the perception of the stressor and the initiation of the response of the organism to stress.

It has been generally postulated that PG as the end neuroendocrine organ of noradrenergic fibres originating from the superior cervical ganglia (Kappers, 1978) expresses its role as a modulator of the endocrine equilibrium in the synchronization of homeostasis to living conditions by transforming exteroceptive neurotropic impulses into polypeptide and indole messages. In case of an initial stress attack (ISA), PG promptly meets secretory demands by the striking extrusion of its active compounds (AC) (Milin et al., 1984). In acute stress, which coincides with the second phase of the alarm reaction of the organism coping with stress, regressive changes in the cytological organization of the gland parenchyma have been accepted as sequels of the pinealocyte secretory exhaustion. Finally, chronic stress-induced progressive cytophysiological alterations of pinealocyte multitude have been understood as a reliable morphodynamic illustration of a new stress-reactive steady state of PG. In this respect, PG as an organ of multidirectional regulative potential has been hypothesized to exert its protective influence in the maintenance and functional stabilization of homeostasis under stress-inducing living conditions (Miline, 1980). In the limelight of this concept, PG may be also regarded as a general tranquillising organ on behalf of homeostatic equilibrium in relationship with changing environmental conditions (Romijn, 1978). But some obscure key questions still demand additional studies to be elucidated. Firstly, whether the domination of PG influence on endocrine equilibrium turnover is established by a prompt initial stress-induced (ISI) discharge of ACs. Secondly, whether all ACs isolated from PG are generated in pinealocytes, or some of them being synthesized somewhere else are only engulfed and stored in pinealocytes. If the second alternative is accepted, it is very likely that ACs exteroglandularly synthesized are accumulated in the case of basal, but not of long-term stimulated PG activity. In this case, it is logical that a prompt PG surge will contain a larger quantity of ACs compared with the secretory content of the long-term activated PG. Thus, the PG capacity probably varies depending on its basal or stably increased activity. Thirdly, whether the promotion of PG of chronically stressed animals into a new steady state increases the capacity of the organism to cope with stress-inducing influences, i.e. favours the inhibition of the function of some endocrine tissues, as well as the neuronal pathways, in order to facilitate the defensive reaction of the organism and to exclude the functions being unnecessary in stress.

Contrary to PG, the involvement of the ACTH-adrenal-corticosteroid axis in the induction of a broad range of systemic modifications of homeostasis has already belonged to the classical endocrinology. However, the finding that ACTH is produced not only in the pituitary but also in the brain neurons (Watson et al., 1982; Saland et al., 1982), as well as the fact that pro-ACTH molecule also represents the precursor of opioid peptides (OPs) (Schwyzer, 1982; Dacheux, 1981), give a new dimension to the consideration of the response of the organism to stress. Indeed, it has been testified that OPs could be those compounds that bring into harmony the metabolic and locomotor, as well as the psychical, responses of the organism to stress.

Ample evidence has shown that PG may decrease the adrenocortical function (Motta et al., 1971; Piva et al., 1973; Vaughan et al.,1972; Devečerski, 1965). The buffering effect of PG on the histophysiology of zona reticularis in chronic stress-affected gravid rats has been also recorded (Milin and Rakić, 1984). PG can also increase the latency to stress (Rivest et al., 1979). The PG effect on the brain OP neurons was reported as well (Kumar et al., 1982). Some pharmacokinetic studies, however, have demonstrated that an acute application of PG ACs has a stimulative effect on ACTH cells (Gromova et al., 1967) making in this case the enigma of the "dual" PG action still current. At any rate, the findings that pinealectomy eliminates some OP effects (Kavaliers, 1982) and that melatonin-induced analgesia is no longer obtainable after naloxone injection (Lakin et al., 1981) suggest that PG could mediate the OP action at least contributively.

We payed special attention to the finding that the pinealocyte elaborative potential was very sensitive to the stimulative effect of ACTH-related compounds (Schotman et al., 1981; Geffard et al., 1981; Levy et al., 1980), or opioid antagonist naloxone (Lowensten et al., 1984) because it pointed to the existence of the PG-ACTH/OP functional link with a probably significant operative repercussion. Furthermore, contrary to the knowledge that PG supresses ACTH secretion in chronic stress, the occurrence of pinealocytes (Milin et al., 1984) and ACTH/OP secretory bursts under ISI demands (de Souza and van Loon, 1982; Guillemin et al., 1977) is especially intriguing because it demands the responses to the following questions: (i) whether PG and ACTH/OP producing structures affect each other under ISA or there is an independent phenomenon related to the increased sympathicotropic tonus, and (ii) whether this parallel outflow is manifested in PG and ACTH/OP synchronous or separate effects on the common target structures. Hence, this study was undertaken to estimate possible involvement of OPs in the generation of a neuroendocrine response of PG upon ISA as a contributive component to ISI noradrenergic impulses. We chose the dynamics of prolactin secretion as an indicator of the possible interactive relationship of OP-PG. The choice was made according to several observations : (i) presence of more than one prolactinotropic stimulative ACs in PG (Kamberi et al., 1971; Blask et al., 1976; White et al., 1974; Pavel, 1979; Padmanabhan et al., 1979), (ii) correlation of ISI neurosecretory discharge of pinealocytes with PRL surge (Milin et al., 1984a), and (iii) dependence of ISI PRL burst also on ISI release of OPs (Ragavan and Frantz, 1982; van Vught et al., 1978).

MATERIAL AND METHODS

3-month-old male Wistar rats were used for the experiment. The animals were housed 3-4 per cage and maintained under laboratory living conditions in the L:D cycle of 14:10h. Food and water were given ad lib.

The pinealectomy was performed after Šćepović-Barbarosa (Šćepović, 1963). ISA, "handling stress", involved the measuring of the animals immediately after their removal from the cage and subsequent single subcutaneous injection of the solution (saline, morphine or naloxone) in a dose of 1 ml/1oo g of body weight.

The manipulation with animals lasted 2o-3o sec., after which they were put back into the cage and left undisturbed until the 1oth min. from the beginning of this procedure, when they were decapitated. The rats were divided into four groups consisting of non-operated and pinealectomized rats. The 1st group comprissed stress-unaffected animals. In order to minimize the stress effects, these animals were decapitated immediately after their removal from the cage. The 2nd group consisted of rats affected by "handling stress" (saline injected). The 3rd group was composed of rats subjected to "handling stress" and injected naloxone (given by the courtesy of DU PONT) in the dose of 1 mg/1ooo g of body weight. The 4th group comprised only non-operated rats which experienced "handling stress" and injected morphine (Alkaloid) in the dose of 1o mg/1ooo g of body weight.

The experiment was carried out in two days (May). On each day, half of each group was sacrificed at the same time, i.e. 7-9 a.m.

Histochemistry and histoenzymology. Lipids were stained with OTAN (Zugibe, 197o). The activity of glucose-6-phosphate and succinate dehydrogenase was examined after the recommended methods (Barka and Anderson, 1975). The number of rats was 5 per group.

Electron microscopy. The fixation of the pineal glands consisted in immersion in 4% glutaraldehyde/0,2 M cacodylate buffer (pH 7,4), whereas the postfixation was in 2% osmic acid/0,2 M cacodylate buffer (pH 7,4). The tissue was embedded in Durcopan-Fluka. The sections were contrasted by means of the usual procedure with uranyl acetate and lead citrate. The examination was performed in JEM loo C electron microscope. The number of rats was 4 per group.

Radioimmunoassay of the plasma PRL. The plasma was separated from trunk blood collected from decapitated rats. It was separated by centrifugation and stored at -20° C until assayed. PRL was determined by the double antibody method using the NIAMDD kits following with minor modifications the directions supplied with the kits. They were created by Dr. A.F. Parlow and provided by the courtesy of NIAMDD (now NIADDK) through the Pituitary Hormone Distribution Program. The results were expressed in the terms of the NIAMDD-Rat Prolactin-RP-1 reference preparation. The number of rats was 5-8 per group.

RESULTS

Histochemistry

Stress-unaffected rats. Usual intracellular distribution of lipid droplets (LDs) nonuniform in size, with sporadic tendency towards their perinuclear agglomeration, was noticeable (Fig. 1 a).

Stress-affected rats. In these animals, significant mobilization of LDs took place. The pinealocytes lined around the pericapillary pathways were almost deprived of LDs (Fig. 1 b).

Stress-affected, morphine-treated rats. The presence of LDs was enormously increased, especially of those unusually gigantic. In the pinealocytes abutting on the pericapillary pathways there were small LDs sometimes pearl-like distributed along the cellular margin (Fig. 1 c).

Stress-affected, naloxone-treated rats. There was a great similarity in the form and the quantity of LDs in comparison with the previous group (Fig. 1 d).

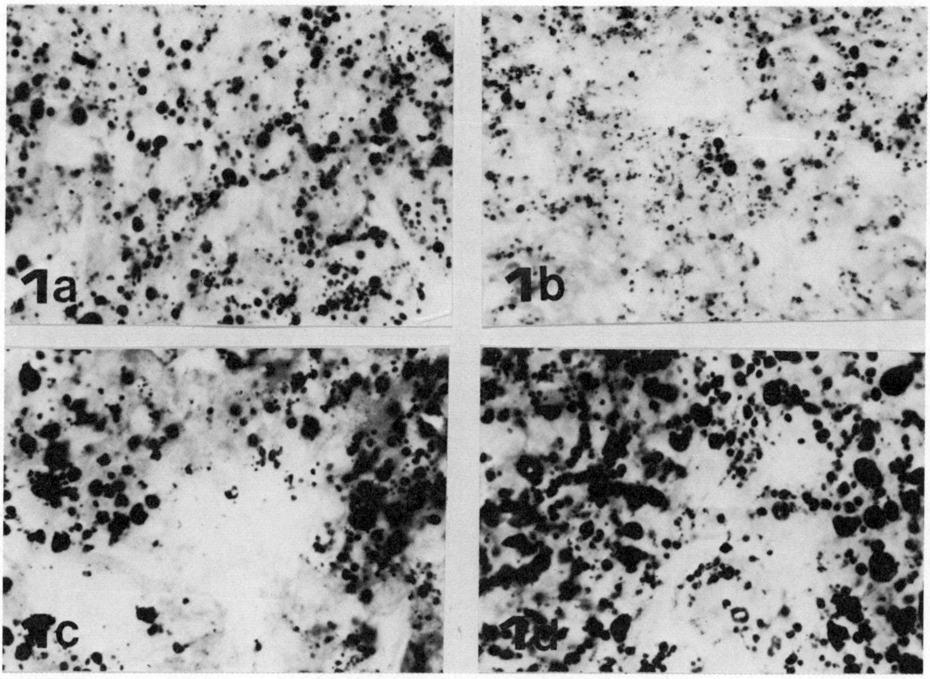

Fig. 1. Lipids. (a) stress-unaffected rat; (b) stress-affected rat; (c) stress-affected, morphine-treated rat; (d) stress-affected, naloxone-treated rat.

Histoenzymology

Stress-unaffected rats. Succinate dehydrogenase activity was found in a relatively homogeneous intracellular dispersion of formazan (Fig. 2 a), whereas in the case of glucose-6-phosphate dehydrogenase it was manifested by a sporadic occurrence of the cells richer in formazan salt (Fig. 3 a).

Stress-affected rats. An increase in the activity of both enzymes was found manifested by the occurrence of many cells with a large quantity of formazan (Figs. 2 b and 3 b).

Stress-affected, morphine-treated rats. The administration of this opiate caused an intensification of the enzymic activity but to a smaller degree than in the previous group. More uniform dispersion of formazan within pinealocytes indicated that this opiate synchronously activated the glandular parenchyma (Figs. 2 c and 3 c).

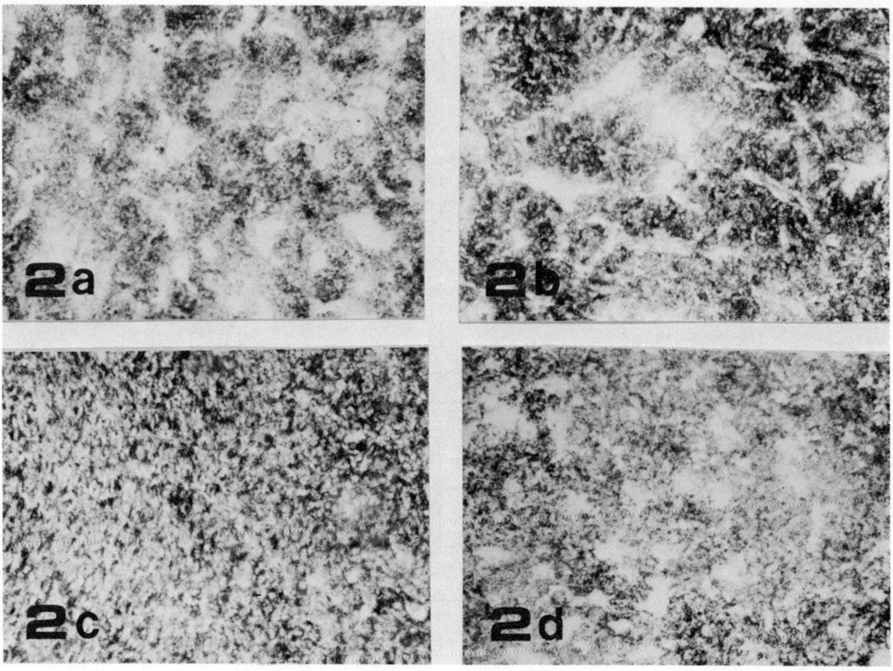

Fig. 2. Succinate dehydrogenase. (a) stress-unaffected rat; (b) stress-affected rat; (c) stress-affected, morphine-treated rat; (d) stress-affected, naloxone-treated rat.

Stress-affected, naloxone-treated rats. The administration of the OP blocker resulted in an evident fall of the enzymic activity compared with all the previous groups. The highest decrease occurred in comparison with saline-injected rats (Figs. 2 d and 3 d). It was interesting to find again the cells with various enzymic activity.

Electron Microscopy

Stress-unaffected rats. Ultrastructural characteristics of PG of the rats housed under physiological living conditions have been already well known (Wolff, 1965; Arstila, 1967; Miline et al., 1968; Rowe et al., 1977), hence this investigation was aimed at studying the morphodynamic properties of PG of experimental animals only.

Stress-affected rats. The gland parenchyma consisted mostly of light pinealocytes (LPis) with polymorphous cell samples, well-noticeable processes and a lucent cytoplasmatic ground. The nuclei of these cells were slightly indented, wholly consisting of euchromatin,

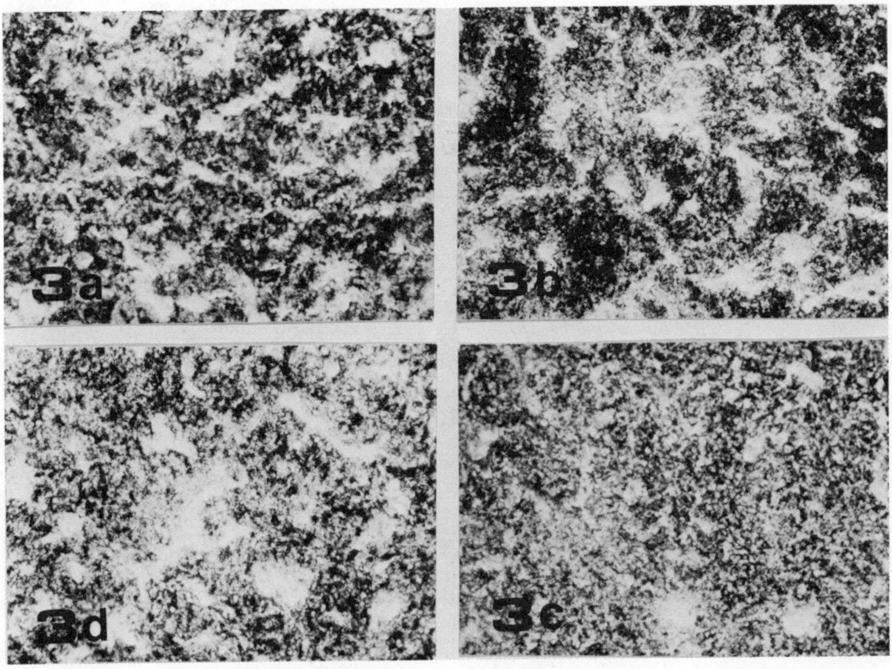

Fig. 3. Glucose-6-phosphate dehydrogenase. (a) Stress-unaffected rat; (b) stress-affected rat; (c) stress-affected, morphine-treated rat; (d) stress-affected, naloxone-treated rat.

whereas nucleoli were enlarged and situated either centrally or peripherally. The abundance of irregularly distributed ribosomes, vesicular profiles (CVPs) and mitochondria, as the basic morphodynamic characteristic of these cells, pointed to their intensified elaborative activity (Fig. 4). The occurrence of CVPs was especially frequent in some LPis (Fig. 5). Omega figures were sporadically found. Some cells were characterized by the fasciculation of the tubuli of the granular endoplasmic reticulum (GER) and the occurrence of grumose bodies, i.e. the structures we called prosecretory granules. The structures classically called LDs were also noticeable, but less frequently, mostly within the area of ribosomes or lined around the cell membrane. The extrusion of these organelles into the intercellular space was not characteristic of PG of these rats. The Golgi apparatus was made up of short but enlarged saccules encircled by vesicles being generated, which merged with the surrounding CVP multitude. Condensed mitochondria were especially numerous. Besides these LPis engaged in the initiation of elaborative activity, we

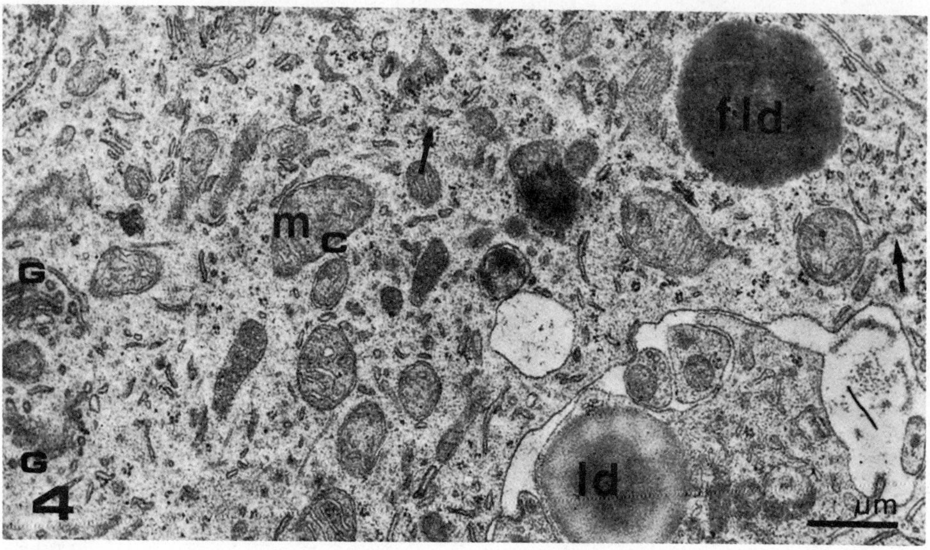

Fig. 4. Stress-affected rat, LPi. Note abundance of uniformly dispersed ribosomes. Tubuli of the granular reticulum (arrow). Golgi apparatus (g). Mitochondria of condensed appearance (m_c). Lipid droplets, characteristic feature (ld) and the organelle in the process of formation (fld).

also noticed LPis with a more compact cytoplasmatic ground, less interwoven with CVPs, less rich in ribosomes, and possessing the Golgi apparatus of an almost quiescent structural organization. Dark pinealocytes (DPis), mostly localized along the pericapillary pathways, had a well-ramified network of GERs (Fig. 6). It is interesting that these cells contained quite a small number of mitochondria.

Stress-affected, morphine-treated rats. The perikaryon of most LPis was enlarged, as well as the processes, which blurred the picture of their polymorphism. It became very difficult to distinguish clearly the cells with a lucent from those with a more compact cytoplasm. The changes in the organization of these structures involved in elaborative processes were more pronounced than those in only stress-affected rats. In the majority of the cells, ribosomes flooded the whole area of the perikaryon and the processes. Within these ribosomal fields, well-dispersed short attenuated or vesicle-shaped GER tubuli were noticeable (Fig. 7). Very attractive was the finding of multilocular dissemination of the Golgi apparatuses in some cells abundantly interwoven with mitochondria but devoid of ribosomes (Fig. 8). It could not be precisely estimated if this was the matter

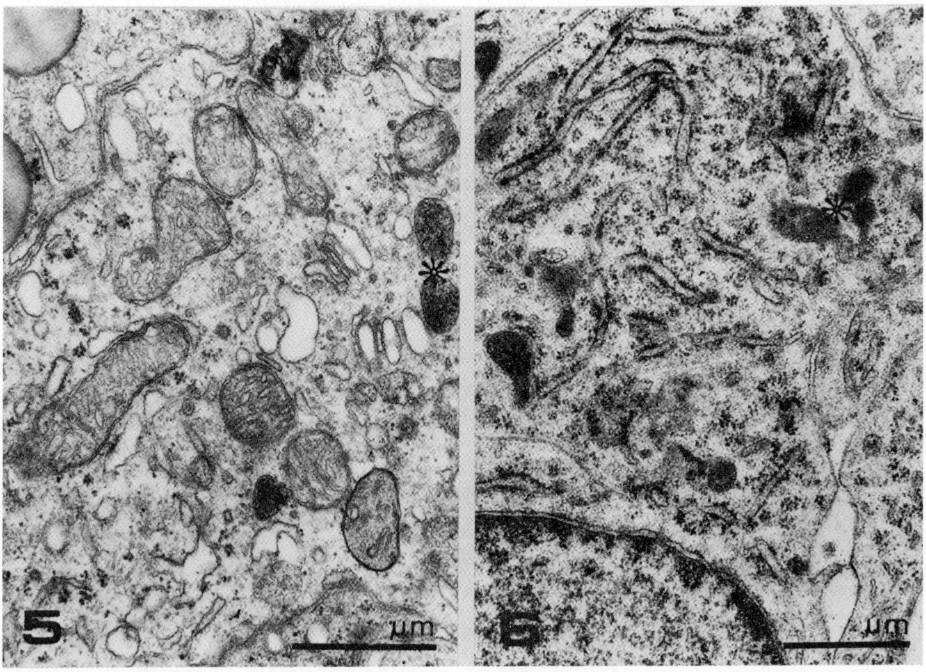

Fig. 5. Stress-affected rat, LPi. Cell sample interwoven with clear vesicular profiles. Prosecretory granules (asterisk)

Fig. 6. Stress-affected rat, DPi. Well-ramified network of GERs. Prosecretory granules (asterisk).

of a ribosomal field- or a Golgi field - dominated cell or of a local phenomenon within the same cell. In the ribosomal field, large structures with a highly condensed matrix, considered to be LDs in generation, were noticeable (Figs. 7 and 9). Their local accumulation, the herniation into the intercellular space and the occurrence of lamellar profiles pointed to their extrusion (Fig. 1o). The quantity of condensed mitochondria with a significantly enlarged outer cistern was enhanced. Some organelles developed lamellar changes. DPis possessed a well-ramified network of GER tubuli, prosecretory granules and a well-developed Golgi apparatus (Fig. 11).

Stress-affected, naloxone treated rats. The area of the perikaryon was nonuniformly and less populated by ribosomes; the presence of short attenuated and vesicle-shaped GER tubuli decreased as well. CVPs were missing. LPis varied in their appearance by the outlook of their mitochondria; while some of them were populated

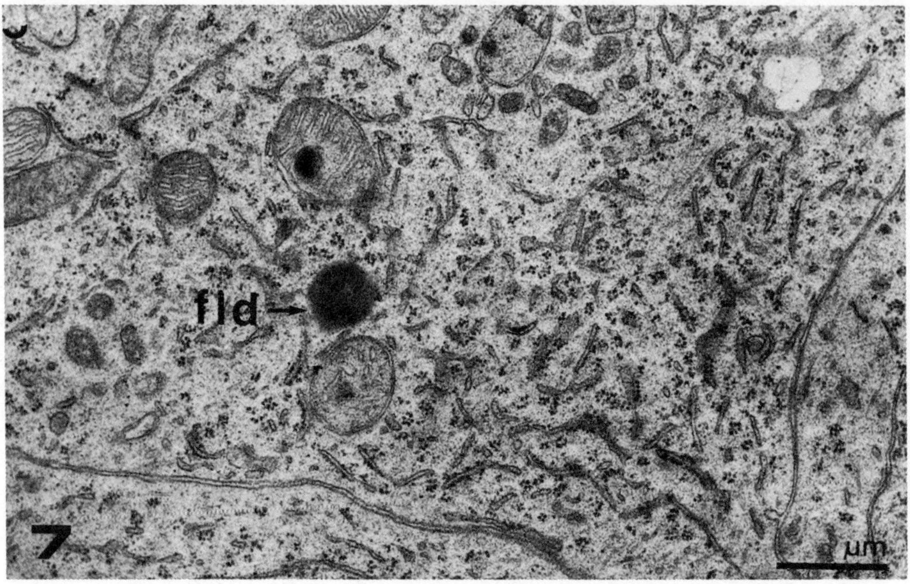

Fig. 7. Stress-affected, morphine-treated rat, LPi. Perikaryon flooded by ribosomes. Lipid droplet in the process of formation (fld).

mostly by usually condensed organelles, the others possessed swollen mitochondria (Fig. 12). The cells containing these mitochondria dominated. The Golgi apparatuses were unequal in size, mostly active. Some cells were characterized by lamellar changes of the Golgi cisterns (Fig. 13). LD accumulations were noticeable within the perikaryon and cell processes (Fig. 14). Their extrusion into the intercellular space was not found.

DPis were still marked by rich ramifications of GER tubuli. Rare mitochondria belonged to the swollen type. Some of them contained gigantic LDs (Fig. 15).

Dynamics of PRL Secretion

Pinealectomy in rats housed under controlled living conditions caused a significant decrease of PRL secretion (Table 1). In ISA-affected rats, the fourfold increase of the plasma quantity of PRL

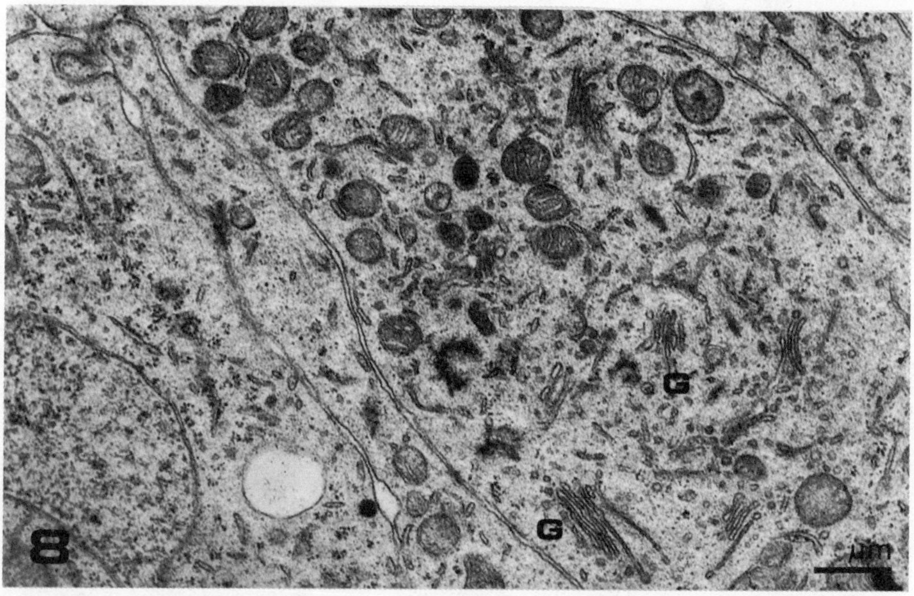

Fig. 8. Stress-affected, morphine-treated rat, LPi. Multilocularly disseminated Golgi apparatuses (G).

took place. In pinealectomized rats, an increase was also found, but it was smaller compared with pinealectomized stress-unaffected rats.

Naloxone injection caused a partial fall of PRL surge upon ISA. In pinealectomized rats, this OP blocker reversed the ISI surge of PRL but statistically insignificantly in comparison with pinealectomized stress-unaffected rats.

DISCUSSION

Morphodynamic Properties of PG Neuroendocrine Parenchyma

Functional evaluation of PG ultrastructural organization in stress-affected rats points to the animation of the elaborative activity of the majority of pinealocytes of both populations. The increase of the enzymic activity is only an additional criterion in the estimation of the increased PG functional turnover. The cytophysiological response to ISA by PG having been in the basal state

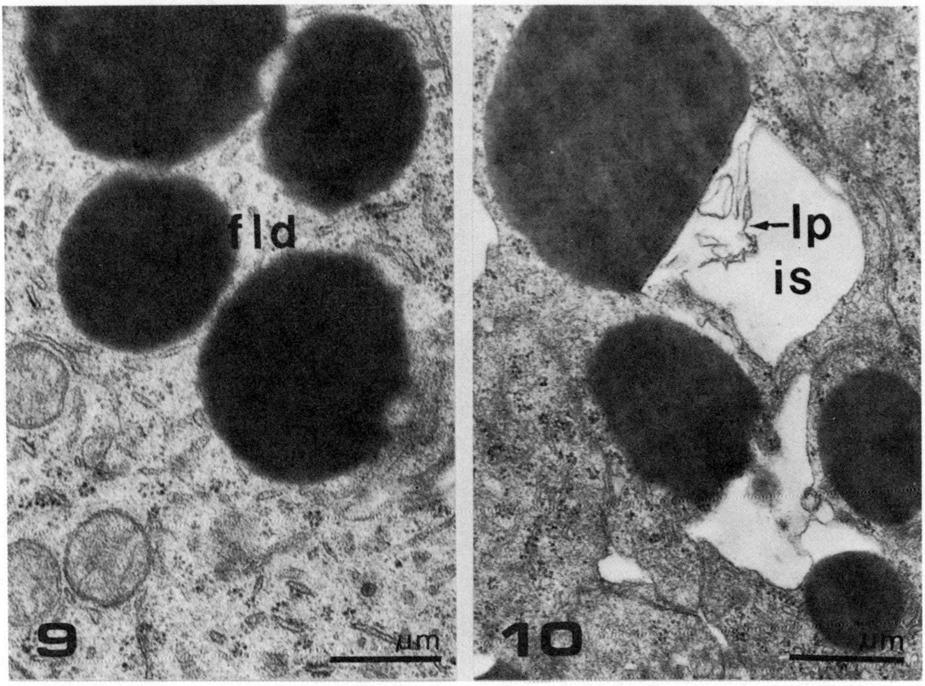

Figs. 9 and 10. Stress-affected, morphine-treated rat; accumulated newly-formed lipid droplets (fld), their herniation into intercellular space (is). Note the concomitant appearance of lamellar profiles (lp) due to the melting of lipid droplet content.

of activity, which took place within the period of time shorter than the studied one (5 min. after ISA),showed the existence of a prompt neuroendocrine outflow of the structures supposed to contain ACs, with the simultaneously initiated gradual disharmonous elaborative activity of both LPis and DPis. Its morphodynamic turnover after ISA application is so evident that two functional analogues of LPis could be distinguished: "dask" and "bright" cells /the latter ones being dominant/ (Milin et al., 1984). In comparison with these results, the present findings offer the evidence that in the time period studied most LPis are engaged in an intensified elaborative activity. The disappearance of LDs and the lack of their massive extrusion point out that the secretory burst is characteristic of

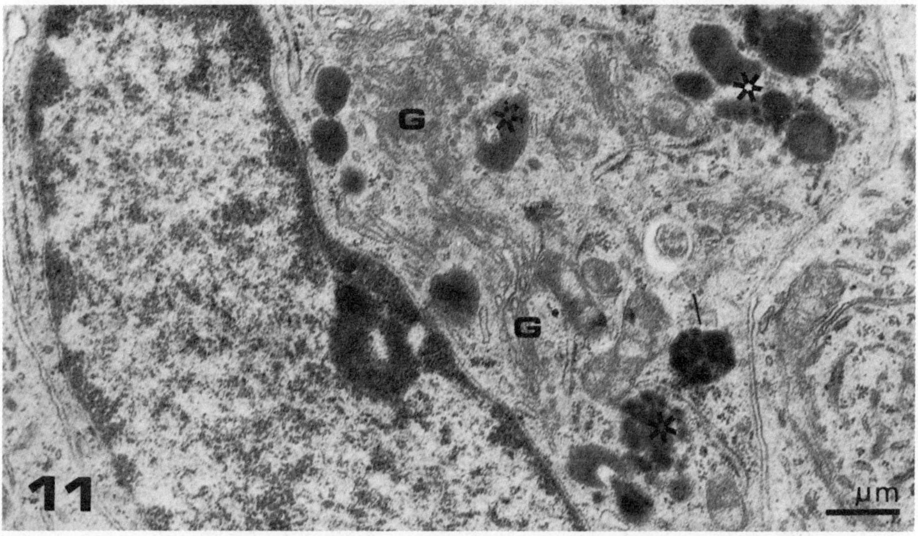

Fig. 11. Stress-affected, morphine-treated rat, DPi. Note well-distended Golgi apparatus (g). Prosecretory granules (asterisk).

the earlier period and that it is related to the very initiation of stress. At present, the data about the time of the equalization of the production and release of ACs after ISA are still not available.

The nonuniformity of the increase of the pinealocyte enzymic activity in the 10th min. after ISA, as well as in the 5th min., represents a further support to the idea of the gradual disharmonious promotion of pinealocytes to the higher level of activity. On the other hand, the relatively uniform occurrence of formazan precipitate in the case of morphine application points to the massive, synchronous and stimulative effect of this opiate on the intensification of PG activity. The difference in enzymic activity between stress-affected rats and those morphine-treated might be a consequence of the interfering effect of morphine upon the already noradrenaline-affected PG functional turnover (see later).

The accumulation of LDs (light microscopy), multilocular dispersion of Golgi apparatuses, enlargement of the ribosomal fields and the concomitant occurrence of LDs in the process of formation provide the evidence that morphine further facilitates PG elabora-

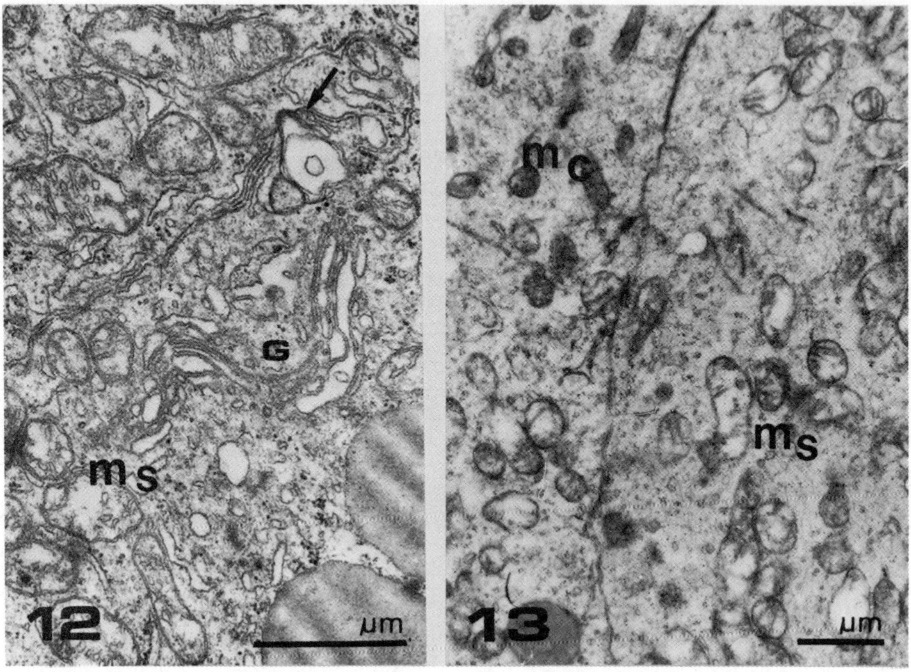

Fig. 12-13. Stress-affected, naloxone-treated rat, LPi. Cell processes populated by condensed (m_c) and swollen mitochondria (m_s). Focal lamellar degeneration of Golgi saccules (arrow) in cell dominated by swollen mitochondria.

tive activity. The finding of pinealocytes having LDs amassed along the cellular margin (light microscopy) and of suspectible LD extrusion (electron microscopy), indicated that morphine-stimulated elaborative activity of pinealocytes had its reflection on the increased AC discharge as well.

Without entering into the polemics whether the rat PG contains one or more pinealocyte populations, we can distinguish two morphologically different AC producing pathways: (i) GER-Golgi-vesicular profiles containing polypeptides and (ii) GER structures containing polypeptides (prosecretory granules). The latter is usually called the ependyme-like secretory process (Pevet, 1981). The observations of a stimulated PG show that the second alternative elaborative pathway may be really reconstructed as GER structures containing polypeptide structures classically recognized as LDs (Milin, 1982). The morphodynamic aspect of AC synthesis seems to be a complex matter

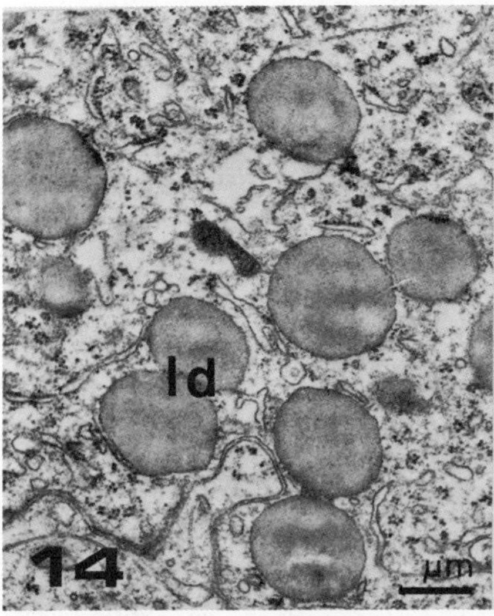

Fig. 14. Stress-affected, naloxone-treated rat, LPi. Accumulated lipid droplets (ld).

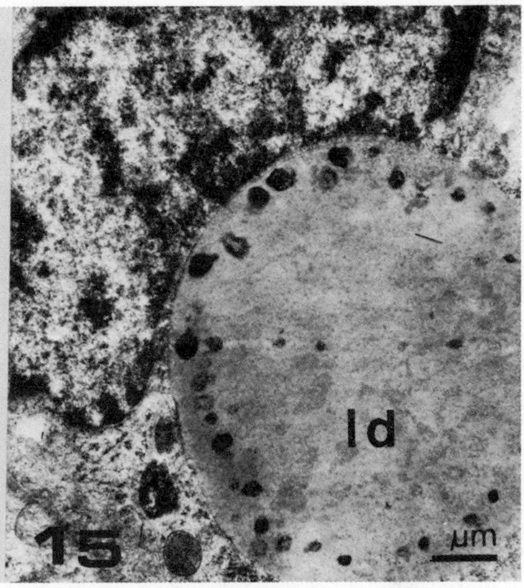

Fig. 15. Stress-affected, naloxone-treated rat, DPi. Cell sample containing gigantic lipid droplet (ld).

since it has been emphasized that melatonin is produced more likely within the cytoplasmatic matrix than inside some profiles belonging to the elaborative structural assemblage (Kappers, 1978; Pevet, 1981). Thus, one cannot rule out the possibility that certain quantity of CVPs represent autochthonous vesicles (non-GER and non-Golgi vesicles) containing this compound. The results obtained show that both elaborative pathways in pinealocytes are stimulated by ISA. Moreover, the opiate applied exerted more pronounced effect on both Golgi- and GER-dependent elaborative potential. This is fully consistent with the pharmacological evidence that OPs facilitate the melatonin and PG polypeptide production (Geffard et al., 1981; Schotman et al., 1981; Nir, 1984).

Naloxone administration caused a considerable decrease of the enzymic activity compared with stress-unaffected rats, but as well with other groups of rats. The lack of LDs being generated, the occurrence of abundant LDs in their usual appearance, but not the finding of their extrusion, indicated that augmented presence of

Table 1. Plasma prolactin levels

state of rat	prolactin, $\bar{x} \pm$ se, ng/ml non-operated	pinealectomized
stress-unaffected	25,91±1,8o[1]	16,52±1,57[2]
stress-affected	109,o5±16,o8[3]	33,28± 7,27[4]
stress-affected naloxone treated	69,54±11,56[5]	12,6o±2,86[6]

1-2 difference p<.ool; 3-4 difference p<.ool;

5-6 difference p<.ool; 1-3 difference p<.ool;

3-5 difference s.n.s.; 2-4 difference s.n.s.;

4-6 difference p<.o5; 2-6 difference s.n.s.

these organelles was rather the consequence of their drug-suppressed discharge than their increased production. Swollen mitochondria and the focal lamellar degeneration of Golgi saccules suggested that naloxone manifested itself not only in the suppression of LD discharge, but also in the alteration of the already impelled activity of the organelles belonging to the elaborative assemblage.

Summarizing, the results obtained substantiate the reliable morphodynamic evidence that OPs exert their stimulative effect, at least contributively, on pinealocyte secretory and elaborative activity at the very initiation of ISA.

Dynamics of Prolactin Secretion

The presence of several prolactinotropic ACs in PG, as well as the diminution of PRL secretion after pinealectomy in rats kept under controlled but non-stress-inducing microclimatic conditions (Relkin, 1972; Rønnenkleiv et al., 1973, 1978; Willoughby, 198o), lead to the conclusion that PG may have a tonic stimulative effect on PRL cell multitude under physiological living conditions. The present results, as well as some previously obtained ones, only confirm the above standpoint.

The increase of the plasma PRL content more than fourfold in initial stress-affected rats is corroborative of the already well-known prompt hormonal surge upon ISA (Euker et al., 1975; Terry et al., 1977), no matter whether it is ended or prolonged (Kawakami et al., 1979). In our case, in pinealectomized rats the ISI hormonal surge was of a slower rate. The occurrence of the prompt ISI neurosecretory discharge of PG being in the basal stage of activity (previous finding), as well as the difference in plasma hormonal content between non-operated and operated initial stress-affected rats (this study) point out that PRL surge in the case of ISA might be related, at least in part, to the action of PG ACs. The immediate but transitory PRL surge in animals affected by ISA or single injected some polypeptide compounds belonging to the AC pool of PG (Blask et al., 198o; Kato et al., 1978) testifies to this. Since melatonin causes somewhat later post-injection PRL release (Kamberi et al., 1971) which lasts longer (Lu et Meites, 1973), it is plausible to conclude that ISI PRL surge is mediated rather by polypeptide than indole compounds. However, an increased PRL release was also characteristic of pinealectomized rats affected by ISA, although to a less degree, which indicates that PG role in the generation of PRL surge is rather of a contributively amplifying character.

The absence of ISI burst of PRL in dexamethasone (Harms et al., 1975; Rossier et al., 198o) or naloxone pre-stress injected rats (Van Vugt et al., 1978; Ragavan and Frantz, 1981; Schin, 1978) points to the key role of OPs in the mediation of ISA demands to which PRL cells are exposed. According to some findings, beta-endorphin might be considered the most potent OP engaged in the regulation of PRL surge after ISA (Ragavan and Frantz, 1981; Nir, 1984). Having in mind that ACTH cells are the dominant source of beta endorphin (Watson et al., 1982), and that ISA causes a considerable fall in the pituitary content of this OP, without any significant changes in its brain content after ISA (Akil et al., 1982), we spontaneously come to the conclusion about the significance of ACTH cells in the supply of OP outflow caused by ISI demands.

In our case, in non-operated "handling" stress-affected rats only a partial suppression of PRL after ISA was found. However, since naloxone was injected after the animals had been weighed, i.e. at the moment of the initiation of the response of the organism to ISA, we may assume that the PRL rise, in comparison with stress-unaffected rats, corresponds to the amount of the hormonal release before the moment the action of the injected OP antagonists is manifested. Naloxone reversed the effect of ISA on PRL burst in pinealectomized rats, which did not happen in non-operated ones. This represents an additional support to the idea that PG modulates ISI PRL cell discharge.

The results obtained, on the whole, suggest that PG might be the "leader" in the mechanism involved in ISI surge of PRL, but only in support to OPs. The fact that naloxone prevented prolactinotropic action of polypeptides belonging to PG (Kato et al., 1978; Blask et al., 198o) corroborates the above statement. According to the evidence that OPs regulate the PRL secretion rather through the suprapituitary structures than directly through the hormone mother cells (Rivest et al., 1977; Grandison et al., 198o; Wardlaw et al., 198o), the present findings indicate that PG may be regarded as an alternative neuroendocrine pathway that mediates (amplifies?) the effect of OPs on the PRL cell multitude.

General outlook. The mechanism of OP effect on PG has not been fully explained as yet. The presence of OP receptor in PG has not been confirmed although it is evident that opiates and their derivates stimulate PG (this study and Geffard et al., 1981). Recent in vitro studies have indicated that beta-endorphin stimulative influence on pinealocytes may be beta-receptor mediated (Nir, 1984). However, with respect to the finding that OPs suppressed an increased nerve stimulation-evoked noradrenaline release (Illes, 1982) and the fact that ACTH reduced the cAMP response to noradrenaline (Kendall, 1982), we may assume that in response to ISA OPs have an inhibitory effect on PG besides a stimulative one. The great likelihood of an inhibitory OP effect on the animation of PG response is of an exceptional importance if we have in mind that the pinealocyte activity is predominantly noradrenaline mediated (Steinberg, 1981). Furthermore, there ensues the question whether the ISI surge of beta-endorphin from PG (Vuolteenaho et al., 1982) should be regarded as (i) an additional support to the regulation of ACTH secretion, (ii) a complementary influence of PG on the structures possessing opiate receptors, or (iii) a "brake" effect on noradrenaline-mediated promotion of pinealocytes to the level of high activity. The connection between stress-induced ACTH secretion and a decrease in beta-adrenergic receptors has been also signalized (Yocca and Friedman, 1984). The finding of a stimulative morphine effect on PG does not contradict with the discussion about the potential dual activity of OPs since the opiate applied also might act through its proper receptor side. Although we are still far from the thorough knowledge about the way OPs affect PG, we may, on the basis of the data discussed, suppose that the balanced OPs and the noradrenergic input keep PG, at least partly, in the basal state of activity, while both the outflow of OPs and noradrenaline evoke the neuroendocrine response of PG. In the case of oversecretion of OP generating structures, with the reflective consequence on the kinetics of OP-noradrenaline interactive action, an inhibitory effect of OPs on noradrenaline release might be manifested. It can be only hypothesized whether this process stabilizes the PG response to exteroceptive impulses in order to buffer the responsiveness of the organism to stress.

On the ground of the data that PG does not contain OP receptors and that naloxone stimulates ACTH release (Ježova et al., 1982), it is logical that naloxone-induced suppression of pinealocyte activity is due to drug-stimulated OP secretion or the consequence of its non-OP receptor-mediated action.

Pharmacological studies have shown that both serotonin and dopamine have their roles in PRL secretion: the former a stimulative, the latter an inhibitory one (Macleod and Lehmeyer, 1974; Collu et al., 1979). It was found that the serotoninergic activation was the more powerful stimulus to the release than the elimination of inhibitory dopaminergic influences (Krulich et al., 1981). Since PG stimulates the turnover of serotoninergic neurons and depresses the turnover of dopaminergic ones (Minneman and Wurtman, 1976), which is similar to opiate effects (Stampinato et al., 1979; van Loon et al., 198o; Enjalbert et al., 1979), the establishment of the PG-OP resultant influence on PRL cell multitude through the PG-OP interactive effect on the multisynaptic neuronal pathways may by no means be neglected.

In the light of the whole discussion, we can emphasize that PG and OP producing structures, from the aspect of their regulative prerogatives, may be only conditionally considered separate variables involved in the ISI PRL cell discharge since PG could be regarded as an alternative neuroendocrine pathway which mediates, at leat in part, the OP effect upon their targets. At the same time, there is no ground for the polemics whether the PG-OP functional link is established through the multisynaptic neuronal pathway as well, with the resultant reflection on the PRL release. Moreover, there still remains to elucidate whether the synchronous interaction between the neuroendocrine and neuronal pathways occurs already at the very beginning of ISA or at a later time some of the two begins to dominate. Finally, it seems reasonable to suppose that by the establishment of the PG-OP functional link, i.e. by the interaction of extero- and interoceptive inputs the overall neuroendocrine and behavioural activities in the organism coping with stress are brought into harmony.

Discussion

LENGUAR: What is a route through which the pineal receives the information of stress?

J. MILIN: Noradrenergic axons arising from the superior cervical ganglia constitute the major part of the PG functional innervation. The existence of the central epithalamo-pineal nerve connection has been verified both morphologically and electrophysiologically, but the neurotransmitter nature of these nerve terminals still has to be elucidated. PG is also an extra blood-brain barrier organ. Hence, it is indisputable that the neural (intraglandular nerve terminals) and humoral (adrenal medulla elaborated) noradrenaline mediates stress-inducing inputs. We are still in the dark about the brain structures involved in the polysynaptic connection between the receptory loci and the superior cervical ganglia. The exception is the retino-pineal tract. Since the superior cervical ganglia are the "final integrative point" of pinealotropic neurons, it is hardly doubtable that individual parts of the retino-pineal tract, primarily the brain stem and spinal cord projections, represent the common neural pathways to other receptor locus-pineal tracts. At the same time, taking into consideration the turnover of the OP producing structures upon ISA, the possibility of an at least contributive engagement of OPs in the generation of PG functional response can by no means be excluded. This is, after all, substantiated by the results of our investigation as well.

LIPOSITS: Have you seen any changes in the number of synaptic ribbons of pinealocytes under stressful conditions?

J. MILIN: The frequent occurrence of synaptic ribbons was noticed in the 5th min. after the animals had been exposed to "handling" stress. This initial increase in synaptic ribbons was not found in the 10th min., when these structures occurred, indeed, very rarely. The initial increase is in accord with the correlation of their occurrence and the noradrenergic turnover. The subsequent decrease in the occurrence of synaptic ribbons is confusing, and is probably due to their instanteous structural disintegration after the transmission of still an enigmatic mediator, naturally if the concept of synaptic ribbons as activating structures is applied. At the same time, we can also take into account the possibility that the ISI surge of OPs may somehow suppress their occurrence. This is indicated by the fact that they occur very rarely in morphine-treated animals.

LIPOSITS: Several neuropeptides have been detected in the pineal gland by RIA, but their presence has not been confirmed by immunocytochemical methods. Could you comment on this discrepancy and have you any data on the origin of these peptides?

J. MILIN: In our previous exposition we mentioned that it was still unclear whether all the polypeptide ACs hitherto isolated from PG were generated in pinealocytes or a number of them were synthetized in other organs and only stored in pinealocytes. The structures containing polypeptide ACs are also still unclarified. In one of our earlier studies we set forth the hypothesis that the organelles classically called LPs really represented "lipidized" structures containing polypeptide ACs. If this concept is plausible, polypeptide ACs could rather exist in the form of a complex molecule (lipoprotein?) than as an integral or cleaved chain. Thus, the antibodies used cannot react with the "masked" polypeptides and hence the failure of the application of immunocytochemical methods.

RAKIĆ: Chronobiology and stressful effects on PG?

J. MILIN: In mammals, the suprachiasmatic nuclei and PG are advocated to be of the major importance in the synchronization of the homeostasis of the organism to environmental inputs, at least photoreceptive ones. It is well known that PG, unlike suprachiasmatic nuclei, does not possess endogenous rhythmicity. Moreover, pinealectomy does not abolish the functional dynamics of suprachiasmatic nuclei, as well as the persistence of the circadian rhythm of some hormone producing cells. Accordingly, PG in a way multiplies the impulses being generated in its superior pacemaker structure in the process of the mediation of circadian and/or circannual photic impulses. Since the function of pinealocytes depends on other environmental impulses as well, it is unquestionable that certain structures in polysynaptic receptor-pineal gland tracts have analytic-integrative properties. It is very interesting that PG, important though it is for the mediation of environmental effects on homeostasis, does not represent an essential organ from the standpoint of chronobiology, at least under physiological living conditions. Ample evidence has demonstrated the morphodynamic turnover of PG in stressed animals. Acute stress disturbs the rhythmicity of the basal activity of pinealocytes. However, it is unclarified whether under chronic stress, when pinealocytes are promoted to the new steady state, any essential disturbance of this rhythmicity of AC synthesis takes place. It is also unclear if stress causes rhythmical disharmony of impulses arising from suprachiasmatic nuclei. At any rate, the progressive changes in PG histophysiology reflected in the changes of the morphodynamics of its target structures show that this brain structure plays an important role in the adaptation of the organism to stressful living conditions. This benefitial influence of PG is manifested primarily in the suppresion of the activity of some functional systems that are not essentially important for survival (reproductive system, but not gravidity) on the occasion of the generalization of an antistressogenic response.

REFERENCES

Akil, H., Shiomi, H., Walker, M., and Watson, S. J., 1982, Characterization of multiple forms of beta-endorphin in pituitary and brain: effect of stress, in: "Regulatory Peptides from Molecular Biology to Function", E. Costa and M. Trabucchi, eds., Raven Press, New York, pp. 61-68.

Arstila, A. U., 1967, Electron microscopic studies on the structure and histochemistry of the pineal gland of the rat, Neuro-endocrin., 2: Suppl. 1.

Barka, T. and Anderson, P. J., 1965, "Histochemistry", Hoeber and Row Publ. Inc., New York.

Blask, D. E., Vaughan, M. K., Reiter, R. J., Johnson, L. Y., and Vaughan, G. M., 1976, Prolactin-releasing and release-inhibiting factor activities in the bovine, rat, and human pineal gland: in vitro and in vivo studies, Endocrinology, 29:152.

Blask, D. E. and Vaughan, M. K., 198o, Naloxone inhibits arginine vasotocin- (AVT) induced prolactin release in urethane-anesthetized male rats in vivo, Neurosci. Lett., 18:181.

Collu, R., de Ruisseau, P., and Taché, Y., 1979, Role of putative neurotransmitters in prolactin, GH and LH response to acute immobilization stress in male rats, Neuroendocrin., 28:178.

Dacheaux, F., 1981, Ultrastructural localization of corticotropin, beta-lipotropin, and alfa- and beta-endorphin in the porcine anterior pituitary, Cell Tiss. Res., 215:87.

Devečerski, V., 1965, "Histofiziološke odlike nadbubrežne žlezde nakon epifizektomije", doktorska disertacija ("Histophysiological characteristics of the adrenal gland after epiphysectomy", doctoral dissertation), Novi Sad.

Dogteron, J., Snijdewint, F. G. M., Pevet, P., and Buijs, R. M., 1979, On the presence of neuropeptides in the mammalian pineal gland and subcommissural organ, Progress in Brain Res., 52:465.

Enjalbert, A., Ruberg, M., Arancibia, S., Priam, M., and Kordon, C., 1979, Endogenous opiates block dopamine inhibition of prolactin secretion in vitro, Nature, 28o:595.

Euker, J. S., Meites, J., and Riegle, G. D., 1975, Effects of acute stress on serum LH and prolactin in intact, castrated and dexamethasone-treated male rats, Endocrinology, 96:85.

Geffard, M., Gaffori, O., Chauveau, J., Muyard, J. P., and Le Moal, M., 1981, Dramatic increase in pineal melatonin levels in the rat after subcutaneous injection of Des-tyrosine-gamma-endorphin, Neurosci. Lett., 27:329.

Grandison, L., Fratta, W., and Guidotti, A., 198o, Location and characterization of opiate receptors regulating pituitary secretion, Life Sci., 26:1633.

Gromova, E. A., Kravs, M., and Krecek, J., 1967, Effect of melatonin and 5-hydroxytryptamine on aldosterone and corticosterone production by adrenal glands of normal and hypophysectomized rats. J. Endocrin., 39:345.

Guillemin, R., Vargo, T., Rossier, J., Minick, S., Ling, N., River, O., Vale, W., and Bloom, F., Beta-endorphin and adrenocorticotropin are secreted concomitantly by the pituitary gland, Science, 1977, 197:1367.

Harms, P. G., Langlier, P., and McCann, S. M., 1975, Modification of stress-induced prolactin release by dexamethasone or adrenalectomy, Endocrinology, 96:475.

Illes, P., 1982, The mechanism of action of opiates in regulating noradrenaline release, in: "Regulatory Peptides from Molecular Biology to Function", E. Costa and M. Trabucchi, eds., Raven Press, New York, pp. 347-352.

Ježova, D., Vigaš, M., and Jurčovičova, J., 1982, ACTH and corticosterone response to naloxone and morphine in normal, hypophysectomized and dexamethasone-treated rats, Life Sci., 31:3o7.

Kamberi, I. A., Mical., R. S., and Porter, J. C., 1971, Effects of melatonin and serotonin on the release of FSH and prolactin, Endocrinology, 88:1288.

Kappers, J. A., 196o, The development, topographical relations and innervation of the epiphysis cerebri in the albino rat, Z. Zellforsch., 52:163.

Kato, Y., Iwasaki, Y., Iwasaki, J., Abe, H., Yanaihara, N., and Imura, H., 1978, Prolactin release by vasoactive intestinal polypeptide in rats, Endocrinology, 1o3:554.

Kavaliers, M., 1982, Pineal mediation of the thermoregulatory and behavioral activating effects of beta-endorphin, Peptides, 3:679.

Kawakami, M., Higuchi, T., Matsuura, M., 1979, Immobilization stress and prolactin secretion in male rats. Neuroendocrin., 29:262.

Kendall, D. A., Duman, R., Slopis, J., and Enna, S. J., 1982, Influence of adrenocorticotropin hormone and yohimbine on antidepressant-induced declines in rat brain neurotransmitter receptor binding and function. J. Pharmacol. Exp. Ther., 222:566.

Krulich, L., MsCann, S. M., and Mayfield, M. A., 1981, On the mode of the prolactin release-inhibiting action of the serotonin receptor blockers metergoline, methysergide, and cyproheptadine, Endocrinology, 1o8:1115.

Kumar, M. S. A., Chen, C. L., Sharp, D. C., Liu, J. M., Kalpa, P. S., and Kalpa, S. P., 1982, Diurnal fluctuations in methionine-enkephalin levels in the hypothalamus and preoptic area of the male rat: effects of pinealectomy, Neuroendocrin., 35:28.

Lakin, M., Miller, C. H., Scott, M. L., and Winter, W. D., 1981, Involvement of the pineal gland and melatonin in murine analgesia. Life Sci., 29:2543.

Levy, R. M., Mefford, I. N., Watson S., Akil, H., and Barchas, J.D., The effect of acute administration of morphine and opiate antagonists on the indole content of the rat pineal gland, in: "Endogenous and exogenous opiate agonists and antagonists", E. L. Way, ed., Pergamon Press, New York, 198o.

van Loon, G. R., Ho, D., Kim, C., 198o, Beta- endorphin-induced decrease in hypothalamic dopamine turnover, Endocrin., 1o6:76.

Lowenstein, P. R., Pereyra, E. N., Solveyra, C. G., and Cardinali, D. P., Effect of naloxone on the nocturnal rise of rat pineal melatonin content, Europ. J. Pharmacol., 98:261, 1984.

Lu, R. H. and Meites, J., 1973, Effects of serotonin precursors and melatonin on serum prolactin release in rats. Endocrinology, 93:152.

Macleod, R. M. and Lehmeyer, J. E., 1974, Studies on the mechanism of the dopamine-mediated inhibition of prolactin secretion, Endocrinology, 94:1o77.

Milin, J., 1982, Ultrastructural characteristics of proteinergic synthesis in the pineal gland, in: "Hormonally Active Brain Peptides", K. W. McKerns and V. Pantić, eds., Plenum Press, New York, pp. 445-466.

Milin, J. and Rakić, M., Histophysiology of the zona reticularis of the adrenal gland in gravid rats affected by noise: role of the pineal gland, Third Congress of Yugoslav Endocrinologists, Novi Sad, 31 May - 2 June 1984, Abstract.

Milin, J., Martinović, J., and Demajo, M., 1984, Morphodynamic response of the pineal gland to initial stress attack, Arch. Anat. micr. Morph. exp. (still going through press).

Miline, R., Krstić, R., and Devečerski, V., 1968, Sur le comportement de la glande pineale dans des conditions de stress, Acta Anat., 71:352.

Miline, R., 198o, The role of the pineal gland in stress, J. Neural Transmiss., 47:191.

Minneman, K. P. and Wurtman R. J., 1976, The pharmacology of the pineal gland, Ann. Med. Pharm., 16:33.

Motta, M., Schiaffini, O., Piva, F., and Martini, L., Pineal principles and the control of adrenocorticotropin secretion, in: "The Pineal Gland", G. E. W. Wolstenholme and J.Knight, eds., Churchill Livingstone, London, 1971, pp. 279-29o.

Nir, I., Can enkephalins be playing a role in pineal function? Third Colloquium of the European Pineal Study Group, Pécs, 1984, Abstracts, pp. 38.

Padmanabhan, V., Convey, E.M., Tucker, H. A., 1979, Pineal compounds after prolactin release from bovine pituitary cells, Proc. Soc. Exp. Biol. Med., 6o:34o.

Pavel, S., 1979, The mechanism of action of vasotocin in the mammalian brain, Prog. Brain Res., 52:445.

Pevet, P., 1981, Ultrastructure of the mammalian pinealocyte, in: "The Pineal Gland", Vol. I, R. S. Reiter, ed., CRC Press, Inc., Boca Raton, Florida.

Piva, F., Schiaffini, O., Mottta, M., and Martini, L., 1973, The role of pineal principles in the control of ACTH secretion, in: "Hormones and Brain Function", K. Lissak, ed., Plenum Press, New York, pp. 231-236.

Ragavan, V. V. and Frantz, A. G., 1981, Opioid regulation of prolactin secretion: evidence for a specific role of beta-endorphin, Endocrinology, 1o9:1769.

Relkin, R., 1972, Rat pituitary and plasma prolactin levels after pinealectomy, J. Endocrinol., 53:179.

Rivest, R. W., Roberts, K. D., and Lepore, F., 1979., The pineal gland and stress: effect of pineal stalk section on the plasma corticosteroid response to cold in rabbits, Psychol. Rep., 44:883.

Romijn, H. J., 1978, The pineal, a tranquillizing organ, Life Sci., 23:2257.

Rønnenkleiv, O. K., Krulich, L., and McCann, S. M., 1973, An early morning surge of prolactin in the male rat and its abolition by pinealectomy, Endocrinology, 92:1339.

Rønnenkleiv, O. K., Krulich, L., and McCann, S. M., 1978, The effect of pinealectomy on the pattern of prolactin secretion in conscious freely moving male rats, Neuroendocrinology, 27:279.

Rossier, J., French, E., Rivier, C., Shibasaki, T., Guillemin, R., Bloom F. E., 198o, Stress-induced release of prolactin blockade by dexamethasone and naloxone may indicate beta-endorphin mediation, Proc. Natl. Acad. Sci. USA, 77:666.

Rowe, V., Neale, E. A., Avins, L., Guroff, G., and Schrier, B. K., 1977., Pineal gland cells in culture. Morphology, biochemistry, differentiation, and co-culture with symphatetic neurons, Exp. Cell Res., 1o4:356.

Saland, L. C., Ortiz, E., and Munger, A. T., 1982, Effect of acute opiate-peptide administration on pro-opiomelanocortin cells of the intermediate lobe of the rat pituitary, Cell Tiss. Res., 225:217.

Shin, S. H., 198o, Blockade of the ether-induced surge of prolactin by naloxone in male rats, J. Endocrinol., 79:397.

Schotman, P., Allart, J., and Gispen, W. H., 1981, Pineal protein synthesis highly sensitive to ACTH-like neuropeptides, Brain Res., 219:121.

Schwyzer, R., 1982, Peptides and the new endocrinology, Naturwissenschaften, 69:15.

de Souza, E. B. and van Loon, G. R., 1982, Stress-induced inhibition of the plasma corticosterone response to a subsequent stress in rats: a non-adrenocorticotropic-mediated mechanism, Endocrinology, 11o:23.

Stampinato, S., Locatelli, V., Cocchi, D., Vincentini, L., Bajusz, S., Ferri, S., and Müller, E. E., 1979, Involvement of brain serotonin in the prolactin-releasing effect of opioid peptides, Endocrinology, 1o5:163.

Steinberg, V., Rome, V., Watanabe, I., and Parr, J., 1981, Effects of norepinephrine and dibutyryl adenosine 3', 5'-cyclic monophosphate on the ultrastructure of pineal cells in monolayer culture, Cell Tiss. Res., 216:181.

Šćepović, M., 1963, Korelativna histofiziologija epitalamo-epifiznog kompleksa nadbubrega, habilitacioni rad, Sarajevo (Correlative histophysiology of the adrenal epithalamo-epiphyseal complex, habilitation thesis).

Terry, L. C., Saunders, A., Audet, J., Willoughby, J. O., Brazeau, P., and Martin, J. B., 1977, Physiologic secretion of growth hormone and prolactin in male and female rats, Clin. Endocrinol., 6:19s.

Vaughan, M. K., Vaughan, G. M., Reiter, R. J., and Benson, B., 1972, Effect of melatonin and other pineal indoles on adrenal enlargement produced in male and female mice by pinealectomy, uni-lateral adrenalectomy, castration and cold stress, Neuroendocrinology, 1o:139.

van Vught, D. A., Bruni, J. F., and Meites, J., 1978, Naloxone inhibition of stress-induced increase in prolactin secretion, Life Sci., 22:85.

Vuolteenaho, O., Leppäluoto, J., and Männistö, P., 1982, Effect of stress and dexamethasone on immunoreactive beta-endorphin levels in rat hypothalamus and pineal, Acta Physiol. Scand., 114:537.

Wardlaw, S. L., Wehrenberg, W. B., Ferin, M., and Frantz, A. G., 198o, Failure of beta-endorphin to stimulate prolactin release in the pituitary stalk-sectioned monkey, Endocrinology, 1o7: 1663.

Watson, S. J., Akil, H., and Barchas, J. D., 1979, Immunohistochemical and biochemical studies of the enkephalins, beta-endorphin, and related peptides, in: "Endorphins in Mental Health Research", E. Usdin, W. E. Bunney, Jr. and N. S. Kline, eds., Macmillan Press, London.

White, W. F., Hedlund, M. T., Weber, G. F., Rippel, R. H., Johnson, E. S., and Wilber, J. F., 1974, The pineal gland: a supplemental source of hypothalamic-releasing hormones, Endocrinology, 94:1422.

Willoughby, J. O., 198o, Pinealectomy mildly disturbes the secretory patterns of prolactin and growth hormone in the unstressed rats, J. Endocrinol., 86:1o1.

Wolfe, D. E., 1965, The epiphyseal cell: an electron-microscopic study of its intercellular relationship and intracellular morphology in the pineal body of the albino rat, Prog. Brain Res., 1o:332.

Yocca, F. D., and Friedman, E., 1984, Effect of immobilization stress on rat pineal beta-adrenergic receptor-mediated function, J. Neurochemistry, 42:1427.

Zugibe, F. T., 197o,"Diagnostic Histochemistry", C. V. Mosby Comp., Saint Louis

EFFECT OF CONSTANT LIGHT AND DARKNESS ON THE DEEP PINEAL OF THE RAT

M. Kecman[1], Lj. Somer[1], M. Matavulj[2]

Dept. of Histol. and Embryol., Fac. of Med.[1]; Inst. of Biol., Fac. of Nat. Scis. and Math.[2], Univ. of Novi Sad Novi Sad, Yugoslavia

INTRODUCTION

Anatomically viewed, the pineal organ of the rat is composed of the superficial pineal, the stalk, and the deep pineal s. lamina intercalaris (Kappers, 1960; Volrath, 1979). The deep pineal represents about 3% of the pineal complex. It lies between the posterior and the habenular commissures, being in the close contact with the third ventricle. Boeckmann (1980) found the identity of pinealocytes of the pineal complex. The innervation of the pineal complex is mainly autonomic (symphatetic, arising from the ganglion cervicale superior and reaching the pineal via nervi conarii), but the commissural and peptidergic fibres, whose origin is still to be elucidated in detail, are also present. Vasopressin and oxitocin fibres are evident in the deep pineal of the rat (Buijs and Pevet, 1980).

The physiological role of the pineal gland still remains to be clarified. As postulated by Miline (1969), the pineal is a sensoneuroendocrine organ. It was reported (Relkin, 1982) that the pineal was affected by light, darkness, noise, heat, olfactory stimuli, magnetic field and affective disturbances. The evidence that the main role of the pineal gland is to mediate light stimuli to the neuroendocrine system (Oksche, 1984) has been increasing. The opposite influence of the light and darkness on the physiology of the pineal, i.e. light - inhibitive, and darkness - stimulative, is well documented by a number of data (Miline, 1957; Rotu et al., 1962; Quay, 1963; Klein and Weller, 1972; Ilnerova et al., 1978, 1982; Levy, 1982).

Despite the structural identity of the cells of the pineal complex, possible dissimilarities in the function between the superficial and deep pineal have been reported (Pevet, 1982). The effects of superficial pinealectomy on the morphometric properties of the deep pineal hitherto reported (Legait, 1979; Heidbuchel and Volrath, 1983; Kecman et al., 1984) are also partly divergent.

The aim of this investigation was to shed more light on the functional and morphological properties of the deep pineal of the rat under two opposite physiological conditions, i.e. constant light and constant darkness, potentiated by the surgical removal of the superficial pineal gland.

MATERIAL AND METHODS

The experiment was performed on male Wistar rats weighing 18o-22o gr. each. Food and water were given ad lib. Experimental animals were divided in two groups consisting of six animals each: 1. intact rats, 2. superficially pinealectomized rats. The total of 12 animals were kept under constant darkness for six weeks. The same number of rats were kept under constant light (12o lux, measured at the bottom of the cage) also for six weeks. The corresponding control group (the total of 1o animals) was housed under natural lighting conditions. The experiment was performed in the period of September-October 1981. Superficial pinealectomy was carried out after Pende-Barbarosa and modified by Šćepović (1963). The animals were decapitated between 9 and 11 a.m. The fixation in Bouin's fluid for 3 weeks was followed by the embedding in paraffin. The serial sections of the whole brain (5 m) in sagital and frontal planes were stained according to Florentin, Gömori-Bargmann and McConail. Stereological methods were used, viz. volume density (Vv) and numerical density (Nv) (Weibel, 1979). We used Weibel's grid M-42. 33 fields per deep pineal were measured under the magnification (1ooo x). The statistical analysis (student T test) was used.

RESULTS

Effects of light. The general appearance of the deep pineal gland region in intact rats under natural lighting conditions is shown in the Fig.1a. The pattern of the pinealocyte distribution is similar to that in the superficial pineal. Superficial pinealectomy leads to an increase of volume (Vv) and numerical (Nv) density, as it is visible in the Hist. 1 and Fig.1b; there are no apparent changes in the relative number of dark pinealocytes.

Constant light did not affect the significative differences in Vv and Nv of the deep pineal in intact rats but in the superficially pinealectomized rats it abolished the significant increase of the same parameters (Hist. 1 and Fig. 2) that occurred under natural

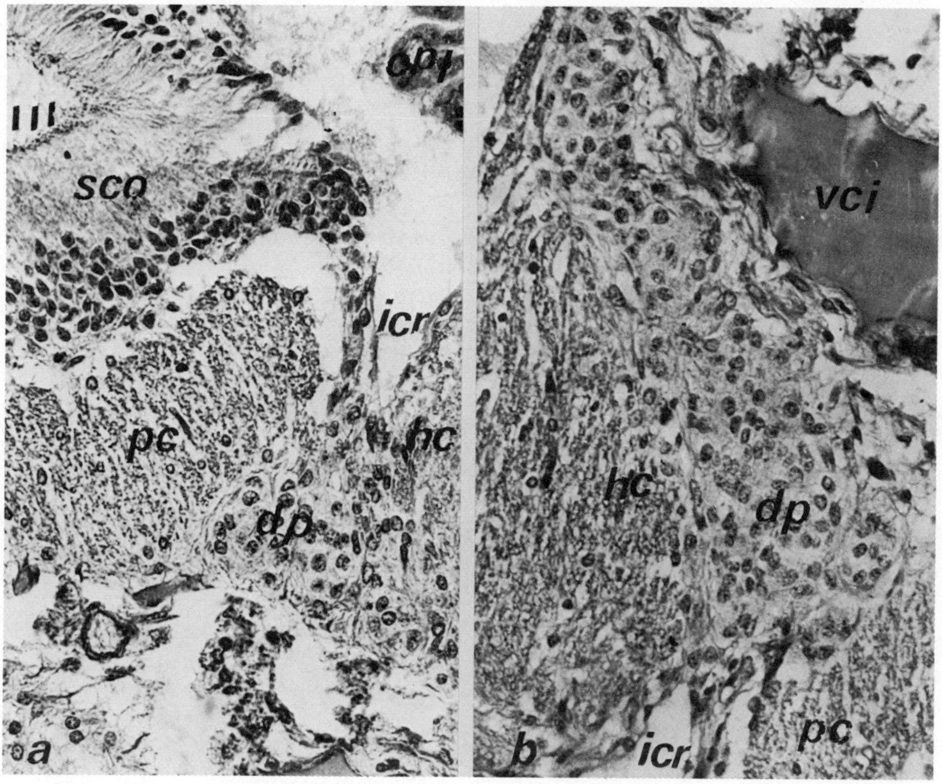

Fig. 1. (a) Region of the deep pineal. Intact rat under natural lighting conditions. Col. Gömori-Bargmann, x 25o. DP - deep pineal; SCO - subcommissural organ; PC - commissura posterior; HC - habenular commissure; ICR - intercommissural recess; III - third ventricle; CPl - chorioid plexus; VCI - vena cerebri interna. (b) Region of the deep pineal. Superficially pinealectomized rat under natural lighting conditions. Col. Gömori-Bargmann, x 25o.

lighting.

Histological analysis of the deep pineal of the superficially pinealectomized rats under constant light revealed that the majority of pinealocytes had the signs of a reduced activity (smaller nuclei and less prominent nucleoli), but there were the cells distributed individually or in small groups with the signs of full activity (Fig. 3a).

Effects of darkness. Under the influence of constant darkness, hyperplasia of the pinealocytes of the deep pineal takes place both

Hist. 1. Deep pineal of the rat. Effect of constant light

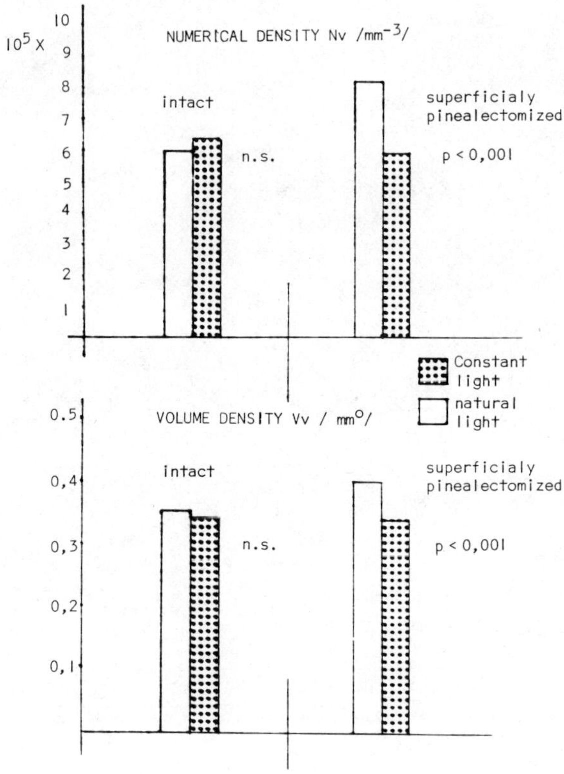

in intact and superficially pinealectomized rats (Hist. 2, Fig. 3b). The increase of Vv and Nv is statistically significant. In the frontal sections of the deep pineal stained after Gömori-Bargmann few neurosecretory fibres on the lateral sides were found (Fig. 3c). Increased chromophilia of pinealocytes was prominent.

DISCUSSION

The results obtained point to the enhancement of the deep pineal activity under the influence of constant darkness and to the decline of the activity under the influence of constant light. This is in agreement with the well-known data about an inhibitive effect of light and a stimulative effect of darkness on the superficial pineal. Therefore, the results obtained indicate a possible concomitant activity of the superficial and deep pineal under different lighting

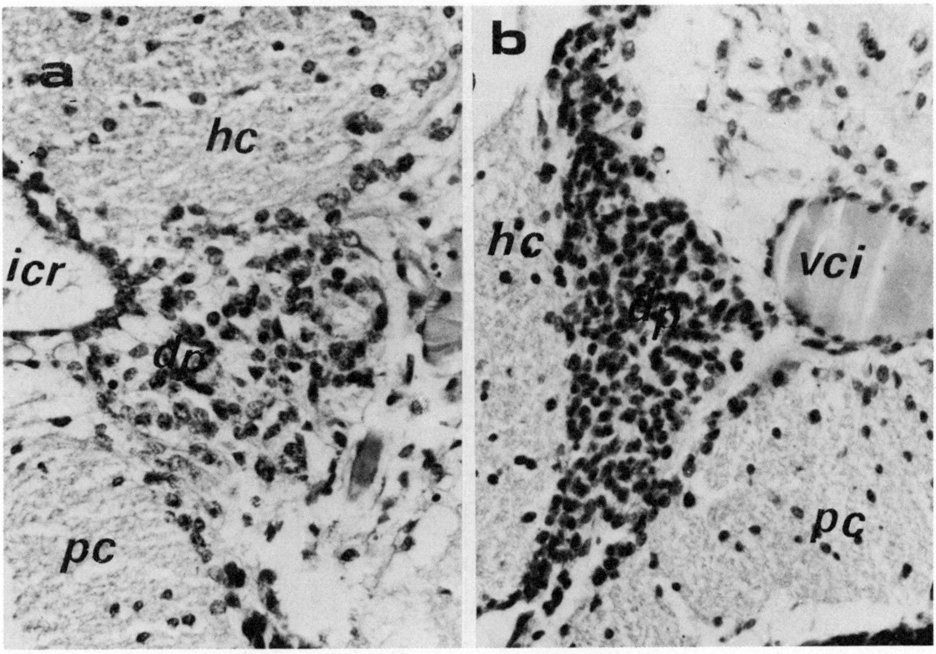

Fig. 2. Region of the deep pineal. Superficially pinealectomized rats. (a) Under constant light. (b) Under constant darkness. Col. Gömori-Bargmann, x 25o. Abbr. under Fig. 1.

conditions. It is likely that the pineal organ reacts as a unit to lighting stimuli. Phylogenetically, the pineal gland of mammals is derived from an ancestral photic receptor, the third eye of amphibians and reptiles. It has been reported about receptor-like cells in the neonatal rat pineal (Clabough, 1973). Melatonin level and N-AT activity are significantly linked to day-night and general light-darkness schedule. All these data strongly suggest that the pineal mainly functions as a mediator (transducer) of light effects.

The possibility that pinealocytes of the superficial pineal differ in some aspects from the cells of the deep pineal was reported by several authors: Wiklund (1974) - differences in serotonin content; Moore (1975) - differences in N-AT and HIOMT activities after sympathectomy and continuous lighting; Vollrath (1981) - differences in the circadian nuclear size changes and possible dissimilarities in the function after osmotic stress. These findings seem to be partly in contrast with our findings. Our sharply divergent experimental conditions are in the main line of the pineal function

Hist. 2. The deep pineal of the rat. Effect of constant darkness

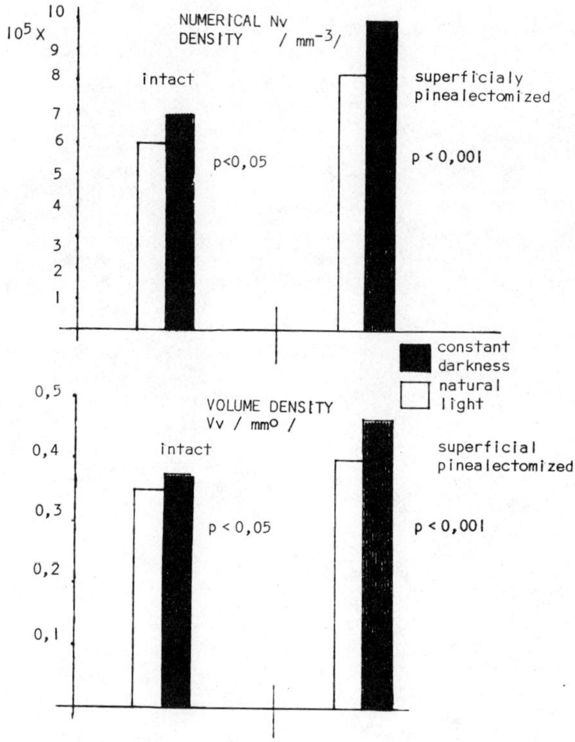

(mediation of light effects), and in connection with the close feedback relationship between the pineal organ and the hypothalamic-pituitary system and other endocrine glands, they could serve as a ground for the explanation of this dissimilarity.

Stereological parameters, numerical (Nv) and volume (Vv) density, when enhanced, indicate, as it is generally assumed, an increased tissue activity and vice versa. Our results are in keeping with the established data about the deep pineal structure. It is difficult to compare different parameters, i.e. Nv and Vv, with the most frequently used histological quantification parameter: nuclear diameter or size. Legait (1979) and Heidbüchel and Vollrath (1983) reported opposite results about the effects of superficial

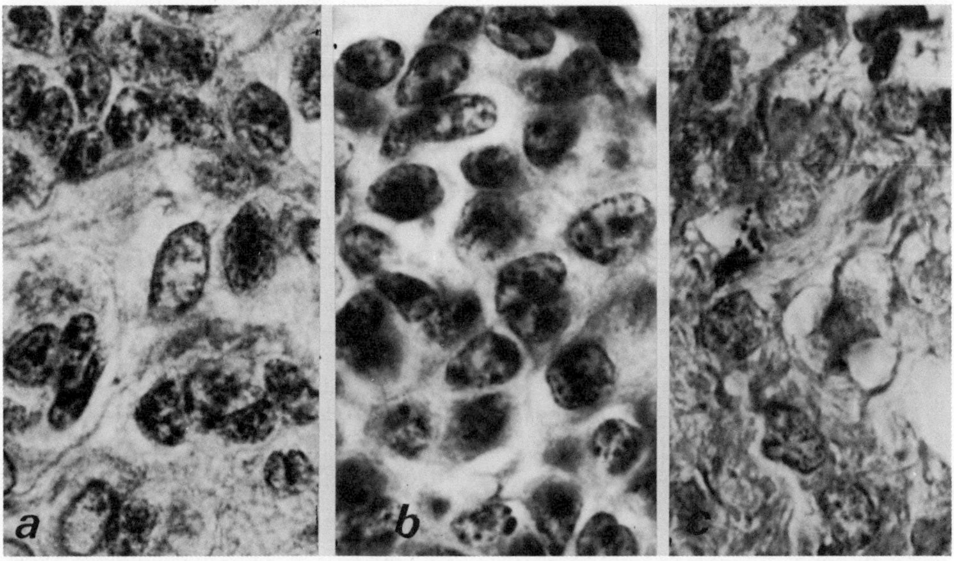

Fig. 3. Deep pineal of superficially pinealectomized rats. (a) Under constant light. (b) Under constant darkness. (c) Under constant darkness - presence of Gömori-positive fibres. Col. Gömori-Bargmann. x 25o.

pinealectomy on the nuclear size of the cells of the deep pineal in the hamster and the rat. Our previous findings (Kecman et al., 1984) of hyperplasia of the deep pineal cells after superficial pinealectomy correspond to the above mentioned results of Legait and are reconfirmed by the present experiments. Keeping in mind the individual diversity of the deep pineal volume and the number of the animals, we did not measure the total volume of the deep pineal.

The innervation pattern of the deep pineal region is severely damaged after superficial pinealectomy, which is manifested by the disappearance of all symphatetic fibres from this region (Reiter, 1976). In contrast, Moore (1975) found an increased habenular serotonin content following ganglionectomy or decentralization of SCG. It is possible that the symphatetic innervation is partly reestablished by the distribution of perivascular nerve fibres. The involvement of the sympathetic nerve fibres from the brain stem also cannot be excluded. The commissural and central fibres that penetrate into the deep pineal connect the mesencephalon with the pineal complex (Korf and Wagner, 198o; Schneider et al., 1981; Möller and Korf, 1983), but specific pathways between the mesencephalon and the suprachiasmatic nucleus (SCN) and other retino-pineal connections still await final definition. Our finding of Gömori-positive peptidergic fibres in the deep pineal stimulated by constant darkness, which fails to be detected in intact animals, are the signs of the engagement of the brain peptidergic system. This is in keeping with Buijs's and Pevet's finding of the presence of vasopressin and oxytocin fibres in the deep pineal gland and the subcommissural organ of the rat.

Having in mind the data about three functionally different types of cells in the pineal of the guinea pig (Semm and Vollrath, 1979, 1981) and rat (Reusss and Vollrath, 1984) in relation to its electrophysiological properties, whose relative number changes during day-night period and different lighting regimen, our findings of morphologically active pinealocytes in the deep pineal of rats under constant light again raise the question of different pineal cell populations. According to Reuss (personal communication), there are no morphological differences between electrophysiologically different cells, and the innervation pattern of the pinealocytes could be a key to this functional difference. The existence of several cell populations was proposed by Tapp and Blomfild (197o) on the criterion of the nuclear diameter of pinealocytes and by Miline (1983) on the basis of cytophysiological characteristics of the pineal gland. Our previous results revealed the presence of the individually distributed pinealocytes (superficial pineal) that escape the inhibitory influence of hypophysectomy (Kecman, 1978).

In conclusion, we could suggest that the deep pineal of the rat is strongly activated in the concomitant answer of the pineal complex to light and darkness stimuli.

REFERENCES

Boeckmann, D., 198o, Morphological investigation of the deep pineal of the rat, Cell Tissue Res., 21o:283.

Buijs, R. M. and Pevet, P., 198o, Vasopressin and oxitocin containing fibers in the pineal gland and subcommissural organ of the rat, Cell Tissue Res., 2o5:11.

Clabough, J. W., 1973, Cytological aspects of pineal development in rats and hamster, Am. J. Anat., 137:215.

Ilnerova, H., Bäckström, M., Sääf, J., Wetterberg, L., and Vangbo, M., 1978, Melatonin in rat pineal and serum; rapid parallel decline after light exposure at night, Neurosci. Lett., 9:189.

Ilnerova, H. and Vanaček, J., 198o, Pineal rhythm in N-acetyltransferase activity in rats under different artificial photoperiods in natural daylight in the course of a year, Neuroendocrinology, 31:316.

Heidbüchel, U. and Vollrath, L., 1983, Pineal complex of rats: Effects of superficial pinealectomy on the deep pineal, Acta anat., 117:165.

Kappers, J. A., 1960, The development, topographical relations and innervation of the epiphysis cerebri in the albino rat. Z. Zellforsch. mikrosk. Anat., 52:163.

Kecman, M., 1978, Histophysiological properties of the pineal gland following hypophysectomy, Doctoral Dissertation, Novi Sad

Kecman, M., Somer, Lj. and Matavulj, M., 1984, Effect of long-term administration of lithium carbonate on superficial and deep pineal of the rat, Third Colloquium of the EPSG, Pécs, Abstracts.

Klein, D. C. and Weller, J. L., 1972, Rapid light-induced decrease in pineal serotonin N-acetyltransferase activity, Science, 177:532.

Korf, H. W. and Wagner, U., 1980, Evidence for a nervous connection between the brain and the pineal organ in the guinea pig, Cell Tissue Res., 209:505.

Legait, E., Legait, H. and Chevalier, C., 1979, Modification de l'epiphyse profonde apres ablation de l'epiphyse superficielle chez Hamster doré, C. r. Seanc. Soc. Biol., 173:725.

Lewy, A., 1982, Biochemistry and regulation of mammalian melatonin production, in: "The Pineal Gland", R. Relkin, ed., Elsevier Biomedical, New York-Amsterdam-Oxford.

Miline, R., 1957, La part de l'epiphyse dans le syndrom d'adaptation, Congr. Nat. des Sci. Med., ed. de l'Akad. Rep. Pop. Roumaine, pp. 421-444.

Miline, R., Devečerski, V. and Krstić, R., 1969, Corpus pineale - glande de nature sensoneuroendocrine, Acad. Sci. and Arts BiH, Radovi, 37:69.

Miline, R., 1982, Peptidergic activity of the pineal gland in stress, in: "Hormonally Active Brain Peptides", K. W. McKerns and V. Pantić, eds., Plenum Press, New York and London.

Möller, M. and Korf, H.-W., 1983, Central innervation of the pineal organ of the Mongolian gerbil, Cell Tissue Res., 230:259.

Moore, R. Y., 1975, Indolamine metabolism in the intact and denervated pineal, pineal stalk and habenula, Neuroendocrinology, 19:323.

Oksche, A., 1984, Comparative aspects in pineal research, Third Colloquium of the EPSG, Pécs, Abstracts.

Quay, W. B., 1963, Cytologic and metabolic parameters of pineal inhibition by constant light in the rat. Z. Zellforsch. mikrosk. Anat., 60:479.

Pevet, P., 1982, Anatomy of the pineal gland of mammals, in: "The Pineal Gland", R. Relkin, ed., Elsevier Biomedical, New York-Amsterdam-Oxford.

Relkin, R., 1982, Miscellaneous effects of the pineal, in: "The Pineal Gland", R. Relkin, ed., Elsevier Biomedical, New York-Amsterdam-Oxford.

Reuss, S. and Vollrath, L., 1984, Electrophysiological properties of the rat pinealocytes: Evidence for circadian and ultradian rhythms, Exp. Brain Res., 55:455.

Reuss, S., 1984, personal communication.

Reiter, R. J. and Hedlund, L., 1976, Peripheral symphatetic innervation of the deep pineal of the golden hamster, Experientia, 32:1o71.

Roth, W. D., Wurtman, R. J., and Altschule, M. D., 1982, Morphologic changes in the pineal parenchyma cells of rats exposed to continuous light or darkness, Endocrinology, 71:888.

Schneider, T., Semm, P., and Vollrath, L., 1981, Ultrastructural observations on the central innervation of the guinea-pig pineal gland, Cell Tissue Res., 22o:41.

Semm, P. and Vollrath, L., 1979, Electrophysiology of the guinea-pig pineal organ: Symphatetic influenced cells responding differently to light and dark, Neurosci. Lett., 12:93

Semm, P. and Vollrath, L., 198o, Electrophysiological evidence for circadian rhythmicity in a mammalian pineal organ, J. Neural Transmiss., 47:181.

Tapp, E. and Bloomfield, M., 197o, The parenchymal cells of the rat t pineal gland, Acta morph. neerld-scand. 8:119.

Vollrath, L., 1979, Comparative morphology of the vertebrate complex, in: "The Pineal of Vertebrates Including Man", J. A. Kappers and P. Pevet, eds., Prog. Brain Res., 52, Elsevier Amsterdam.

Vollrath, L., 1981, The Pineal Organ. Handbuch der mikroskopischen Anatomie des Menschen, Vol. 7, Springer Verlag, Berlin.

Weibel, E. R., 1979, Stereological Methods, Vol. I, Practical Methods for Biological Morphometry, Acad. Press, London-New York-Toronto-Sydney-San Francisco.

Wiklund, L., 1974, Development of serotonin-containing cells and symphatetic innervation of the habenular region in the rat brain, Cell Tissue Res., 155:321.

THE RELATIONSHIP BETWEEN STRESS AND ACUPUNCTURE ANALGESIA

Zhang Chong-Li and Feng Bei-Yuan

Department of Endocrinology, Institute of Zoology
Academia Sinica,
Beijing, China

INTRODUCTION

Although it is known from clinical practice and animal experiments that the nervous system could be involved in acupuncture analgesia (Chang, 1978), the facts indicate that the acupuncture anaesthesia requires an induction period of about 20-30 minutes and its analgesic effect can be retained for a certain period of time. Furthermore, under acupuncture, the patients' physiological condition is not affected and the anti-inflammatory effect is also not detected or observed. It is, therefore, suggested that there might be a factor or factors other than the nervous system being involved. It is well known that some corticosteroids have analgesic and sedative effects (Lee and Pfeffer, 1951; Winter and Flataker, 1951; Woodbury, 1958). People are familiar with the fact that under stress human beings or animals show great pain endurance. Acupuncture anaesthesia, therefore, might implicate a kind of stress and if so, the hypothalamo-pituitary-adrenal system would likely be involved. The researches reported here were undertaken to investigate the role of corticosteroids in acupuncture analgesia with an established animal model in order to elicite the underlying mechanism of acupuncture analgesia.

A. ANIMAL EXPERIMENTS

In animal experiments, the first thing is to establish a suitable animal model. After many attempts we finally established a suitable animal model by using conscious albino rats. The rat was placed into a fixing case and then a series of square waves were given through an electro needle placed under the tail skin to evoke pain. The squeakings were taken as the signal of pain. Bilateral electro needles were inserted at the base of the earlobe to induce analgesia. Consistent results were obtained through repeated experiments and morphine (3 mg/kg) was used to assure the validity of the model. Figure 1 shows the effect of electro acupuncture upon the pain threshold of rats. Figure 2 demonstrates the electro analgesic effect in the same animal two months later. According to these results, this model is considered to be reliable and could be used to study the relationship between corticosteroids and acupuncture analgesia.

I. Correlation between stress and endogenous corticosteroids in analgesia

The prominent increment of plasma corticosteroids is commonly

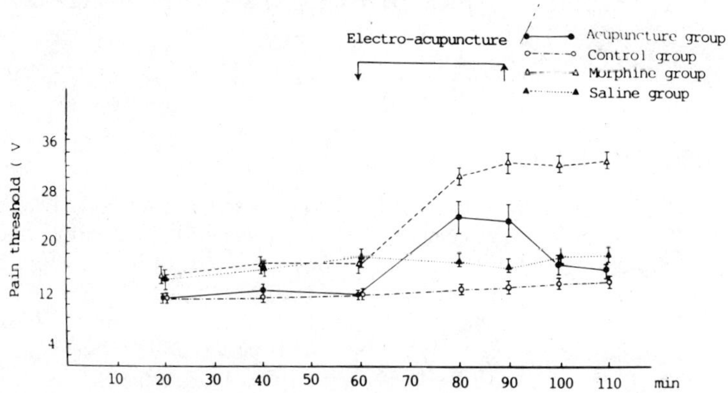

Fig. 1. The effect of electro-acupuncture (frequency : 6 HZ) on the pain threshold in rats (28)

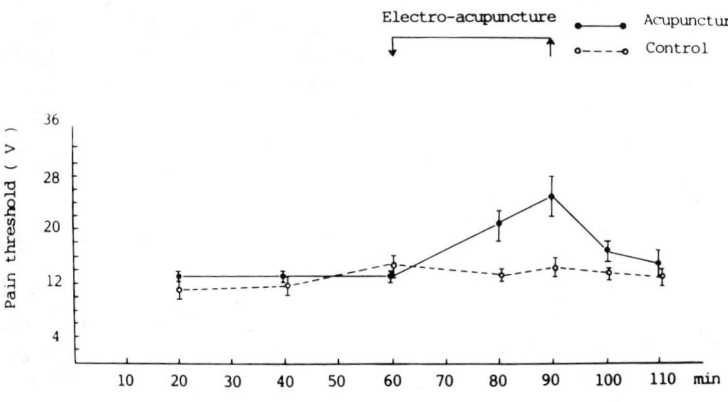

Fig. 2. The effect of electro-acupuncture on part of animal in rats in fig. 1 after two months

regarded as an indication of stress (Knigge, Penrod and Schindle, 1959). Would the process of operation such as placing the rats into the fixing case and electro-stimulation of tail skin cause stress? Figure 3 shows the amount of plasma corticosterone of rats that had been placed in cases for varying periods. The corticosterone was measured by a fluorimetric method (Zenker and Bernstein, 1958). The results show that the corticosterone rose rapidly within 30 minutes and stayed at a high level extended over 2 hours. It is apparent that changing the environment itself could produce stress. Since blood was collected from the caudal vein through cutting off the tail skin, we were uncertain if this manipulation could be responsible for the increase of plasma corticosterone. The rats were then gently placed into a case without any other maneuver and plasma corticosterone were assayed as before. It was found that the plasma corticosterone reached its peak in 60 minutes. The dotted line denotes that plasma corticosterone had reached a peak at 60 minutes after placing into the case. It is, therefore, concluded that a change of environment alone could cause an increase in hormonal level and the tail-cutting did not further augment this effect. Figure 4 shows a dose correlation between stress and analgesia. Even though the plasma corticosterone rose when the rats were placed in the case for 40 minutes, the pain threshold did not change. In order to find out if other factors such as the pain caused by cutting the tail skin or squeezing the blood vessel would affect the pain threshold, we carried out another experiment as illustrated in Figure 5. This demonstrates that with repeated blood collecting up to seven times, pain threshold remained stable. It indicates clearly that the results represented in Figure 4 are likely to be the true pain threshold and are not influenced by bleeding. Through this set of experiments, it is evident that, in rats, endogenous corticosteroid bear no relation to analgesia and therefore stress is not involved in analgesia.

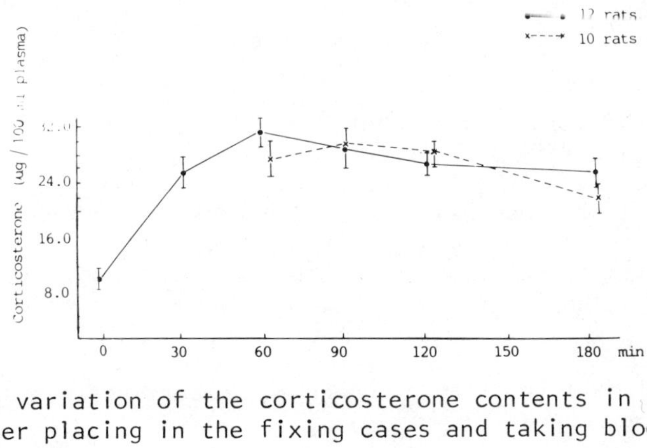

Fig. 3. The variation of the corticosterone contents in rat plasma after placing in the fixing cases and taking blood from the tail

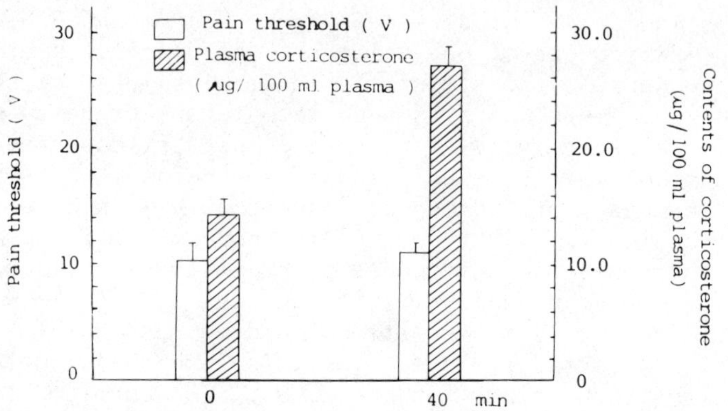

Fig. 4. The relationship between the contents of plasma corticosterone and pain threshold after the rats were placed in the fixing cases after 40 min. (21 rats)

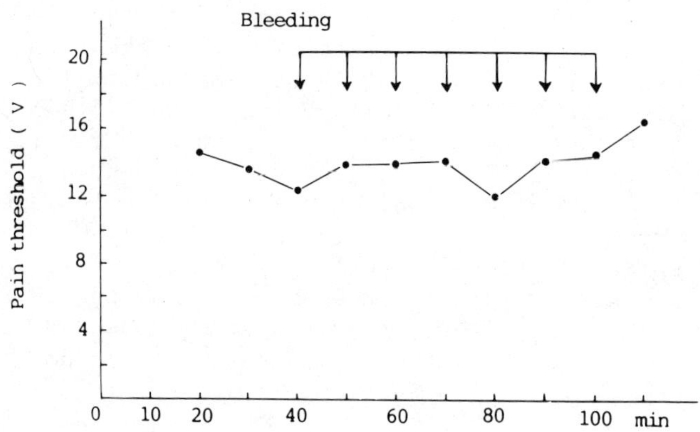

Fig. 5. The effect of bleeding at tail on the pain threshold (5 rats)

Most of the animal experiments and clinical studies are carried out following a brief rest period. This is the period that the corticosterone level usually remains high. One must make sure if corticosteroids are responsible in this respect. For this purpose, the following three experiments were carried out: 1. Effects of exogenous corticosteroids on acupuncture analgesia; 2. Ablation of adrenal glands; and 3. Effect of Dexamethasone - a corticosteroid antagonist.

II. The relationship between exogenous glucocorticosteroid and acupuncture analgesia

Some workers had reported that exogenous cortisone and hydrocortisone raise the pain threshold and improve acupuncture analgesia (Lee and Pfeffer, 1951; Winter and Flataker, 1951; Woodbury, 1958). This is not confirmed by the following experiments as shown in Fig. 6. Exogenous hydrocortisone acetate given intraperitoneally and observed continuously for 6 hours after injection, showed no change in the pain threshold. The result was also not different from that of the saline control. Corticosterone is the main corticosteroid in the rat. We therefore performed a second experiment by injecting exogenous corticosterone, as shown in Fig. 7. It is well known that after intraperitoneal injection, corticosterone moves rapidly into the blood stream producing a plasma level 3 times higher than before injection and staying at a high level beyond one hour. This level was far higher than those occurring during stress. The pain threshold is shown in Fig. 8, indicating that the pain threshold was not changed one hour after injection and there was no effect compared with the vehicle control. It is evident that both corticosterone and hydro-

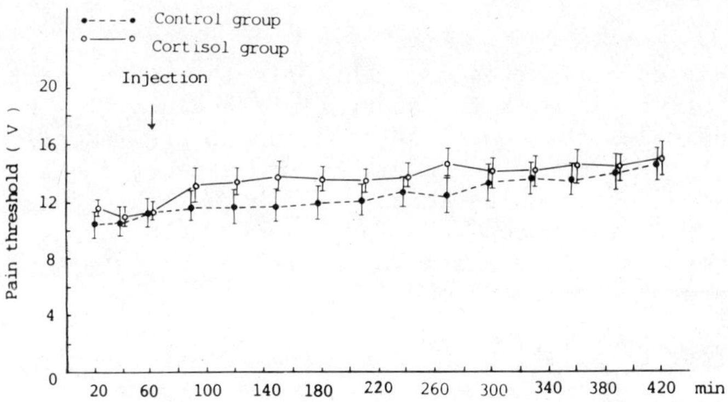

Fig. 6. The effect of cortisol on pain threshold in rats (12 rats)

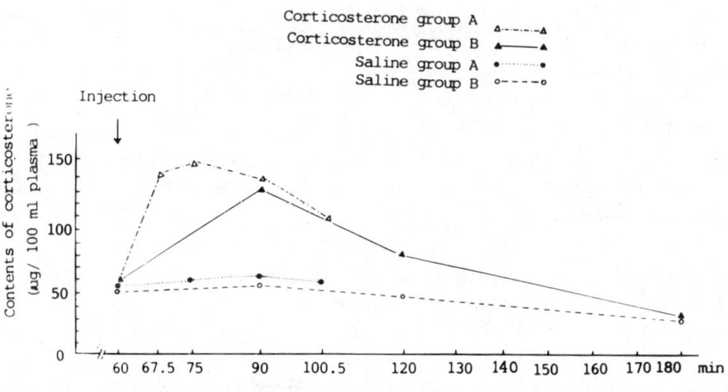

Fig. 7. The effect of exogenous corticisterone on the contents of plasma corticosterone in rats (4)

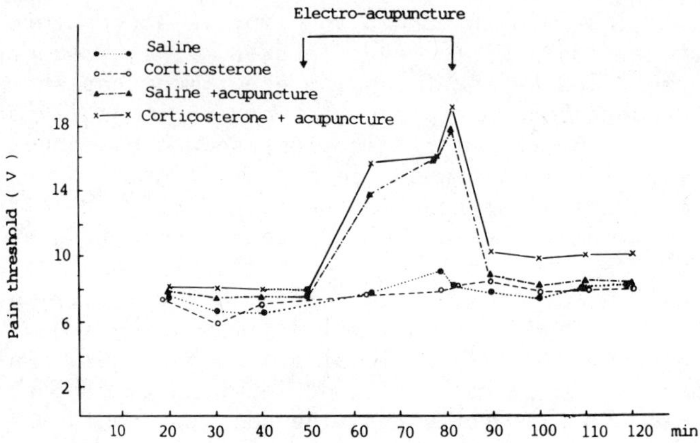

Fig. 8. The effect of exogenous corticosterone on acupuncture analgesia in rats (15)

cortisone exerted no influence on the pain threshold. But do they bear any relationship with the acupuncture analgesia? The solid line in Fig. 8 indicates that when electro acupuncture induction was introduced at the time of the corticosterone peak, the analgesic effect remained unchanged as compared with the vehicle control. The same is true with the group that had a lower level of hormone. The findings suggest that glucocorticoids are not mediators of analgesia in acupuncture.

III. The effect of bilateral adrenalectomy upon acupuncture analgesia

The experiment with exogenous hormone does not eliminate the possibility of the involvement of endogenous hormone produced by the adrenal glands. We next performed bilateral adrenalectomy without corticosteroid supplement in order to investigate further the role of endogenous corticosteroid upon analgesia. Fig. 9 shows that the electro acupuncture displayed a noticeable analgesic effect in the absence of adrenal glands. No difference in pain threshold or electro acupuncture analgesic effect was found compared to the pre-operational stage. Meanwhile their plasma corticosterone had dropped to a very low level. At this time, neither placing the animal in the case, cutting the tail skin, nor electro acupuncture stimuli showed any effect upon plasma corticosterone concentration. This experiment provided a sustaining proof that corticosteroids had no effect upon either analgesia or acupuncture analgesia. The next question is: would the trauma caused by the operation of bilateral adrenalectomy affect acupuncture analgesia? A sham operation was performed. Figure 10 shows no difference in pain threshold and electro acupuncture analgesia between pre- and post sham operations. The after-effects of acupuncture analgesia were the same in those two groups; all disappeared 10 minutes following the withdrawal of the needle.

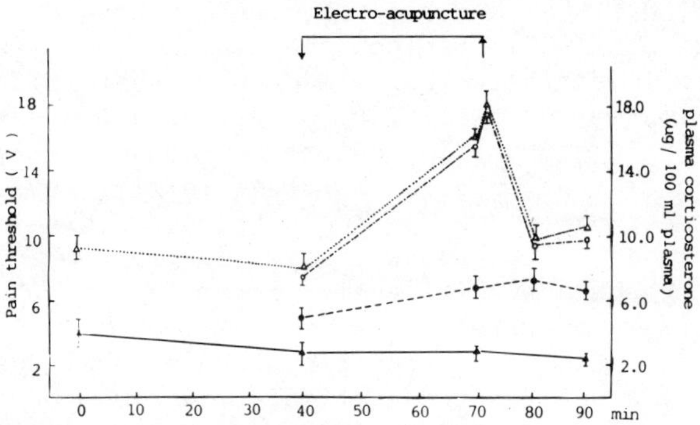

Fig. 9.
The effect of corticosterone on the pain threshold in rats before and after adrenalectomy and the contents of plasma corticosterone after operation (26 rats)
●-----● The native fluctuation of pain threshold
△·····△ After operation
○-·-·-·-○ Before operation
▲———▲ Contents of corticosterone after operation

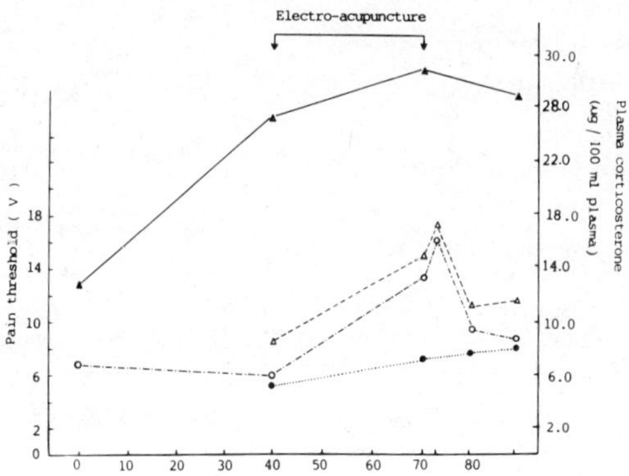

Fig. 10.
The effect of acupuncture on the pain threshold before and after pseudo-surgery and the contents of plasma corticosterone after pseudo-surgery
●-----● The native fluctuation of pain threshold
○-·-·-·-○ After operation
△------△ Before pseudo-surgery
▲———▲ Contents of corticosterone after pseudo-surgery

However, the plasma corticosterone concentration rose markedly during stress and during electro acupuncture induction in sham-operated rats. Thus, operational trauma could raise plasma corticosterone level, but did not influence acupuncture analgesia.

IV. The effect of hypothalamo-pituitary-adrenal axis blocked by Dexamethasone on acupuncture analgesia

As we have seen from the above experiments the adrenal gland and its corticosteroids had shown neither an inhibitory effect on analgesia nor an improvement of acupuncture performance. The next question is: whether the hypothalamo-pituitary-adrenal system participates in acupuncture analgesia? We used dexamethasone (de

Wied, 1964; Russell, Dhariwal, McCann and Yates, 1969; Sirett and Gibbs, 1969) to block the hypothalamo-pituitary-adrenal axis in order to investigate the role of this system in the acupuncture analgesia. Figure 11 shows: 1. Prior to the administration of dexamethasone, corticosterone concentration rose markedly. The corticosterone concentration dropped to the initial level following dexamethasone treatment. However, no difference in pain threshold was found in either of the above cases. 2. Electro acupuncture elevated pain threshold significantly, regardless of whether dexamethasone was given before or after stress stimulation. 3. The electro acupuncture did not influence the corticosterone level when the dexamethasone was given before stress stimulation. On the other hand, the electro acupuncture elevated the corticosterone to a high level. Pain threshold was increased, nevertheless, in both cases by electro acpuncture. The finding provided further evidence to show that the corticosteroids and hypothalamo-pituitary-adrenal system are not involved in analgesia or acupuncture analgesia.

It is thus clear that no matter whether the adrenal glands were present or not, no matter what the level of plasma corticosterone was, or whether the stress response was blocked or not, the analgesic performance remained unchanged. Glucocorticosteroid is demonstrated not to participate in acupuncture analgesia.

B. CLINICAL STUDY

From animal studies, it was concluded that corticosteroids are not involved in acupuncture analgesia. Is the same situation true for human beings? We have investigated: 1. the relationship between changes of endogenous corticosteroids and the outcome of acupuncture performance in patients subjected to lobectomy, and 2. the effects of exogenous corticosteroids on the performance of acupuncture analgesia

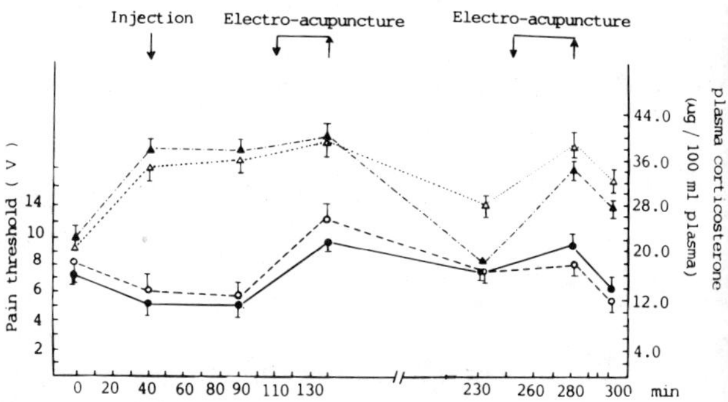

Fig. 11. The effect of Dexamethasome on the pain threshold of acupunture and the variation of contents of plasma corticosterone in rats (17)

●——● Pain threshold of Dexamethasone

○-----○ Pain threshold of phosphate buffer

▲-·-·-▲ Contents of plasma corticosterone of Dexamethasone group

△·····△ Contents of plasma corticosterone of phosphate buffer group in patients under the operation of tubal ligation.

I. The relationship between changes of endogenous corticosteroids and the outcome of acupuncture performance during lobectomy

Changes of plasma 11-hydroxycorticosteroid were measured during lobectomy under acupuncture anaesthesia. A modified method of de Moore et al, 1960, was used. Figure 12 shows that: 1. The patients' plasma corticosteroid rose markedly regardless of the outcome of acupuncture anaesthesia. This result may indicate that the patients were already under stress as soon as they entered the operation room. 2. There was no change in the concentration of plasma corticosteroid before and after induction, indicating that the outcome of acupuncture anaesthesia does not correlate with plasma corticosteroid concentration. Therefore, corticosteroids do not play an important role in mediating the effect of acupuncture anaesthesia. 3. Surgical trauma alone could increase the plasma corticosteroid concentration significantly but this had no relationship whatsoever with acupuncture anaesthesia.

Based on physiological and psychological considerations, the patients' emotional states could be divided into stable and tensional types. Clinical trials shows that when patients entered the operation room, the plasma hydroxycorticosteroid level of the tensional patients increased significantly as compared with those of the stable type. Table 1 shows that the plasma hydroxycorticosteroid is 5.5 ± 1.5 µg/ 100 ml plasma in the stable type and 10.3± 1.3 µg/100 ml plasma in the tensional type; an increase of 153.3% and 209% respectively as compared with the basic concentration. Figure 13 shows the performance of acupuncture in patients under the lobectomy. In Grade I (excellent group) the performance is 62% in the stable type and 3% in the tensional type. In Grade III (moderate group) the order is reversed: 71% in tensional type and only 16% in stable type. So the

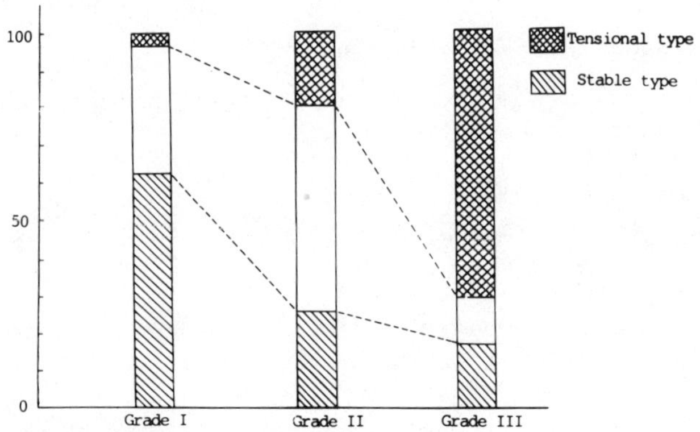

Fig. 12. The relationship between emotional state and acupuncture anaesthesia (101 cases)

Table I. The relationship between the changes of 11-hydroxycorticosteroid and emotional type

Type	Case	Alterative value of corticosteroid (mean ± S.E.) µg/100 ml plasma	Alterative percentage $(\frac{\text{content of entering room}}{\text{basic content}} \times 100)$
Stable	19	5.5 ± 1.5	153.3%
Tensional	16	10.3 ± 1.3	209 %

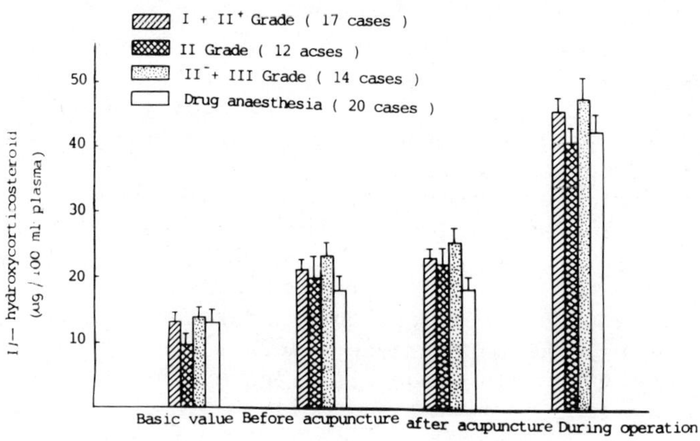

Fig. 13. The variation of contents of plasma hydroxycorticosteroid during lobectomy under acupuncture and drug anaesthesia

patients' emotional states may be used as an indicator for the effect of acupuncture anaesthesia.

II. The effects of exogenous corticosteroids on the performance of acupuncture analgesia in patients under the operation of tubal ligation

Clinical studies in patients receiving exogenous corticosteroids provide further evidence to sustain the above conclusion. No influence of the outcome of acupuncture analgesia was observed in those patients undergoing tubal ligation who took orally hydrocortisone sodium succinate (150 mg/person) before surgery (see Table 2).

Table II. The effect of cortisol on the performance of acupuncture analgesia during tubal ligation

Grade	Drug Group (case)	Control group (case)	X^2	P
I (Excellent)	19	18		
II (Good)	14	19		
III (Moderate)	7	1	6.18	>0.05
IV (Failing)	1	0		
Total	41	38		

X^2 value P 0.05 = 7.81

CONCLUSION

From animal experiments it was found that no matter whether the adrenal glands were present or not, no matter what the level of plasma corticosterone or whether stress was blocked or not, there was no influence upon the analgesic effect. Corticosteroids, especially glucocorticosteroid, do not participate in acupuncture analgesia. Through the clinical studies, evidence was obtained to suggest that during acupuncture anaesthesia or acupuncture analgesia, corticosteroids do not act as mediators and that the involvement of stress is also not involved.

We thank Prof. C. Y. Chang for his reading of the manuscript.

REFERENCES

Chang, Hsiang-tung (1978): Neurophysiological basis of acupuncture analgesia. Scientia Sinica 21 (6):829-846.

Knigge, K.M.; Penrod, C.H. and Schindler, W.J. (1959): In vitro and in vivo adrenal corticosteroid secretion following stress. Amer. J. Physiol.196(3):579-582.

Lee, R.E. and Pfeffer, C.C. (1951): Effects of cortisone and 11-dexosycortisone on pain threshold in man. Proc. Soc. Biol. and Med.77:752-754.

de Moore, P.; Steeno, O.; Raskin, M. and Hendrikx, A. (1960): Flourimetric determination of free plasma 11-hydroxycorticosteroids in man. Acta Endocrionol.33:297-307.

Russell, S.M.; Dhariwal, A.P.S.; McCann, S.M. and Yates. F.E. (1969): Inhibition by dexamethasone of the in vivo pituitary response to corticotropin-releasing factors (CRF). Endocrinol.85:512-521.

Sirett, N.E. and Gibbs, F.P. (1969): Dexamethasone suppression of ACTH release: Effects of the interval between steroid administration and application of stimuli known to release ACTH.Endocrinol. 85:355-359.

de Wied, D. (1964): The site of the blocking action of dexamethasone on stress-induced pituitary ACTH release. J. Endocrinol.29:29-37.

Winter, C.A. and Flataker, L. (1951): The effect of cortisone, desoxycorticosterone and adrenocorticotrophic hormone upon the response of animals to analgesic drugs. J. Pharmacol. and Exp. Therap. 103(1):93-105.

Woodbury, D.M. (1958): Relations between the adrenal cortex and central nervous system. Pharmacol. Rev. 10(2):275-357.

Zenker, N. and Bornstein, D.E. (1958): The estimation of small amounts of corticosterone in the rat plasma. J. Biol. Chem. 231: 695-701.

ACTH NEURONS, STRESS AND BEHAVIOR: A SYNTHESIS

John M. Stewart

Department of Biochemistry
University of Colorado School of Medicine
Denver, Colorado 80262

INTRODUCTION:

Recent discoveries in the field of neuropeptides have made it clear that these molecules play many important roles in regulation of brain function (Krieger, 1983). Although it had been suggested as early as 1953 by Lembeck that substance P (SP) may be a neurotransmitter, progress in the neuropeptide field was slight until the major impetus provided in 1975 by the discovery of enkephalins and endorphins. Since that time the literature has been filled with a flood of often confusing data from which, however, much important new information can be gleaned. Progress in the opioid area has been particularly rapid. It is now well established that ß-endorphin and adrenocorticotropic hormone (ACTH) are synthesized together in one protein precursor (Mains et al., 1977), and that the brain contains a set of ACTH-endorphin (ACTH-End) neurons completely distinct from the pituitary (Watson et al., 1978b). Although there has been considerable speculation about the role or roles of this brain ACTH-End system, only recently has it become possible to synthesize from the available data a reasoned hypothesis as to what that role may be. In this paper it is proposed that the brain ACTH-End system is a major regulator of central nervous system (CNS) activity, and that its action can be bimodal, principally through its influence on the midbrain monoamine systems. In certain circumstances it appears that this system can stimulate higher brain centers to more effective function, while under other circumstances it can cause the higher, cortical centers to be turned off, or else disconnected, so that the organism functions under the control of the evolutionarily ancient midbrain centers. It is proposed that whereas ACTH in the periphery is a major mediator of the biochemical response to stress, the CNS ACTH-End system is a major mediator of the behavioral response to stress.

MacLean has suggested (1973) that although the ancient midbrain centers (the reptilian, or R-complex) have been functionally superseded by the more dominant paleomammalian (limbic system) and neomammalian (cortical) brain areas in the course of evolutionary accretion, the reptilian brain remains functional and can become dominant under certain conditions, such as during acute stress. It is proposed here that this "switch-off" of the higher centers appears to be accomplished by a massive burst of activity of the norepinephrine (NE)-producing neurons whose cell bodies are primarily in the locus ceruleus of the midbrain. The brain serotonin (Ser) system, whose perikarya are located in the midbrain Raphe nuclei, and the mesolimbic dopamine (DA) system, whose cell bodies are in the interpeduncular nucleus, may also participate in this "switch-off". The brain ACTH-End neurons appear to make up the "trigger" which activates this "switch". Neurons which release vasopressin (VP), corticotropin releasing factor (CRF) and substance P (SP) appear to participate by acting either directly on the monoamine systems or indirectly via the ACTH-End neuronal system.

This hypothesis concerning a role of the brain ACTH-End system is based upon and supported by recent discoveries in peptide neuroanatomy and neuroendocrinology, studies of the effects of peptides on behavior, learning and memory and on the development of opiate tolerance and dependence. Information on the apparent evolution of biologically important peptides has played an important role. Throughout the development of the hypothesis a major clue has been provided by evidence of stimulation of sexual function in situations where CNS levels of ACTH are high, such as acute stress, in opiate withdrawal, in paradoxical (rapid eye movement - REM) sleep, and following central administration of ACTH or CRF.

The brain enkephalin and ACTH-End systems are totally distinct (Watson et al., 1978a). Enkephalin perikarya occur at many different places in the CNS, and with but few exceptions have short axons. In general it can be said that enkephalin neurons appear to serve local modulatory functions, principally inhibitory in nature. The fact that they may modulate functions of other neurons involved in a variety of processes undoubtedly leads to much of the multiplicity of actions of opiates. In sharp contrast, the brain ACTH-End system comprises a single set of perikarya located in the arcuate nucleus of the hypothalamus. The long axons of these cells proceed first rostrally and dorsally through several limbic areas where some fibers terminate, then caudally to terminate on midbrain and reticular formation nuclei. ACTH-End terminals have been described on such limbic areas as the amygdala, septum, nucleus accumbens and periventricular nucleus of the thalamus, and on the midbrain Ser-producing cells of the Raphe nuclei and the NE-producing cells of the locus ceruleus (LC). ACTH related peptides have been shown to stimuate NE turnover in brain (Versteeg, 1973).

An important question is the nature of the signals or events which trigger activity in the brain ACTH-End neurons. While this is still an open question, several lines of evidence suggest that central VP and CRF neurons may be important in this role, and that there may be parallels between stimulation of ACTH release in the CNS and in the periphery. After many years of debate, it now appears that vasopressin does indeed have a physiological role as a component of hypothalamic corticotropin releasing factor. Gillis and Lowry showed (1979) that an extract of hypothalamic median eminence possessing high CRF activity can be separated chromatographically into three components, each of which possesses some CRF activity. The sum of these separated activities did not equal the total activity of the original extract. However, if the three separated components were recombined, the total activity of the original extract was regenerated. One of the isolated components of the mixture has been identified as the 41-residue peptide CRF (Vale et al., 1981) and a second as vasopressin; since synthetic CRF has become available it has been shown conclusively that VP potentiates the ACTH-releasing action of CRF (Beny & Baertschi, 1982). The other component has not yet been firmly identified, although certain other peptides are known to affect ACTH release. The neuropeptide PHI is a candidate, since it also potentiates the action of CRF (Tilders et al., 1984). Angiotensin II also stimulates release of ACTH (Capponi et al., 1982), and may also be a natural component of this system.

The VP and CRF which stimulate release of ACTH from the anterior pituitary arise from cells in the paraventricular nucleus (PVN) of the hypothalamus. Axons from the PVN cells terminate upon the vascular region of the median eminence, where they are ideally situated to secrete VP, CRF, and other peptides into the pituitary portal system for delivery to the anterior pituitary. If CRF and VP (and perhaps other peptides from the hypothalamus) function to release ACTH in the anterior pituitary, might they not also function to stimulate the ACTH-producing cells of the arcuate nucleus of the brain? Immunohistochemical studies have shown VP and CRF nerve terminals on or near the ACTH-producing perikarya in the arcuate nucleus (Sofroniew and Weindel, 1978; Seino et al., 1982; Swanson et al., 1983). Thus anatomical evidence supports the proposed roles for these peptides as transmitters of stimuli to the brain ACTH neurons. Behavioral effects of CRF and VP may not be mediated only via the ACTH-End neurons. Many terminals containing these peptides, as well as CRF cell bodies, have been found in midbrain and limbic areas (Swanson et al., 1983; Buijs,

Vasopressin: Cys-Tyr-Phe-Gln-Asn-Cys-Pro-Arg-Gly-NH_2

DGAVP: Cys-Tyr-Phe-Gln-Asn-Cys-Pro-Arg

ACTH(4-10): Met-Glu-His-Phe-Arg-Trp-Gly

Substance P: Arg-Pro-Lys-Pro-Gln-Gln-Phe-Phe-Gly-Leu-Met-NH_2

Fig. 1. Structures of some peptides which enhance learning.

1980). Intraventricular administration of CRF increases firing of LC neurons, although it is not clear at this time if this is a direct effect or may be mediated by brain ACTH; the arcuate nucleus is readily accessible to the ventricular system (Valentino et al., 1983). In addition to the anatomical evidence, circumstantial support for this hypothesis comes from studies of the effects of peptides on behavior and on learning and memory as well as upon opiate tolerance and dependence.

PEPTIDES AND LEARNING

Work pioneered by the group of de Wied has shown that several peptides related to vasopressin and ACTH have potent effects on learning and memory (de Wied, 1977; Garrud et al., 1974). Structures of several of these peptides are given in Fig. 1. Vasopressin, des-glycinamide vasopressin (DGLVP) and certain peptides related to the sequence of residues 4-10 of ACTH inhibit the extinction of learned behavior in several paradigms. Facilitation of acquisition of a behavior has also been demonstrated (Bohus et al., 1973; Sandman et al., 1980) These activities are clearly not related to any antidiuretic hormone (ADH) activity, for DGLVP has no ADH activity, nor are they related to to steroidogenic activity in the case of the ACTH peptides, for the short ACTH fragments have no ability to release glucocorticoids *in vivo* (Smotherman and Levine, 1980). Evidence presented by the de Wied group and others suggests that these are distinct, centrally-mediated effects of the peptides not involving any peripheral endocrine functions. ACTH has also been shown to be responsible for "imprinting" in newly-hatched ducklings (Martin, 1978). In contrast to these actions of DGLVP and ACTH fragments to stimulate retention of learned behavior, oxytocin, its carboxyl-terminal tripeptide amide (Pro-Leu-Gly-NH_2, also characterized as melanotropin release inhibiting factor, MIF) and the ACTH(4-10) fragment in which the phenylalanine residue at position 7 was of the abnormal D-configuration were reported to have opposite effects (Bohus and de Wied, 1966; Garrud et al., 1974). They promoted extinction of learned behavior in certain paradigms. More recently substance P and certain of its metabolite fragments have been found to have remarkable effects on learning and memory (Gaffori et al., 1984). The integration of SP neurons into the proposed functioning of the system will be discussed later.

In the learning experiments, ACTH-related peptides appeared to have immediate, but short-lasting, effects, while the action of vasopressin and DGLVP was characterized by delayed onset and longer duration (Bohus et al., 1973). While it is by no means conclusive evidence nor the only possible interpretation, one explanation of these observations is that ACTH-related peptides are directly or proximally affecting the centers involved in memory while vasopressin may be acting more distally, or indirectly. It may possibly be acting to stimulate the release of ACTH in the brain. One brain role of vasopressin might then be quite analogous to its role in the anterior pituitary.

OPIATE TOLERANCE AND DEPENDENCE

Twenty years ago it was postulated (Cohen et al., 1965) that certain analogies exist between learning and the development of tolerance to opiates such as morphine. If this is true, then substances which affect learning and memory should also similarly affect the development of tolerance to opiates. Ten years after his original proposal of the learning-tolerance analogy, Krivoy showed that DGLVP does, in fact, facilitate the development of tolerance to morphine in mice (Krivoy et al., 1974). De Wied and Gispen (1976) then showed that Brattleboro rats, genetically lacking vasopressin, do not develop tolerance to morphine at a normal rate, and Walter et al. (1979) showed that oxytocin, MIF and related peptides inhibit the development of tolerance to and physical dependence upon morphine. Most recently we have shown that [D-Phe]-ACTH(1-10)-amide can inhibit development of tolerance to morphine. (Stewart et al., 1980), and Szekely et al. (1979) showed that α-MSH inhibits development of morphine tolerance and dependence.

Recent evidence has led to a more complete understanding of the mechanisms involved in development of opiate tolerance and physical dependence. The principal brain area involved appears to be the locus ceruleus (Gold et al., 1979). Microapplication of opiates to the LC inhibits firing of these neurons in naive animals but not in tolerant animals. Administration of the opiate antagonist naloxone to tolerant-dependent animals causes a spasm of hyperactivity of the LC neurons, but has litle effect on the LC of naive animals. This hyperactivity is blocked by administration of the drug clonidine, which is currently receiving wide clinical application for blocking the opiate withdrawal syndrome (Aghajanian, 1978). Clonidine is a catecholamine agonist specific for the presynaptic NE receptors whose function is to inhibit release of NE from the neuron, the α_2 receptors. Binding of clonidine to these α_2 receptors on LC neurons prevents release of NE from their terminals, even during the acute and massive stimulation due to opiate withdrawal. We then understand physical dependence on opiates to be due to hypersensitivity of the LC which develops during prolonged and increasing inhibition of this organ (development of tolerance) by exogenous opiate. The physical manifestations of opiate withdrawal are due to hyperstimulation of certain brain areas innervated by NE neurons from the LC.

Further support for the description of the morphine withdrawal syndrome (MWS) as a massive central outpouring of NE from the LC cells comes from the "quasi-morphine withdrawal syndrome" (QMWS) studied by Collier (1980). He has shown that large doses of methyl xanthines such as caffeine or the more potent isobutylmethylxanthine will reproduce the entire MWS in drug-naive animals and humans. Since these drugs act by inhibiting the phosphodiesterase which destroys cyclic adenosinemonophosphate (cAMP) and since the central actions of NE are generally mediated by adenylate cyclase-linked ß-receptors, we can now understand the basis of the QMWS. Methyl xanthines and opiate withdrawal produce a similar behavioral end result by stimulating different links of the same central pathways involving NE neurons from the LC. Withdrawal causes the LC neurons to fire excessively, causing excess cAMP to be synthesized in the post-synaptic cells innervated by NE neurons. The methyl xanthines, by preventing destruction of cAMP, cause normal activity of the NE neurons to build up excessive levels of cAMP in the target postsynaptic neurons and thus produce similar results.

Jacquet (1978) has shown that microinjection of ACTH into the central grey area of the brain of naive rats will reproduce the complete MWS. She proposed that the brain contains two types of opiate receptors, stereospecific and non-stereospecific (Jacquet et al., 1977). While morphine acts upon both these postulated receptor types, she suggested that the normal endogenous ligand for the non-stereospecific receptors is ACTH. ACTH is known to combine with some opiate receptors to a certain degree (Terenius, 1976). Jacquet proposed that the two receptors are linked, and that administration of exogenous opiate causes supression of the cells containing the ACTH receptors, causing them to become hypersensitive. Withdrawal of opiate or administration of opiate antagonist causes hyperactivity of the cells containing these ACTH receptors. We propose that these cells are the NE-producing neurons of the locus ceruleus.

Recent discoveries have also clarified the mechanisms

involved in opiate-induced analgesia. Work of Basbaum and Fields (1978) and of Yaksh et al. (1979) has shown that centrally-mediated opiate analgesia depends upon activity of the serotonin-producing cells in the Raphe nuclei of the midbrain. Axons of these cells descend the spinal cord to liberate serotonin at appropriate sites. The serotonin-producing cells possess opiate receptors and may be stimulated by exogenous opiate or by the conditions which produce stress-induced analgesia. This latter condition evidently involves delivery of enkephalin or endorphin-like peptides to receptors on the Raphe cells or on Raphe-stimulating interneurons.

Peripheral ACTH levels are elevated by normal diurnal cycles and in response to stress. We now know that ß-endorphin is also synthesized and liberated along with ACTH. Since CRF- and vasopressin-producing neurons are a common feature of both the pituitary and brain ACTH-producing systems, we can postulate that stress will also cause liberation of ACTH and ß-endorphin from central synapses of the brain ACTH-End neurons, probably via the mediation of CRF and VP release. Recent papers have described increases in cerebrospinal fluid of vasopressin following anesthesia stress (Simon-Opperman et al., 1983) and CRF following footshock (Britton, et al., 1984). We can then search for evidence to support this hypothesis.

Returning to centrally-mediated analgesia and opiate tolerance and dependence, we can now propose an overall neuronal circuitry to explain these phenomena. The essential elements are shown in Fig. 2. We suggest that in stress the brain ACTH-End neurons deliver ACTH and ß-endorphin to the cells of the Raphe and the LC. If the stress is elicited by peripheral noxious sensory input (e.g., pain), the message is evidently transmitted to the brain by SP neurons in the spinal cord and relayed to the arcuate nucleus either directly or via certain thalamic nuclei. The thalamic neurons which innervate the arcuate nucleus for this function may be cholinergic, but the evidence on this point is not clear. If, on the other hand, the stress is elicited by auditory, visual or psychic stimuli, relay of the stress message apparently involves mediation by VP and/or CRF. We suggest that the serotonin producing cells of the Raphe contain stimulatory receptors for ß-endorphin, and that action of this peptide on these cells causes release of serotonin from their terminals to produce analgesia. We suggest that cells of the LC contain both inhibitory ß-endorphin receptors and stimulatory ACTH receptors; these latter are the "non-stereospecific" receptors of Jacquet. Delivery of ß-endorphin to the LC will cause supression, but simultaneous delivery of ACTH will cause a continuous "micro-withdrawal" and prevent any net rapid supression and consequent hypersensitivity of the LC from developing. Administration of exogenous opiate, on the other hand, will not only stimulate the Raphe to produce analgesia, but will

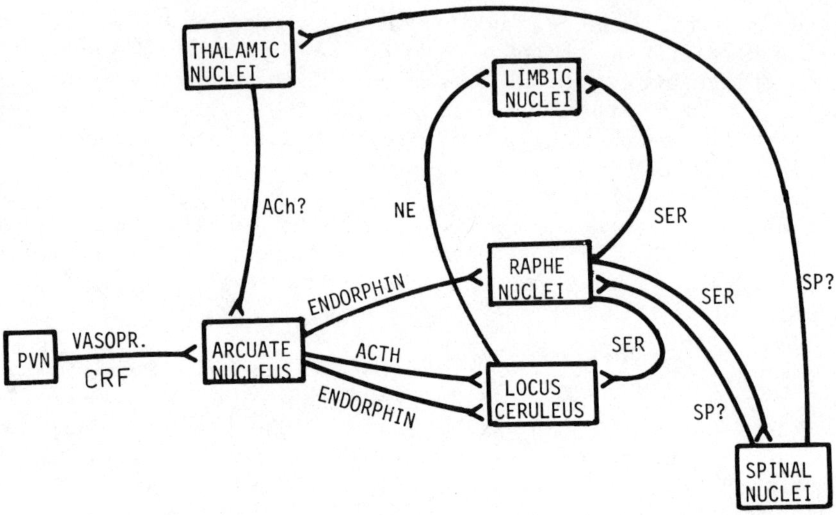

Fig. 2. Proposed neuronal circuitry involved in stress-induced analgesia. PVN = paraventricular nucleus of the hypothalamus. Neurotransmitters are indicated along the courses of the axons.

also inhibit the LC and allow hypersensitivity to develop in the absence of any counterbalancing ACTH. This hypersensitivity constitutes physical dependence. Consistent with this proposed mechanism is the fact that electrical stimulation of the arcuate nucleus or application of morphine there causes inhibition of firing of LC neurons (Strahlendorf et al., 1980). ACTH also probably regulates the opiate receptor synthesis involved in development of tolerance. We can now understand how exogenous ACTH related peptides may affect tolerance and dependence by acting directly on the midbrain nuclei, while vasopressin-related peptides probably stimulate the brain ACTH-End system by acting upon its cells in the arcuate nucleus.

Hosobuchi et al. (1980) have shown that large doses of dietary tryptophan will retard the development of tolerance in patients on chronic opiates. We can understand this observation when we know that increased dietary tryptophan can increase the concentration of this amino acid, which is the precursor for serotonin, in the brain, and also can increase stores of serotonin, the ultimate analgesic. In the presence of such abnormally high levels of serotonin, analgesia may still be provided by the reduced stimulation available during morphine tolerance. It is not known if this treatment also reduces physical dependence.

Different kinds of analgesia-producing stimulation may activate different circuitry. For example, the fact that tolerance can develop to electrically-induced analgesia ("electroacupuncture") may suggest that this type of stimulation does not evoke release of adequate amounts of midbrain ACTH. Moreover, all stress-induced analgesia is not mediated by endogenous opioids. It is well known that in animals generally chronic stress evokes opioid-mediated analgesia (that is, it can be blocked by opiate antagonists such as naloxone), while brief, acute stress evokes analgesia which is non-opioid and cannot be blocked by naloxone (Lewis et al., 1980).

CENTRAL ACTH AND SEXUAL BEHAVIOR

With this understanding of central mechanisms of analgesia, tolerance and physical dependence, we may turn to other aspects of central ACTH function. Many lines of evidence suggest that ACTH may play a role in central regulation of sexual function, and examination of several aspects of this area may provide many clues to lead us to a greater understanding of brain regulation.

Peptide Evolution

Several peptides important in sexual function appear to have evolved from the "active core" of ACTH (Stewart and Channabasavaiah, 1979). One such is luteinizing hormone releasing hormone (LRH), which is physiologically essential for reproduction as a releaser of pituitary luteinizing hormone and follicle-stimulating hormone. LRH is also important for the behavioral aspects of reproduction. It stimulates mating behavior in males (Dorsa and Smith, 1981) and produces the lordosis response in females (Moss et al., 1975) to facilitate mating. LRH-containing neurons terminate on the septum and the amygdala, limbic brain areas known to be important for sexual behavior (Kozlowski et al., 1980; Willoughby and Martin, 1978). Fig. 3 gives the amino acid sequences of the "active core" of ACTH (the N-terminal 13 amino acid residues, which also comprises the sequence of α-melanocyte stimulating hormone (α-MSH)) and LRH, and shows the surprising homology between the structures of these two peptides. The sequence homology is made even more striking if a tripeptide segment of ACTH is transposed "upstream" by four residues, as indicated in the second structure of the figure. This transposition could occur as the result of three successive unequal "crossing over" events. Once this transposition had occurred, only simple point mutations were necessry to yield the amino acid sequence of LRH. The pyroglutamyl residue is derived from a glutamine sequence in the peptide. The yeast peptide is a mating pheromone for one of the haploid forms of *Saccharomyces cerevisiae*. It is synthesized and secreted by the alpha type cells

```
ACTH(1-13):  Ser-Tyr-Ser-Met-Glu-His-Phe-Arg-Trp-Gly-Lys-Pro-Met-

Trans ACTH:  Glu-His-Phe-Ser-Tyr-Ser-Met-Arg-Trp-Gly-Lys-Pro-Met-

LRH:        <Glu-His-Trp-Ser-Tyr-Gly-Leu-Arg-Pro-Gly-amide
              1       1           1   1       2

Alpha Factor:   His-Trp-Leu-Gln-----Leu-Lys-Pro-Gly-Gln-Pro-Met-Tyr
                        1   2           1           1
```

Fig. 3. Amino acid sequences of ACTH(1-13), hypothetical "transposed" ACTH(1-13), Luteinizing hormone releasing hormone and the Saccharomyces alpha mating factor peptide. The numbers under amino acid symbols indicate the number of base changes required to evolve that residue from the one above it. <Glu = pyroglutamyl. The sequence of dogfish ACTH is shown; mammalian ACTH has Val at position 13.

and attracts the A type cells. It also stops the cell cycle of growth in the A cells to prepare them for mating. It appears to have arisen from LRH by a further simple series of mutations. These mutations must have taken place very early on the evolutionary scale. The numbers and types of mutations suggest that the order of evolution was ACTH-LRH-α-factor (or the reverse). Since ACTH has recently been found in the single-cell eukaryote Tetrahymena (LeRoith et al., 1982), it is apparent that ACTH is also a very old peptide.

A well-established principle of comparative biology is that structure follows function. That is, if two different organisms possess a morphologically similar structure, that structure can be presumed to be involved in a similar function in both organisms. Since morphology depends upon the amino acid sequences of the structural proteins and enzymes involved in the creation of structure, it is logical to extend this principle to amino acid sequences. It is also logical to suggest that since LRH and the α-factor are involved in sexual behavior, this function might extend to ACTH. A surprisingly large body of evidence suggests that this is the case. Let us examine that evidence.

ACTH and Sexual Stimulation

Although the functioning of the CNS in sexual behavior is still largely a mystery, some progress is being made (Sandler and Gessa, 1975). There are remarkable interactions between the brain ACTH system and sexual function. Spontaneous erection and orgasm are common features of the opiate withdrawal syndrome, whether it is produced by abstinence in dependent individuals, by the QMWS, or by microinjection of ACTH into the central grey area of the brain (Mintz et al., 1974; Bertolini et al., 1969). These types of sexual responses have been considered to be mediated by spinal cholinergic and adrenergic reflexes, respectively, and their spontaneous occurrence probably indicates release from descending central inhibitory pathways. Recent evidence implicating the neuropeptides VIP and substance P in erection (Virag et al., 1982; Gu et al., 1983) suggests that this process is very complex. Since we understand the withdrawal syndrome to be due to hyperactivity of the LC, it is not surprising that clonidine, which inhibits LC function, inhibits erection and orgasm. On the other hand, yohimbine, a catecholamine α_2-antagonist which stimulates the LC, produces orgasm when microinjected into the LC and is well known as a classical aphrodisiac (Clark et al., 1984). Yohimbine has also been used clinically in the treatment of impotence (Morales et al., 1981). Also consistent with this general scheme are the facts that morphine and endorphin inhibit sexual behavior (Mintz et al., 1974; Gessa et al., 1979), whereas the specific morphine antagonist naloxone stimulates mating behavior. The orgasm-like "rush" of cocaine administration is likely due to its producing hyperstimulation of central NE neurons; it inhibits presynaptic reuptake of NE and like methyl xanthines greatly increases the effects of firing of NE neurons. Much of the popularity of cocaine use is said to be due to the sexual stimulation which it produces. This description of centrally mediated sexual stimulation is surely over-simplified. For example, there is also evidence that dopamine systems are involved in sexual function (Stefanick et al., 1982).

Stress and Sexual Stimulation

Like the effects of stress on pain response, two different types of sexual response to stress can be distinguished. While chronic stress inhibits sexual behavior and performance, apparently due to elevated endorphin levels, acute stress produces sexual stimulation. When the tail of a male rat is pinched, he will make one of two responses. If a sex partner is available, he will copulate; if a partner is not available, he will eat. Switching or flogging has long been known to be a concomitant of human sexual behavior, and is said to be stimulating to both the actor and the recipient. A recent scientific paper (Antelman and Caggiula, 1980) reproduces an illustration of sexual flogging from an early edition of the well-known erotic novel "Fanny Hill" and cites this as application of the tail pinch phenomenon to humans.

Massive release of ACTH occurs in stress. Some kinds of extreme stress produce spontaneous erection and orgasm - the so-called "agonal orgasm." Asphyxiation is particularly effective in producing this response; it is a "humoral stress." Agonal orgasm is reputed to have been an important factor in the popularity of public hangings when they were common. Habitual use of hanging to induce orgasm apparently leads to the accidental death of many persons annually, mostly men. A recent study sponsored by the US Federal Bureau of Investigation (Hazelwood et al., 1983) found that at least 500 persons per year in the United States probably die from accidental autoerotic death. Frequent newspaper articles report deaths due to such hangings, often of youths who have apparently not developed their techniques for this practice to the point where rescue is automatic (The Denver Post, April 2, 1981). A finding of accidental autoerotic death, rather then suicide or murder, is usually returned if there is no suicide note and there is evidence of habitual hanging with a provision for recovery and prevention of physical injury. Items having sexual connotation are often present. Stress-induced sexual stimulation is depicted in such works of literature as Samuel Beckett's "Waiting for Godot", John Hersey's "The War Lover", and the works of de Sade. There is anecdotal evidence of stress-induced orgasm under less traumatic circumstances. In the British university system where the final examination determines the total outcome of the course, a student entering the examination was under such stress he could remember nothing -- which further increased the stress. He experienced a spontaneous orgasm, the stress was relieved, and he could then remember clearly the information he needed for the examination.

Some individuals can perhaps achieve orgasm only under acute stress, and this fact may contribute, in addition to accidental autoerotic death, to some of the antisocial violence of our times as manifested in such actions as rape, arson and sadism.

It is not a purpose of this writer to contest or minimize the interpretation of rape as an act of anti-female violence. However, the intrinsic sexual stimulation involved in the act should not be overlooked, and is in actuality most likely the critical point in the rapist's choice of a means of expression of his rage and aggression. Many vehicles other than rape are available for expression of violence; indeed, the woman-beater probably is sexually stimulated by his acts of battery. The rapist, on the other hand, may often be a person who is genetically or psychogenically unable to achieve orgasm as a result of normal stimuli and must (or believes he must) have the added violence (stress) of rape to enable him to achieve orgasm (Valzelli, 1981).

Arson, when not done for revenge or collection of fire insurance, is well known to be sexually linked (Macdonald, 1977). The pyromaniac will often be found by the police masturbating as he watches the flames. Many persons who would never consider burning buildings for pleasure confess to being sexually stimulated by fire. A recent well-publicized, but misinterpreted, case of sexually linked arson in the United States was the burning of the Hilton hotel in Las Vegas. Like the rapist, the pyromaniac may have discovered his need of (or uncontrollable pleasure in) the acute stress of arson as a sexual adjunct. Bombers evidently also fall within this same general category.

While rape and arson are generally male aberrations, a female counterpart may be found in kleptomania. The sexual nature of kleptomania is described in the psychiatric literature (Stoller, 1975). Most kleptomaniacs are women, and they have often reported experiencing orgasm as they commit their acts of theft.

The phenomena associated with these types of sexually linked antisocial acts strongly implicate ACTH as a mediator of, or adjunct to, these behaviors. Records show that these individuals may not be able to function sexually in modes considered normal but use these stressful behaviors to enable them to function sexually or as a substitute for normal sexual functioning. If these defects are indeed brought on or aggravated by a deficiency of central ACTH functioning, perhaps peptide research can yield an orgasm-evoking drug which would protect women and property in the future. Such a hypothetical drug was described many years ago as "soma" by Huxley (1979) in "Brave New World".

In addition to the sexually-related pathology discussed above, another pathological condition, that of multiple personality disorder, probably represents an aberration of the brain ACTH system and its function (Braun, 1984). In the multiple personality syndrome two or more personalities exist within the same individual, and they can appear either at the will of the subject or when triggered by external events. These personalities may have drastically different characteristics and have associated with them distinct physiological and endocrine characteristics. The classic case of multiple (double) personality was represented in literature by "Dr. Jekyll and Mr. Hyde" (Stevenson, 1964), who showed typical extremes of personality characteristics. The abrupt "switching" probably depends for its origin and repetition on the brain ACTH neurons and their connections to the NE system. Persons with multiple personality disorder were subjected repeatedly in childhood to severe abuse, usually of a sexual nature. This abuse has been described in the well-known case of Sybil (Schreiber, 1973). The "switching" off of the higher brain centers described above evidently took, in these individuals, an extreme and variant form, probably due to genetic characteristics of the individual and the nature and repetition of the stress. It is of interest that treatment of male mice with ACTH or vasopressin after a defeat increases future submissiveness (Roche and Leshner, 1979). Production of permanent changes in behavior by repeated stresses may have some analogy with "kindling" of the limbic system (Livingston and Hornykiewicz, 1978).

Venoms of the spider _Phoneutria nigriventer_ and the scorpion

Leiurus quinquestriatus produce erection and orgasm as well as massive hypertrophy of the adrenal cortex (Efrati, 1978; Schenberg and Pereira Lima, 1978). These peptide venoms, when they are fully characterized, may well be found to mimic actions of ACTH or CRF, possibly due to the presence of homologous amino acid sequences in their proteins.

Since synthetic CRF has become available there has already been some investigation of its effects on behavior of rodents (Morley and Levine, 1982) and monkeys (Kalin, 1983) when administered centrally. CRF clearly evokes behavior reminiscent of many stress responses; sexual stimulation was a concomitant of these responses. It is not clear at this time whether these responses to CRF are mediated via brain ACTH or if they are produced directly by CRF. As was mentioned earlier, there are CRF terminals in several limbic brain areas.

Circadian ACTH Secretion

Sexual stimulation is also associated with the diurnal rhythm of ACTH secretion. ACTH and VP are secreted in bursts during episodes of paradoxical sleep (PS) or rapid eye movement (REM) sleep, which are always accompanied by sexual stimulation (Williams and Karacan, 1978). In men with properly functioning physiological systems, penile erection always occurs during each PS episode. Orgasm may or may not accompany these episodes. In women, vaginal temperature and lubrication increase during PS. The dramatic sexual content of PS dreams has often proved disturbing to persons who have not understood that this is normal. Much needless anxiety and expenditure of money for psychiatrists has been a result. Widespread education on this matter is clearly needed.

Sleep is regulated by endogenous timers, or pacemakers, evidently located in the suprachiasmatic nucleus (Moore-Ede, et al., 1983). These timers are responsible for the 90-minute "ultradian" cycle which regulates much of the body's endocrine function (e.g., secretion of hypothalamic and anterior pituitary hormones) as well as sleep. During the 90-minute sleep cycle the sleeper goes first through the stages of slow-wave sleep (SWS, deep sleep), and then switches into PS. During the course of a normal night's sleep, each successive sleep cycle contains progressively more PS, so that the last cycle of the night is predominantly PS. Spontaneous awakening, either during the night or in the morning, usually occurs at the end of a PS period. Although in normal individuals PS can only occur following SWS, different pacemakers control the different types of sleep and the hormonal events associated with them. SWS is controlled by the so-called "pacemaker Y", while PS is controlled by "pacemaker X". Following a clock shift, such as is involved in west-east jet travel or shift-work schedule changes, the Y pacemaker resets immediately, while the X pacemaker may be totally reset only after two weeks in some individuals. This slow resetting of the X pacemaker leads to the mental dissociation of jet-lag or other rapid clock shift. It has recently been reported that male rats routinely have spontaneous orgasms during sleep (M. L. Stefanick and J. M. Davidson, personal communication). When the light-dark clock cycle was shifted by 12 hours, the frequency of orgasm was markedly diminished, and did not return to the normal value until about two weeks had passed.

Growth hormone is secreted principally during SWS, leading to the concept that the function of SWS is regeneration of the body. On the other hand, PS is thought to be necessary for regeneration of the mind, since memory consolidation (Cohen, 1980; Corner et al., 1980) and juvenile brain development (Corner et al., 1981; Jouvet, 1980) appear to occur principally during PS. The fact that normal circadian secretion of vasopressin and ACTH occurs only during PS strongly suggests that they may have a role in regulation of brain function related to sleep. ACTH secretion recovers only slowly after a shift in clock cycles (Rubin, 1975; Weitzman et al., 1975).

Vasopressin secretion is regulated by several factors. The best understood of these is the hydroosmotic balance of the body; vasopressin causes reabsorption of water in the renal tubules and thus reduces urine excretion. In addition to its secretion in response to dehydration, vasopressin is also secreted during stress and during periods of PS. A significant population of vasopressin cell bodies is located in the suprachiasmatic nucleus (Buijs, 1980) and may be associated with the endogenous X pacemaker. Axons from these VP neurons terminate upon the septum, which is important in sexual behavior, and upon the habenula, which contains cell bodies of the substance P neurons which stimulate the dopamine cells of the ventral tegmental area. These DA neurons supply the mesolimbic system, which is important in regulation of perception and behavior.

Vasopressin, CRF and ACTH work together physiologically to facilitate uninterrupted sleep. ACTH, by stimulating cortisol secretion, causes conversion of protein to glucose to maintain brain function during the overnight fast and to prevent the necessity of feeding during this period. Vasopressin not only functions during PS as a corticotropin releasing substance, but also inhibits water excretion, thus minimizing the need for awakening to urinate during the night. Morning urine is very concentrated, and the excess water retained during the night is then excreted during the early hours of the day.

PS is also characterized by hyperactivity of certain NE-producing neurons of the LC, while other LC neurons are turned off (Chu and Bloom, 1974). Other features of PS, such as loss of thermal regulation, muscular atonia, variable heart rate, blood pressure and respiration and retention of body water suggest that the normal physiological control mechanisms are not functioning in their usual way. These facts are consistent with the proposal that the body is under control of the ancient reptilian brain during PS. Although the present literature on vasopressin levels in PS is conflicting, the water retention suggests stimulation of the magnocellular hypothalamic neurons which produce this peptide during PS. When regulation of secretion of CRF is studied, it will also surely be found to be secreted selectively during PS.

Sagan (1977) has suggested in "The Dragons of Eden" that PS dreams represent a recall of our evolutionarily ancient reptilian sleep. It appears now that there is neurophysiological evidence to support a position somewhat related to his proposal.

There has been much research and discussion on the central mechanisms regulating the sleep cycles. A currently popular view is that of McCarley and Hobson (1975), who propose that the LC is "turned off" during PS. They have addressed principally the triggering of the PS cycle, while we are concerned here principally with the functioning of the LC during PS. All the evidence (including a careful reading of the paper of Chu and Bloom (1974) on activity of LC neurons in PS) is consistent with the contrary proposal that the LC is very active in PS. PS is blocked by clonidine (Kleinlogel et al., 1975), which "turns off" the LC, and by the adrenergic beta-antagonist propranolol (Lanfumey and Adrien, 1981), which blocks NE receptors in the brain. On the other hand, the LC stimulant yohimbine increases PS (Kafi and Gaillard, 1981).

These facts are all consistent with activation of the brain VP-ACTH-LC system during PS, and suggest that it may be playing an important role in the evident "disconnection" of body functions from normal control mechanisms during PS. One might suggest that the higher centers are thus liberated to conduct other important functions, such as the consolidation of memory, which take place during PS and which are enhanced by exogenous stimulants of this system.

The new understanding of "disconnection" of higher brain centers during PS and knowledge of the persistence of PS cycles for several days have major implications for life style, particularly with respect to persons who undergo abrupt shifts in work schedules. One can anticipate that immediately following the schedule shift the worker will not be able to perform mental tasks with his usual clarity during those times when he would have otherwise been in a period of PS. The events at the nuclear power plant at Three Mile Island in Pennsylvania are a dramatic demonstration of this. The emergency alarms were functioning properly, but the operator, who had just come onto the night shift, was looking at them with his higher brain centers disconnected. Therefore he failed to perform the emergency procedures in which he had been well trained. Indeed, clock shift produces retrograde amnesia (Tapp and Holoway, 1981). Nurses and other health care workers who are now routinely subjected to frequent work schedule shifts are also required to make rapid decisions involving the lives of their patients. A recent rash of train accidents during the early morning hours may also indicate that this phenomenon is at work there as well. Ironically, the usual schedule of shift changes (to advance the clock time of the worked hours in successive one or two-week periods) seems designed to be the worst possible. The endogenous clock has a normal period of about 25 hours when free-running. Hence every day the entrainment to a 24-hour schedule involves a one-hour advance from the spontaneous rhythm. Additional clock advance is then more difficult and stressful than clock delay. This appears to be the reason why adaptation after west-east jet travel (clock advance) is more difficult than after east-west travel (clock delay). "Blue Monday" may be partly due to the relaxation of time schedules toward the spontaneous rhythm during the week-end, with subsequent painful re-advance on Monday morning. Work performance has been shown to improve when shifts are changed by clock delay rather than advance (Czeisler et al., 1982) and when the changes occur less frequently. Clearly, current work practices in this area need revision.

It is not clear at this time why sexual stimulation should always occur in PS. It has been suggested that this represents "exercise" to insure that an important physiological function will be operable when needed. In any event, erection during PS provides a useful diagnostic tool in cases of impotence (Marshall et al., 1981). It probably serves some other function whose exact nature is not yet apparent. It is also not clear why ACTH should have been utilized as the stimulus for erection, but it has been suggested that erection is a primordial aggression signal. Several species of male animals as well as primitive tribes go into combat with penises erect. Certain tribes in New Guinea even construct a long sheath to cover the penis in battle, the combination being held in the erect position by a string about the waist. Thus a function which may have been lost in evolution is maintained symbolically for its usefulness in aggression signalling.

If PS is represented as "disconnection" of the higher centers, then acute stress is probably best represented as massive inhibition of the higher centers. One might present a teleological argument for an advantage for survival in turning off the higher, deliberative, centers and returning control of the organism to the older centers which mediate instinctive behavior. While such instinctive stress-mediated behaviors may have had survival value, they may have lost their appropriateness in our contemporary culture. That this "Switch-off" still functions is demonstrated by the memories each of us carries of often embarassing inability to think during acute stress. When the stress is exacerbated by the effects of clock advance, the "switch-off" is even more complete. Although behavioral aspects of both PS and acute stress may be brought about principally by stimulation of the brain ACTH neuronal system, there are clearly great differences between them, suggesting participation of other major regulatory systems in the brain.

The stimulation of learning by mild stress and the roles of brain peptides in stimulating learning and memory apparently represent a third phase or type of activation of the brain VP-ACTH-NE system. Present ideas of the mechanisms involved in learning and memory suggest that at least four phases can be identified: 1) acquisition and storage in short-term memory, which has a maximum persistence of about one day, 2) consolidation, which apparently involves function of the hippocampus or amygdala, 3) storage in the long-term "engram" and 4) retrieval of the learned information. While neuropeptides and amine transmitters may influence all of these stages, the consolidation event apparently functions well only if PS occurs within one day of the learning event. This observation has led to the concept that the events of consolidation take place during PS and may be influenced by the high levels of vasopressin and ACTH peptides present in the CNS at that time. Our own practical experience tells us that mild stress facilitates learning; we learn more effectively if we know the examination is tomorrow and not next month. If, however, we study all night and fail to obtain our quota of PS, the "learned" material may disappear immediately after the examination.

The implied paradox of stimulation of higher brain centers by ACTH can however be understood in the light of new understanding of brain regulatory mechanisms. Actions of several neurotransmitters or neuromodulators have been found to show a biphasic response; a low amount of the substance may produce one effect, while a high dose may produce the opposite effect. For example, a low concentration of NE was found to facilitate an evoked response in a hippocampal preparation (Mueller et al., 1981) and in cerebellum (Basile and Dunwiddie, 1984) while a high concentration inhibited the responses. These changes appear to be due to different sensitivities of α and β receptors for NE. Stimulation of brain adenylate cyclase (and consequent cAMP production) by calcium has been shown to have an "inverted U" shaped concentration-response curve (Wolff, et al., 1977). Substance P applied in low amounts inhibited a monosynaptic spinal reflex in the cat, while higher amounts facilitated the response

(Krivoy et al., 1979). Actions of SP and other neuropeptides on nociception and other behaviors are frequently seen only within a narrow dose range of the peptide; a higher dose may produce the opposite effect, or no effect (Frederickson, et al., 1978, Stewart et al., 1982). Surprisingly, an "inverted U" shape dose-effect curve has been seen at the level of pure enzymes. ACTH stimulates adrenal cortex glucose-6-phosphate dehydrogenase, but only within a narrow concentration range; higher and lower concentrations of the hormone have less or no effect (Criss and McKerns, 1968). It was proposed that ACTH binds to the enzyme protein and affects its activity allosterically. Given then the complex brain systems regulating the phenomena discussed in this paper, one can comprehend that low stress or low amounts of certain peptides or monoamines may facilitate higher brain function, while intense stress or large amounts of the neurotransmitters or neuromodulators may completely inhibit higher centers. It can also be appreciated that the conditions of "disconnection" of the higher centers seen in PS may represent a third type of functioning of the same system in the CNS where a different set of auxiliary regulators or modulators has been brought into play.

SUBSTANCE P AND BEHAVIOR

In recent years it has become apparent that the neuropeptide substance P is involved in many CNS processes in addition to its effects on smooth muscles and blood vessels in the periphery of the body (Pernow, 1983; Skrabanek and Powell, 1983). SP and some related peptides show remarkable effects on learning and memory processes, and it interacts with stress responses. SP is perhaps best known for its evident role as a stimulus for dopamine release in both the nigro-striatal and mesolimbic-mesocortical systems. Different kinds of interactions between SP and the endogenous opioid peptides have been demonstrated (Hall and Stewart, 1983). It also has a role as a neurotransmitter in certain sensory neurons, especially those having to do with pain sensations. At the same time, exogenously administered SP can evoke antinociception.

This apparent paradox in actions of SP on pain seems to be due to selective processing of endogenous SP by enzymes in the brain to yield fragments which produce opposite effects in a given behavior paradigm (Hall and Stewart, 1983). Proposed enzymatic processing of SP in the brain is outlined in Fig. 4. The metalloendopeptidase which cleaves SP between the phenylalanine residues at positions seven and eight (Benuck and Marks, 1975; Lee et al., 1981) has been described as a SP-inactivating enzyme. It does inactivate SP for actions on classical SP receptors, where the intact C-terminal pentapeptide is the minimum structure with any activity, and N-terminal fragments have no activity at all.

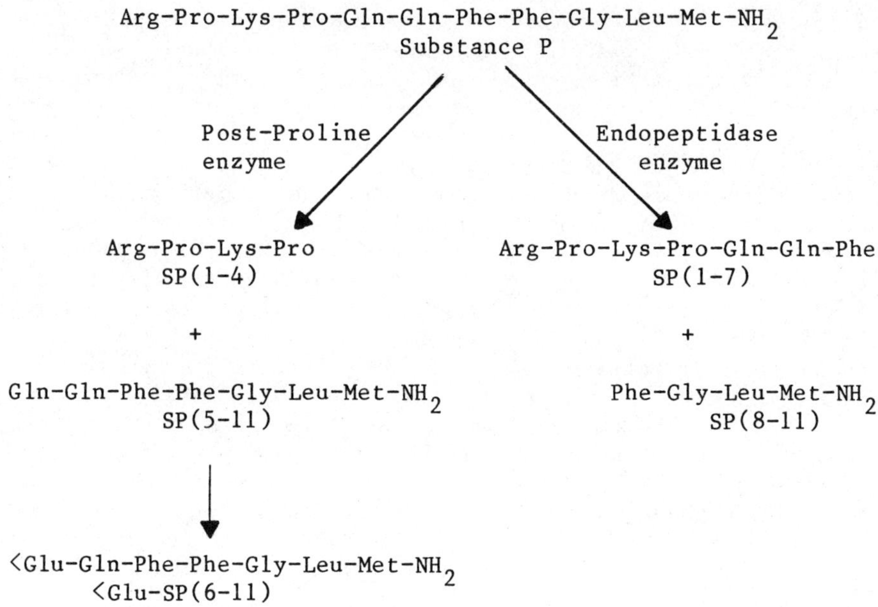

Fig. 4. Proposed processing of substance P in brain.
<Glu = Pyroglutamyl

However, the SP(1-7) which this enzyme produces evokes a range of behaviors when administered exogenously (either peripherally or centrally), and its presence has been demonstrated in brain (Stewart et al., 1982) and in cerebrospinal fluid (Rimon et al., 1984). The other SP-processing enzyme shown, the post-proline cleaving enzyme, produces SP(1-4) and SP(5-11) (Friedman et al., 1984). The N-terminal glutamine residue of SP(5-11) is unstable and probably cyclizes rapidly *in vivo* to the pyroglutamyl peptide (pyroglutamyl-SP(6-11)). This latter and related C-terminal fragments, which are agonists for peripheral SP receptors, also evoke a range of behavioral responses when administered to animals peripherally or centrally. In general, these effects are opposite to those produced by SP(1-7) (see Table 1) and can be interpreted as enhancing stress-like behaviors in rodents. In contrast, actions of SP(1-7) can be interpreted as minimizing stress and enhancing normal behaviors.

Several different kinds of interactions of SP and related peptides with endogenous opioid systems have been demonstrated. The early observation that the antinociception evoked by SP or SP(1-7) could be blocked by pretreatment of the animals with the opiate antagonist naloxone is consistent with the recent observation that SP stimulates release of methionine-enkephalin

Table 1. Effects of Substance P and Fragments on Behavior

Biological Effect	Peptide Structure		
	SP	SP-N	SP-C
Hot plate test (analgesia)	Analgesic Nx reverses	Analgesic Nx reverses	(Pain transmitter)
Stress-mediated analgesia:			
Immobilization	Blocks analgesia	No effect	Blocks anal.
Footshock	No effect	No effect	No effect
Aggression (isol. induced)	Inhibits Nx potentiates	Inhibits Nx no effect	Stimulates Nx blocks
Grooming	Increases	Inhibits	Increases
Rearing/leaning	Mixed	Increases	Reduces
Learning/memory			
Peripheral adm.	Enhances	?	?
N. accumbens	Inhibits	Enhances	Inhibits

SP-N is SP(1-7); SP-C is Pyroglutamyl-SP(7-11); Nx = Naloxone.

(Del Rio et al., 1983). Substance P and its C-terminal fragment block the opioid form of stress-induced analgesia (Hall and Stewart, 1983), while SP has been reported to inhibit many of the deleterious effects of chronic stress (Oehme et al., 1982). Inhibition by naloxone of the aggression-stimulating action of the C-terminal fragment of SP suggests a different kind of interaction of SP with endogenous opioid systems. In this latter experiment, aggression was measured in the isolated male mouse, where brain serotonin levels have been shown to be decreased. These results suggest that the N-terminal fragment of SP stimulates release of endogenous opioids, and that the C-terminal fragment may either stimulate or inhibit release of opioids, depending upon the experimental situation. Additional research is needed to clarify these points.

Exogenously administered substance P enhances performance in the one-trial passive avoidance paradigm; this effect can be interpreted as an enhancement of learning and memory (Schlesinger et al., 1983). Microinjection of SP into the lateral hypothalamus has been reported to enhance learning, while injection of SP into

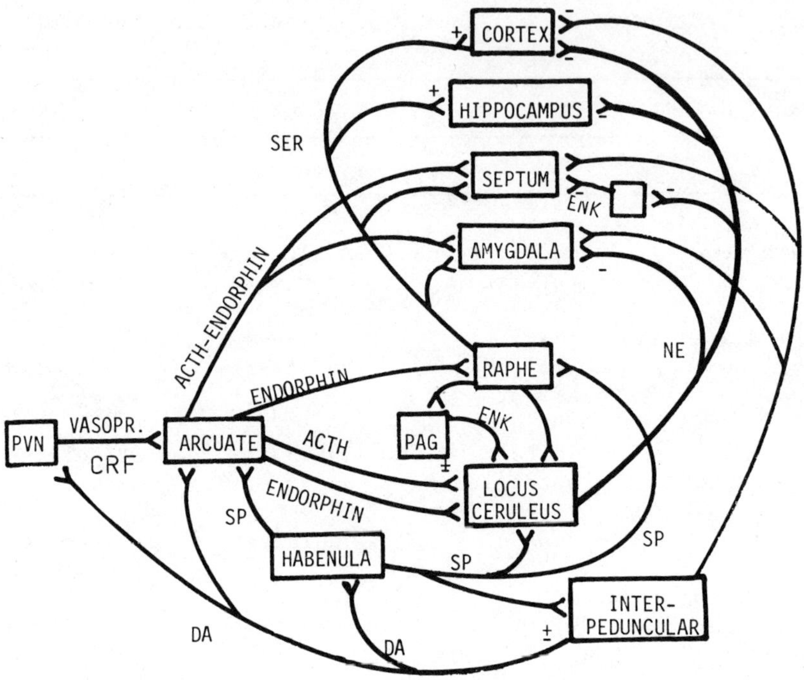

Fig. 5. Proposed neuronal circuitry mediating the effects of stress on behavior. Presumed excitatory and inhibitory effects are indicated by + and -, respectively, although biphasic effects are proposed in some cases. PVN = paraventricular nucleus; PAG = periacqueductal grey matter.

the amygdala was reported to impair learning (Huston and Staubli, 1979). More recently, microinjection of the N-terminal and C-terminal fragments of SP into the nucleus accumbens has been reported to enhance or abolish learning, respectively, in a similar paradigm (Gaffori et al. 1984).

While there is no firm evidence at the present time that these actions of SP on behavior are mediated through the brain ACTH-End system, our present knowledge of SP neuroanatomy is consistent with such an interpretation (Porter and O'Connor, 1982). A simplified version of the relevant neuroanatomy which integrates the various kinds of evidence discussed in this paper is presented in Fig. 5. The neuroanatomy represented there suggests that SP may exert its actions directly on the locus ceruleus and raphe, by acting upon the ACTH cells of the arcuate nucleus of the hypothalamus (Hisano et al., 1984), or via the mesolimbic-mesocortical dopamine system. The cell bodies of this latter system are in the interpeduncular nucleus, and microinjection of SP into this area produces profound effects on behavior (Kelley et al., 1979). Extrahypothalamic terminals of CRF neurons are not indicated in Fig. 5, but may be important in mediating these behaviors, as suggested above. Also not shown are the vasopressin axons from hypothalamus which terminate on SP cells in the habenula (Buijs, 1980). Axons of the norepinephrine neurons originating in the locus ceruleus and terminating on various limbic brain areas are indicated by heavy lines, since these neurons appear to be of prime importance in mediating the behaviors discussed here.

These suggestions concerning roles for central ACTH-endorphin neurons and associated peptidergic and aminergic circuitry integrate and extend evidence from many different kinds of observations. The hypothesis set forth in this paper was first described in public in 1979, and a brief account appeared in 1981 (Stewart, 1981). Those presentations summarized the supporting literature evidence at that time. Since then much additional support for the hypothesis has appeared in the literature; many of the literature references herein are to recent papers. This increasing body of supporting evidence attests to the general correctness of these proposals. There probably are significant errors in the assessments and predictions made here due to the inadequacy of our present knowledge of function and interactions of peptidergic neurons. Nevertheless, these proposals provide the basis for a wide variety of experiments to test the hypotheses presented and may well open the way for greatly increased understanding of brain function and behavior.

ACKNOWLEDGMENT

Work on substance P reported here was supported by grant NS-18531 from the NINCDS-NIH.

REFERENCES

Aghajanian, G. K., 1978, Tolerance of locus coeruleus neurones to morphine and suppression of withdrawal response by clonidine, Nature, 276:186.

Antelman, S. M., and Caggiula, A. R., 1980, Stress-induced behavior: chemotherapy without drugs, in: "Psychobiology of Consciousness," J.M. Davidson and R.J. Davidson, eds. Plenum, New York.

Basbaum, A. I., and Fields, H. L., 1978, Endogenous pain control mechanisms: Review and hypothesis, Ann. Neurol., 4:451.

Basile, A. S., and Dunwiddie, T. V., 1984, Norepinephrine elicits both excitatory and inhibitory responses from Purkinje cells in the in vitro rat cerebellar slice, Brain Res., 296:15.

Benuck, M., and Marks, N., 1975, Enzymatic inactivation of substance P by a partially purified enzyme from rat brain, Biochem. Biophys. Res. Comm., 65:153.

Beny, J. L., and Baertschi, A. J., 1982, Synthetic CRF needs AVP for full corticotropin releasing activity, Experientia, 38:1078.

Bertolini, A., Ferrari, W., Fratta, W., Gessa, G. L., Merew, G. P. and Tagliamonte, A., 1975, Sexual arousal in male animals: a central effect of ACTH-like peptides in mammals, in "Peptides: Chemistry Structure Function," R. Walter and J. Meienhofer, eds., Ann Arbor Science Pub., Ann Arbor, MI.

Bohus, B., and de Wied, D., 1966, Inhibitory and facilitatory effect of two related peptides on extinction of avoidance behavior, Science, 153:318.

Bohus, B., Gispen, W, and de Wied, D., 1973, Comparison of ACTH(4-10) and LVP on acquisition of conditioned avoidance response, Neuroendocrinol., 11:139.

Braun, B. G., 1984, Towards a theory of multiple personality and other dissociative phenomena, Psychiat. Clin. North America, 7:171.

Britton, K. T., Lyon, M., Vale, W. and Koob, G. F, 1984, Stress-induced secretion of corticotropin releasing factor immunoreactivity in rat cerebrospinal fluid, Soc. for Neurosci. Abst., 10:94 (Part I).

Buijs, R. M., 1980, Immunocytochemical demonstration of vasopressin and oxytocin in the rat brain by light and electron microscopy, J. Histochem. Cytochem., 28:357.

Capponi, A. M., Faviod-Coune, C. A., Gaillard, R. C. and Muller, A. F., 1982, Binding and activation properties of Angiotensin II in dispersed rat anterior pituitary cells, Endocrinology, 110:1043.

Chu, N.-S. and Bloom, F. E., 1974, Norepinephrine-containing neurons: changes in spontaneous discharge patterns during sleep and waking, Science, 179:908.

Clark, J. T., Smith, E. R. and Davidson, J. M., 1984, Enhancement of sexual motivation in male rats by yohimbine, Science, 225:847.

Cohen, D. B., 1980, The cognitive activity of sleep, Prog. Brain Res., 53:307.

Cohen, M., Keets, A., Krivoy, W. A. and Unger, G., 1965, Effect of actinomycin D on morphine tolerance, Proc. Soc. Exp. Biol. Med., 119:381.

Collier, H. O. J., 1980, Cellular site of opiate dependence, Nature, 283:625.

Corner, M. A., Mirmiran, M., and Bour, H., 1981, On the role of active (REM) sleep in ontogenesis of the central nervous system, in "Sleep 1980, 5th. Eur. Cong. Sleep Res.

Amsterdam", W. P. Koella, ed., Karger, Basel.

Corner, M. A., Mirmiran, M., Bour, H. L. M. G., Boer, G. J., van de Poll, N. E., van Oyen, H. G. and Uylings, H. B. M., 1980, Does rapid-eye-movement sleep play a role in brain development?, Prog. Brain Res., 53:347.

Criss, W. E. and McKerns, K. W., 1868, Activation of cow adrenal glucose 6-phosphate dehydrogenase by adrenocorticotropin, Biochemistry, 7:2364.

Czeisler, C. A., Moore-Ede, M. C., and Coleman, R. M., 1982, Rotating shift work schedules that disrupt sleep are improved by applying circadian principles, Science, 217:460.

de Wied, D., and Gispen, W. H., 1976, Impaired development of tolerance to morphine analgesia in rats with hereditary diabetes insipidus, Psychopharmacologia, 46:27.

de Wied, D., 1977, Behavioral effects of neuropeptides related to ACTH, MSH and ß-LPH, Ann. N.Y. Acad. Sci., 297:263.

del Rio, J., Naranjo, J. R., Yang, H.-Y. T., and Costa, E., 1983, Substance P-induced release of met5-enkephalin from striatal and periaqueductal gray slices, Brain Res., 279:121.

Dorsa, D. M. and Smith, E. M., 1981, Facilitation of mounting behavior in male rats by intracranial injection of LRH, Regul. Peptides, 1:147.

Efrati, P., 1978, Epidemiology, symptomatology and treatment of Buthinae stings, Handb. Exp. Pharm., 48:312.

Frederickson, R. C. A., Burgis, V., Harrell, E., and Edwards, J. 1978, Dual actions of substance P on nociception: Possible role of endogenous opioids, Science, 199:1359.

Friedman, T. C., Orlowski, M., and Wilk, S., 1984, Prolyl endopeptidase: Inhibition in vivo by N-benzyloxycarbonyl-prolyl-prolinal, J. Neurochem., 42:237.

Gaffori, O., Stewart, J. M., and de Wied, D., 1984, Influence of sustance P and fragments on passive avoidance behavior, Experientia, 40:89.

Garrud, P., Gray, J. A., and de Wied, D., 1974, Pituitary adrenal hormones and extinction of rewarded behavior in the rat, Physiol. Behav., 12:109.

Gessa, G. L., Paglietti, G., and Quaranotti, B. P., 1979, Induction of copulatory behavior in sexually inactive rats by naloxone, Science, 204:203.

Gillies, G., and Lowry, P., 1979, Corticotropin releasing factor may be modulated vasopressin, Nature, 278:463.

Gold, M. S., Byck, R., Sweeney, D. R., and Kleber, H. D., 1979, Endorphin-locus coeruleus connection mediates opiate action and withdrawal, Biomedicine, 30:1.

Gu, J., Polak, J. M., Probert, L., Islam, K. N., Marangos, P.J., Mina, S., Adrian, T. E., McGregor, G. P., O'Shaughnessy, D. J., and Bloom, S. R., 1983, Peptidergic innervation of the human male genital tract, J. Urol.,

130:386.

Hall, M. E., and Stewart, J. M., 1983a, Substance P and behavior: Opposite effects of N-terminal and C-terminal fragments, Peptides, 4:763.

Hall, M. E., and Stewart, J. M., 1983b Prevention of stress-induced analgesia by substance P, Behav. Brain Res., 10:375.

Hazelwood, R. R., Dietz, P. E., and Burgess, A. W., 1983, "Autoerotic Fatalities", Heath, Lexington, MA.

Hisano, J., Okamura, Y., and Daikoku, S., 1984, Synaptic regulation of hypothalamus neurons containing ACTH by substance P, Brain Res., 308:162.

Hosobuchi, Y., Lamb, S., and Baskin, D., 1980, Reversal of tolerance to opiates by oral tryptophan, Pain, 9:161.

Huston, J. P., and Staubli, V., 1979, Post-trial injection of substance P into lateral hypothalamus and amygdala, respectively, facilitates and impairs learning, Behav. Neural Biol., 27:244.

Huxley, A., 1979, "Brave New World", Harper-Row, New York.

Jacquet, Y. F., 1978, Opiate effects after adrenocorticotropin or ß-endorphin injection in the periaqueductal gray matter of rats, Science, 201:1032.

Jacquet, Y. F., Klee, W. A., Rice, K. C., Iijima, I., and Minamikawa, J., 1977, Stereospecific and nonstereospecific effects of (+)- and (-)- morphine: Evidence for a new class of receptors? Science, 198:842.

Jouvet, M., 1980, Paradoxical sleep and the nature-nurture controversy, Prog. Brain Res., 53:331.

Kafi, S., and Gaillard, J.-M., 1981, Pre- and postsynaptic effect of yohimbine on rat paradoxical sleep, in "Sleep 1980: 5th Eur. Congr. Sleep Res., Amsterdam", W. P. Koella, ed., Karger, Basel.

Kalin, N. H., 1983, Associated endocrine, physiological and behavioral changes in rhesus monkeys following intravenous CRF administration, Peptides, 4:211.

Kelley, A. E., Stinus, L., and Iversen, S. D., 1979, Behavioral activation induced in the rat by substance P infusion into ventral tegmental area: Implication of dopaminergic A10 neurones, Neurosci. Lett., 11:335.

Kleinlogel, H., Scholtysik, G., and Sayers, A. C., 1975, Effects of clonidine and BS 100-141 on the EEG-sleep pattern in rats, Eur. J. Pharmacol., 33:159.

Kozlowski, G. P., Chu, L., Hostetter, G., and Kerdelhue, B., 1980, Cellular characteristics of immunolabeled leutinizing hormone releasing hormone (LHRH) neurons, Peptides, 1:37.

Krieger, D. T., 1983, Brain peptides: What, where, and why?, Science, 222:975.

Krivoy, W. A., Couch, J. R., Henry, J. L., and Stewart, J. M., 1979, Synaptic modulation by substance P, Federation Proc., 38:2344.

Krivoy, W. A., Zimmermann, E., and Lande, S., 1974, Facilitation of development of resistance to morphine analgesia by desglycinamide[9]-lysine vasopressin, Proc. Nat. Acad. Sci., 71:1852.

Lanfumey, L., and Adrien, J., 1981, Effects of a noradrenergic agonist on sleep in the rat, in "Sleep 1980, 5th. Eur. Congr. Sleep Res., Amsterdam", W. P. Koella, ed., Karger, Basel.

Lee, C., Sandberg, B., Hanley, M. and Iversen, L., 1981, Purification and characterization of a membrane-bound substance P degrading enzyme from human brain, Eur. J. Biochem., 114:315.

LeRoith, D., Liotta, A. S., Roth, J., Shiloach, J., Lewis, M. E., Pert, C. B., and Krieger, D. T., 1982, Corticotropin and ß-endorphin-like materials are native to unicellular organisms, Proc. Natl. Acad. Sci., 79:2086.

Lewis, J. W., Cannon, J. T., and Liebeskind, J. C., 1980, Opioid and non-opioid mechanisms of stress analgesia, Science, 208:623.

Livingston, K. E., and Hornykiewicz, O., eds., 1978, "Limbic Mechanisms", Plenum, New York.

Macdonald, J. M., 1977, "Bombers and Firesetters", Thomas, Springfield, IL.

MacLean, P. D., 1973, "A Triune Concept of the Brain and Behavior", Univ. of Toronto Press, Toronto.

Mains, R. E., Eipper, B. A., and Ling, N., 1977, Common precursor to corticotropin and endorphins, Proc. Nat. Acad. Sci., 74:3014.

Marshall, P., Surridge, D., and Delva, N., 1981, The role of nocturnal penile tumescence in differentiating between organic and psychogenic impotence: The first stage of validation, Arch. Sex Behav., 10:1.

Martin, J. T., 1978, Imprinting behavior: Pituitary-adrenocortical modulation of the approach response, Science, 200:565.

McCarley, R. W., and Hobson, J. A., 1975, Sleep cycle oscillation: Reciprocal discharge by two brainstem neuronal groups, Science, 189:55.

Mintz, J., O'Hare, K., O'Brien, C. P., and Goldschmidt, J., 1974, Sexual problems of heroin addicts, Arch. Gen. Psychiat., 31:700.

Moore-Ede, M. C., Czeisler, C. A., and Richardson, G. S., 1983, Circadian timekeeping in health and disease, N. Engl. J. Med., 309:469; 309:530.

Morales, A., Surridge, D. H., and Marshall, P. G., 1981, Yohimbine for treatment of impotence in diabetes, N. Engl. J. Med., 305:1221.

Morley, J. E., and Levine, A. S., 1982, CRF, grooming and ingestive behavior, Life Sci., 31:1459.

Moss, R. L., McCann, S. M., and Dudley, C. A., 1975, Releasing hormones and sexual behavior, Prog. Brain Res., 42:37.

Mueller, A. J., Hoffer, B. J., and Dunwiddie, T. V., 1981, Noradrenergic responses in rat hippocampus: Evidence for mediation by α and ß receptors in the *in vitro* slice, *Brain Res.*, 214:113.

Oehme, P., Hecht, K., Piesche, L., Hilse, H., and Rathsack, R., 1982, Relations of substance P to stress and catecholamine metabolism, *in* "Substance P in the Nervous System", Ciba Fdn. Symp. #91, R. Porter and M. O'Connor, eds., Pitman, London.

Pernow, B., 1983, Substance P, *Pharmacol. Rev.*, 35:85.

Porter, R., and O'Connor, M., eds., 1982, "Substance P in the Nervous System" Ciba Fdn. Symp. #91, Pitman, London.

Rimon, R., LeGreves, P., Nyberg, F., Haikkila, L., Salmela, L., and Terenius, L., 1984, Elevation of substance P-like peptides in CSF of psychiatric patients, *Biol. Psychiat.*, 19:509.

Roche, K. E., and Leshner, A. I., 1979, ACTH and vasopressin treatments immediately after a defeat increase future submissiveness in male mice, *Science*, 204:1343.

Rubin, R. T., 1975, Sleep-endocrinology studies in man, *Prog. Brain Res.*, 42:73.

Sagan, C., 1977, "The Dragons of Eden", Random House, New York.

Sandler, M., and Gessa, G. L., eds., 1975, "Sexual Behavior: Pharmacology and Biochemistry", Raven, New York.

Sandman, C. A., Beckwith, B. E., and Kastin, A. J., 1980, Are learning and attention related to the sequence of amino acids in ACTH/MSH peptides?, *Peptides*, 1:277.

Schenberg, S. and Pereira Lima, F. A., 1978, Venoms of *Ctenidae*, *Handb. Exp. Pharmacol.*, 48:217.

Schlesinger, K., Lipsitz, D. U., Peck, P. L., Pelleymounter, M. A., Stewart, J. M., and Chase, T. N., 1983, Substance P enhancement of passive and active avoidance conditioning in mice, *Pharmacol. Biochem. Behav.*, 19:655.

Schreiber, F. R., 1973, "Sybil", Warner Books, New York.

Seino, S., Sakurai, H., Kazuya, H., Tsuda, K., Tanigawa, K., Takahashi, K., Seino, Y., and Imura, H., 1982, Immunocytochemical localization of CRF in ovine hypothalamus, *Peptides*, 3:183.

Simon-Oppermann, C., Gray, D., Szczepanska-Sadowska, E., and Simon, E., 1983, Vasopressin in blood and third ventricle CSF of dogs in chronic experiments, *Am. J. Physiol.*, 245:R541.

Skrabanek, P., and Powell, D., eds., 1983, "Substance P Dublin", Boole Press, Dublin, Ireland.

Smotherman, W. P. and Levine, S., 1980, ACTH-(4-10) affects behavior but not plasma corticosterone levels in a conditioned taste aversion situation, *Peptides*, 1:207.

Sofroniew, M. V., and Weindl, A., 1978, Projections from the parvocellular vasopressin- and neurophysin-containing neurons of the suprachiasmatic nucleus, *Am. J. Anat.*,

153:391.

Stefanick, M. L., Smith, E. R., Clark, J. T., and Davidson, J. M., 1982, Effects of a potent dopamine receptor agonist, RDS-27, on penile reflexes and seminal emission in intact and spinally transected Rats, Physiol. Behav., 29:973.

Stevenson, R. L., 1964, "Dr. Jekyll and Mr. Hyde", Prentice-Hall, New York.

Stewart, J. M., 1981, Brain ACTH-endorphin neurons as regulators of central nervous system activity, in "Peptides 1980", K. Brunfeldt, ed., Scriptor, Copenhagen.

Stewart, J. M. and Channabasavaiah, K., 1979, Evolutionary aspects of some neuropeptides, Federation Proc., 38:2302.

Stewart, J. M., Chipkin, R. E., Channabasavaiah, K., Gay, M. L., and Krivoy, W. A., 1980, Inhibition of development of tolerance to morphine by a peptide related to ACTH, in "Neural Peptides and Neuron. Commun.", E. Costa and M. Trabucchi, eds., Raven Press, New York, 1980.

Stewart, J. M., Hall, M. E., Harkins, J., Frederickson, R. C. A., Terenius, L., Hokfelt, T., and Krivoy, W. A., 1982, A fragment of substance P with specific central activity: SP(1-7), Peptides, 3:851.

Stoller, R. J., 1975, "Perversion", Pantheon, New York.

Strahlendorf, H. K., Strahlendorf, J. C., and Barnes, C. D., 1980, Endorphin-mediated inhibition of locus ceruleus neurons, Brain Res., 191:284.

Swanson, L. W., Sawchenko, P. E., Rivier, J., and Vale, W. W., 1983, Organization of ovine CRF immunoreactive cells and fibers in the rat brain: an immunohistochemical study, Neuroendocrinol., 36:165.

Szekely, J. I., Miglecz, E., Dunai-Kovacs, Z., Tarnawa, I., Ronai, A. Z., Graf, L., and Bajusz, S., 1979, Attenuation of morphine tolerance and dependence by α-melanocyte stimulating hormone (α-MSH), Life Sci., 24:1931.

Tapp, W. N., and Holloway, F. N., 1981, Phase shifting circadian rhythms produces retrograde amnesia, Science, 211:1056.

Terenius, L., 1976, Somatostatin and ACTH are peptides with partial antagonist-like selectivity for opiate receptors, Eur. J. Pharmacol., 38:211.

Tilders, F., Tatemoto, K., and Berkenbosch, F., 1984, The intestinal peptide PHI-27 potentiates the action of CRF on ACTH release from rat pituitary fragments in vitro, Endocrinology, 115:1633.

Vale, W., Spiess, J., Rivier, C., and Rivier, J., 1981, Characterization of a 41-residue ovine hypothalamic peptide that stimulates secretion of corticotropin and ß-endorphin, Science, 213:1394.

Valentino, R. J., Foote, S. L., and Aston-Jones, G., 1983, CRF activates noradrenergic neurons of the locus ceruleus, Brain Res., 270:363.

Valzelli, W., 1981, "Psychobiology of Aggression and Violence",

Raven, New York.

Versteeg, D. H. G., 1973, Effect of two ACTH analogs on norepinephrine metabolism in rat brain, Brain Res., 49:483.

Virag, R., Ottesen, B., Fahrenkrug, J., Levy, C., and Wagner, G., 1982, VIP release during penile erection in man, Lancet, 2:1166.

Walter, R., Ritzmann, R. F., Bhargava, H. N., and Flexner, L. B., 1979, Prolyl-leucyl-glycinamide, cyclo(leucylglycine), and derivatives block development of physical dependence on morphine in mice, Proc. Natl. Acad. Sci., 76:518.

Watson, S. J., Akil, H., Richard, C. W., III, and Barchas, J. D., 1978a, Evidence for two separate opiate peptide neuronal systems, Nature, 275:226.

Watson, S. J., Richard, C. W., III, and Barchas, J. D., 1978b, ACTH in rat brain: Immunocytochemical localization in cells and axons, Science, 200:1180.

Weitzman, E. D., Boyer, R. M., Kapen, S., and Hellman, L., 1975, The relationship of sleep and sleep stages to Neuro-endocrine secretion and biological rhythms in man, Rec. Prog. Hormone Res., 31:399.

Williams, R. L., Karacan, I., eds., 1978, "Sleep Disorders", Wiley, New York.

Willoughby, D. O., Martin, J. B., 1978, The role of the limbic system in neuroendocrine regulation, in "Limbic Mechanisms", H. E. Livingston, and D. Hornykiewicz, eds., Plenum, New York.

Wolff, D. J., Brostrom, M. A., and Brostrom, C. O., 1977, Divalent cation binding sites of CDR and their role in the regulation of brain cyclic nucleotide metabolism, in "Calcium Binding Proteins and Calcium Function", R. H. Wasserman, R. A. Corradino, E. Carafoli, R. H. Kretsinger, D. H. MacLennan, F. L. Siegel, eds, North Holland, New York.

Yaksh, T. L., and Tyce, G. M., 1979, Microinjection of morphine into the periaqueductal gray evokes the release of serotonin from spinal cord, Brain Res., 171:176.

SOME ENDOCRINE AND METABOLIC CONSEQUENCES OF THE STRESS FOLLOWING HIGH LEVEL SPINAL CORD SECTION

Kalina I. Vaptzarova and Panteley G.Popov

Regeneration Research Laboratory
Bulgarian Academy of Sciences
Sofia-1431, Bulgaria

INTRODUCTION

The important role of glucocorticoids in the stress pathogenesis is characterised by two main points: a rise in plasma concentration of glucocorticoids (GC) and protection against stress by glucocorticoid hormones. Yet, the mechanism of these effects is poorly understood.

Among the possible causes of the stress-elevated concentration of GCs could be considered: an increase of consumption of GCs induced by stress accompanied by a switch-off (or a new setting at a higher point of the glucocorticoidostat in hypothalamus) and/or a lowered responsiveness of body cells to GCs with a compensatory rise in secretion. The latter alternative suggests a new possibility for regulation of the effects of GCs along with the variation in concentration, namely changes in responsiveness of the cells to the corticosteroids. Experimental data in this respect are almost lacking. The plasma glucocorticoid antagonizing factor (GAF) discovered by Berry (1980) is the first indication for the possibility of the regulation of the responsiveness to GCs. GAF is induced in macrophages under the influence of endotoxin. No data for the possible physiological role of GAF are presented till now. The presence of a macromolecular modulator inhibiting the nuclear binding of estrogen receptors was proposed recently in in vitro experiments (Sato et al., 1983).

In this paper we report that decentralisation of the liver by high level (C_7) transection of the spinal cord (HLTSC) brings about a dramatic decrease of responsiveness to the GCs in the liver. It is well known that HISCS leads to a transitory state of areflexia under the level of transection, designated as spinal shock, accompanied by a pronounced decrease of sympathetic tonus. Along with the spinal shock HLTSC brings about a severe stress.

Glucocorticoid hormones are inducers of several hepatic enzymes, the best studied being tryptophan oxygenase (TO) and tyrosine aminotransferase (TAT). A new RNA and protein biosynthesis is a prerequisite for the induction of TO and TAT by GCs.

The influence of the central nervous system (CNS) on the biosynthesis of macromolecules is comparatively little studied. As a model for studying the effect of CNS on the biosynthesis of macromolecules and the responsiveness to hormones we have chosen the GC induction of TO and TAT in vivo in rats with HLTSC. This paper represents a survey summarizing our experimental results, some of which appeared as preliminary communications or in detail elsewhere (Vaptzarova et al., 1969, Vaptzarova et al., 1973a,b, Vaptzarova and Hanoune 1976, Vaptzarova et al., 1980a,b).

MATERIALS AND METHODS

All the experiments were carried out on male albino "Wistar" rats, weighing 120-180 g. Some of the animals were adrenalectomized translumbarly under light ether anaesthesia and used in experiments on the fourth day after operation. Hypophysectomies were performed transauricularly as described by Strashimirov (1967). Transection of the spinal cord at C_7 or L_3 level was carried out under light ether anaesthesia. Sham operation consisted in exposing spinal cord without incision. The operations were performed during the time of the lowest circadian activity, i.e. between 8 and 9 a.m. for the 4th h group and between 12 a.m. and 1 p.m. for the 24th and 48th h group, except the 12th h group which was killed at 9 p.m. TAT activity was determined according to the method of Canellakis and Cohen, as modified by Rosen et al. (1963) and TO activity - according to Knox et al. (1966). The results obtained for both enzymes are expressed as units per gram wet weight, one unit defined as the amount of enzyme yielding 1 micromol product after incubation for 1 h at 37°. The data presented in this paper both for TAT and TO refer to the total enzyme activity after activation of the latent forms of this enzymes by preincubation with the cofactors of TAT and TO. Adenylate cyclase activity was measured as described by Hanoune et al. (1975). Results are expressed in pmol cAMP formed per mg protein for 10 min at 30°. The activity of cyclic nucleotide phosphodiesterase was determined according to the method of Thompson and Appleman (1971), as modified by Vaptzarova and Hanoune (1976). Results are expressed in nmol of cAMP transformed per mg protein for 10 min at 37°. Radioimmunoassay of cyclic nucleotides was performed as described by Vaptzarova and Hanoune (1976). The plasma corticosterone concentration was determined fluorimetrically according to Silber et al. (1958). The blood glucose concentration was determined with the Boehringer test for determination of the true glucose (glucose oxidase-peroxidase method), and plasma insulin concentration - as described by Vaptzarova et al. (1980). The steroid binding capacity of rat liver cytosol glucocorticoid reseptors (GCR) was determined by the method of Baxter and Tomkins (1971). Scatchard (1949) plots were constructed with 5 dilutions of the labelled dexamethasone (DM) and experimental points were fitted according to a linear regression equation. Nuclear binding was studied as follows: nuclei from adrenalectomized both control and C_7-chordotomized rats, isolated by the method of Dabeva (1976) were incubated with labelled hormone-receptor complexes (HRC) from either control or C_7-chordotomized animals for 15 min at 25°. After chilling, centrifugation (600 xg for 5 min at 4°) and 3 washes with buffer the radioactivity (RA) of HRC bound to the nuclei was measured in a toluene-triton X-100 based liquid scintillation cocktail. The DNA content of the nuclei suspension was determined according to Burton (1956). In vivo labelling experiments with ^{3}H-DM were performed as follows: ^{3}H-DM with a specific activity 20 Ci/mmol was injected i.p. in a dose of 44 μ Ci per rat both in control and in C_7-chordotomized animals. The rats were killed 30 min, 1, 2, 3 and 4 h after the administration of the labelled steroid. Liver cytosol and nuclei were isolated as described above and their RA was estimated. The RA of cytosol was measured after treatment with charcoal-dextran in order to eliminate the unbound labelled DM. All substances administered in vivo were injected intraperitoneally. A microcrystalline suspension of hydrocortisone acetate (G.Richter, Budapest) was applied in a dose of 100 mg/kg body weight. Actinomycin D (Serva) was dissolved in 1,2-propylene glycol and injected i.p. at a dose of 1,0 mg/kg. Cycloheximide (Sigma), freshly dissolved in saline was administered by the same rout at a dose of 1,6 mg/kg.

RESULTS

The rise in plasma corticosterone level is the first easily demonstrable biochemical manifestation of the stress.

As shown in Fig.1 sham operation brought about a 2,7-fold increase increase in the level of the corticosterone 2,5 h after the operation as compared to intact controls. This rise in corticosterone level can be ascribed to the operation stress. C_7-level sectioned animals showed much more pronounced (4,1-fold) elevation of plasma corticosterone level at the same time after the operation. Therefore, the C_7-level section of the spinal cord causes a severe stress and cannot prevent the stress rise in plasma corticosterone. It is interesting to note that 24 h after C_7-level section the plasma corticosterone level was still 2,6 times higher than the controls, whereas in sham operated rats the corticosterone concentration was nearly normal. It is well known that glucocorticoids selectively stimulate de novo synthesis of tyrosine aminotransferase (EC 2.6.1.5.) and tryptophan oxigenase (EC 1.11.1.4.) in liver. Maximal response of these two hepatic enzymes can be seen 4-5 h after i.p. administration of the

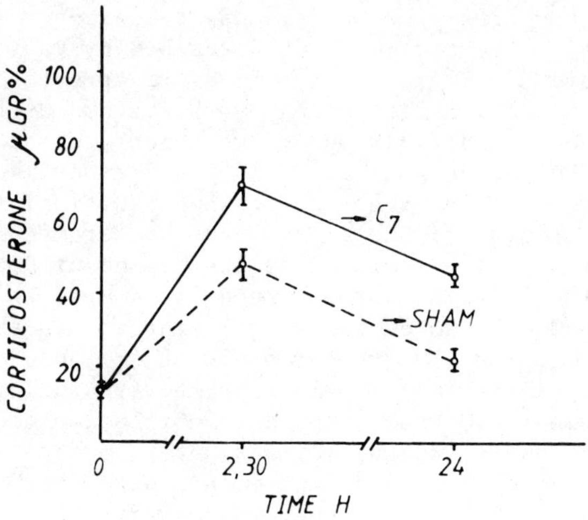

Fig. 1. Effect of C_7-level spinal cord section on the plasma corticosterone level. Abscissa, time after surgery; ordinate, corticosterone concentration in µ g per 100 ml blood. Each experimental group consisted of 7 to 12 animals. Each value is the mean ± s.e.m.

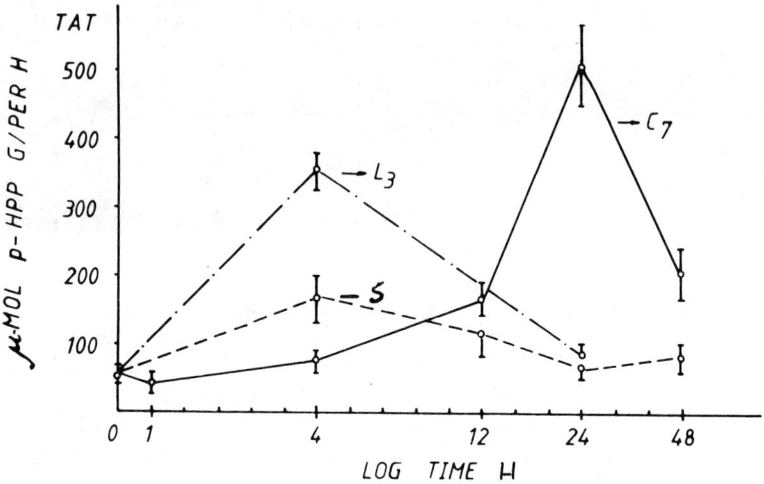

Fig. 2. TAT activity after C_7- and L_3-level spinal cord section and sham operation: a time response study in non-adrenalectomized rats. Abscissa, log time after surgery; ordinate, enzyme activity. Each experimental group consisted of 5 to 17 animals. Each value is the mean ± s.e.m.

hormone. The changes in tyrosine aminotransferase that follow the section of the spinal cord at the level of C_7 or L_3 and sham operation in different terms after the surgery in non-adrenalectomized rats are shown in Fig.2.

The pattern of enzyme activity in sham operated animals shows an increase only at 4th h after the intervention,followed by marked decrease at the 12th h and return to normal level at 24th h. These changes correspond to those obtained with stress agents or following application of the glucocorticoids. Spinal cord section at L_3-level (i.e. below the segments innervating the liver) resulted in a pattern of the enzyme changes similar to that of the sham operated animals but more pronounced. Section of the spinal cord at C_7-level (i.e. above the segments which innervate the liver), gives a quite diffe - ent enzyme pattern. The stress rise at the 4th h after the operation, seen in sham operated and L_3 sectioned rats, is lacking in this group, despite the four-fold rise in corticosterone plasma concentration. Therefore, TAT does not respond to the increased corticosterone concentration. At the 24th h after C_7-level spinal cord section, contrary to sham-operated and L_3-sectioned rats, we found out a nine-fold rise of TAT activity which could be seen, although less pronounced, in adrenalectomized rats, too.

It might be supposed that high section of the spinal cord would block the stress reaction of the adrenals by cutting off the abnormal impulses coming from the body below the lesion. The assay of plasma corticosterone level showed that it was not the case. Then we studied the induction of liver TAT activity by hydrocortisone administration to spinal cord sectioned rats. Hydrocortisone was injected immediately after the spinal cord section and enzyme assay was performed 4 h and 24 h after the operation. Both intact and adrenalectomized rats were used in these experiments. From Fig. 3A and 3B is evident that spinal cord section at C_7-level blocked the inducing effect of hydrocortisone at the 4th h both in intact and adrenalectomized rats, the inhibitory effect being more clearly seen in adrenalectomized rats. L_3-section of the spinal cord not only did not blocked the inducing effect of hydrocortisone, but even enhanced it. The influence of hydrocortisone at 24 h has disappeared - the characteristic C_7-induction is seen undiminished and in intact and L_3-sectioned animals enzyme activity is back to normal.

TO is another glucocorticoid inducible enzyme. It was interesting therefore to know what would be the effect of C_7-level section of the spinal cord on the glucocorticoid induction of TO.

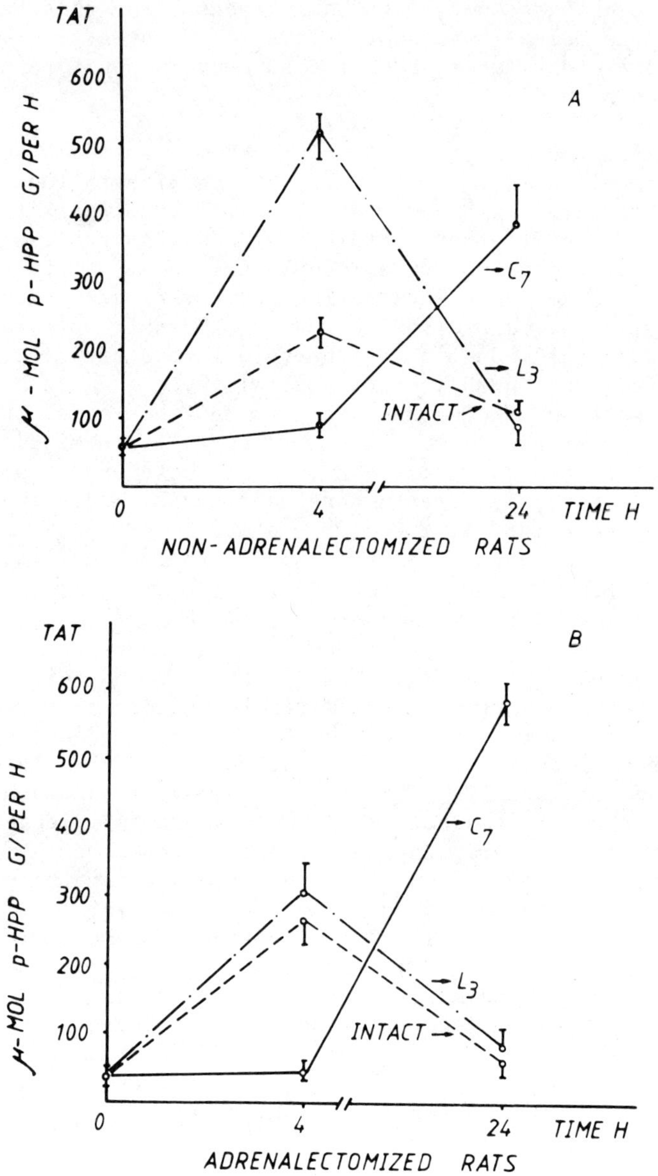

Fig.3 A. Hydrocortisone induction of TAT activity in rats with intact or transectioned at C_7- or L_3-level spinal cord. Enzyme activity is assayed 4 h or 24 h after the operation and hydrocortisone administration. Non-adrenalectomized rats. Each experimental group consisted of 5 to 10 animals Each value is the mean + s.e.m.

B. Hydrocortisone induction of TAT activity in rats with intact or transectioned at C_7- or L_3-level spinal cord. Adrenalectomized rats.

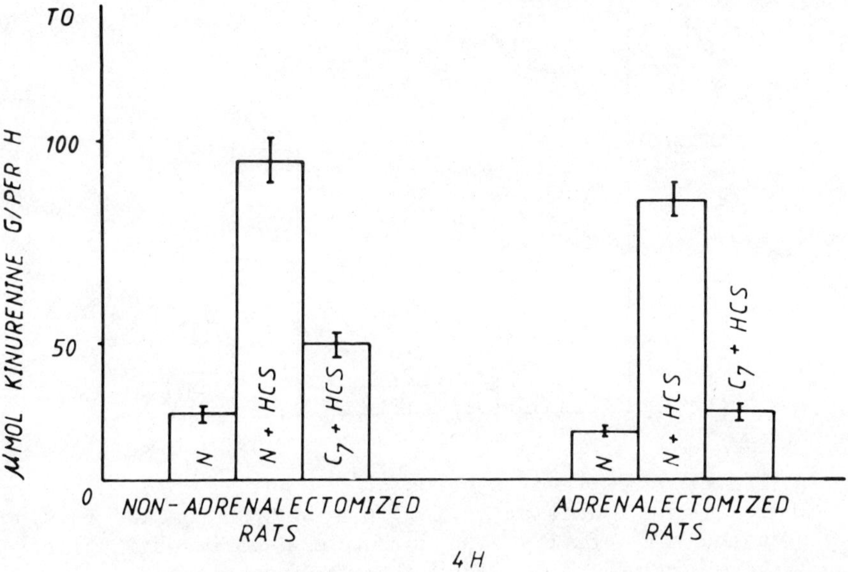

Fig. 4. TO activity after hydrocortisone induction in intact and spinal cord sectioned rats. Ordinate, enzyme activity. Each experimental group consisted of 5-12 animals. Each value is the mean ± s.e.m.

As shown in Fig. 4, the glucocorticoid induction of TO is depressed after C_7-section of the spinal cord, similarly to TAT, the inhibition being more pronounced in adrenalectomized rats, too. The phenomenon of unresponsiveness to the hydrocortisone after C_7-level section of the spinal cord can not be attributed to disturbances in absorption of hydrocortisone, since experiments with labelled hydrocortisone and dexamethasone did not reveal a decreased peritoneal absorption. Experiments with ^3H dexamethasone showed that the labelled glucocorticoid reached the hepatocytes nuclei unhindered. These experiments and the absence of the stress induction at 4th h showed clearly that the liver TAT and TO systems became refractory both to endogenously and exogenously elevated glucocorticoids at the 4th h after C_7-section of the spinal cord.

A series of experiments were performed in order to elucidate the mechanism of unresponsiveness of TAT and TO system to glucocorticoids after high level spinal cord section. Harding and Rosen (1963) confirmed by Kenney (1967), Shapiro (1968) and others found that growth hormone lowered TAT activity in the liver of hypophysectomized rats. These data gave us foundation to suppose a probable involvement of the hypophysis in the observed inhibition of hydrocortisone induction of TAT after C_7-level spinal cord section.

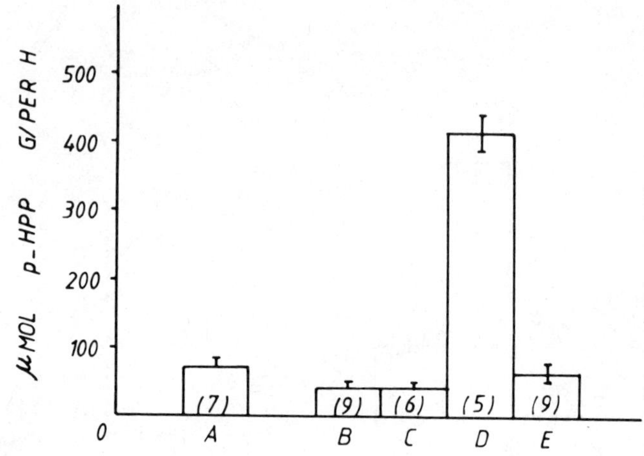

Fig. 5. Effect of C_7-level section of the spinal cord on the hydrocortisone induction of TAT in hypophysectomized rats. Ordinate, TAT activity. The number of experimental animals is given in brackets. Each column represents mean value ± s.e.m. A, controls with intact hypophysis; B, hypophysectomized rats; C, sham-operated hypophysectomized rats; D, hypophysectomized rats 4 h after hydrocortisone injection; E, hypophysectomized rats with C_7-level section of the spinal cord at 4th h after hydrocortisone injection.

However, as it can be seen in Fig. 5, the unresponsiveness of TAT to high level spinal cord section is observed both in animals with intact hypophysis and in hypophysectomized rats. Therefore we cannot ascribe the unresponsiveness of TAT to hydrocortisone to enhanced secretion of growth (or whichever hypophyseal) hormone following spinal cord section.

Hanoune et al. (1971) observed the involvement of glucose in regulation of TAT activity. They found that the administration of large quantities of glucose inhibits to some extent the glucocorticoid induction of TAT. We studied the blood glucose level and glucose content of the liver after C_7-section of the spinal cord. In Fig. 6 can be seen that this operation brought about a decrease in the levels of glucose in blood and liver. Therefore, the unresponsiveness of TAT to glucocorticoids after high level spinal cord section cannot be explained by the changes in glucose level.

It was interesting to know if there was any change in the concentration of insulin after C_7-level spinal cord section. As shown in Fig. 7 the insulinemia after sham operation was raised significantly at the 5th min, reaching peak value (47% increase) at the 15th min after the operation. Half an hour after the sham operation the blood insulin level fell (insignificantly) below the normal

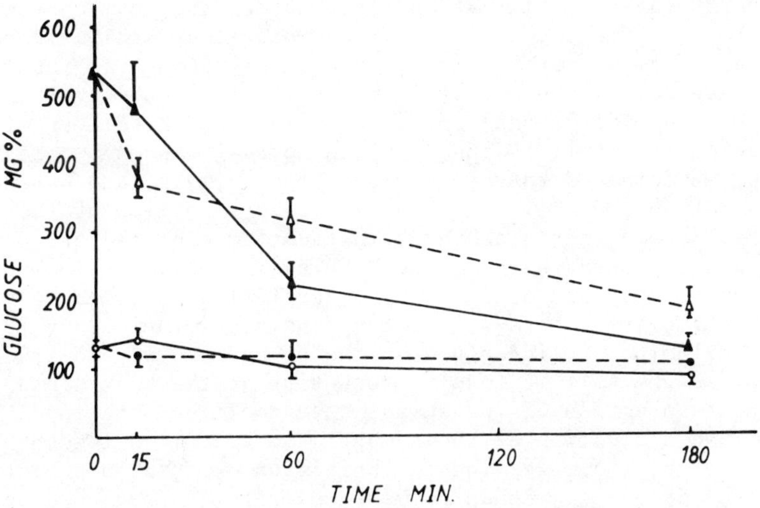

Fig. 6. Effect of C_7-level section of the spinal cord on the glucose level in blood and glucose content of liver. o——o, blood glucose level in C_7-sectioned rats; •------•, blood glucose level in sham-operated rats; ▲——▲, glucose content in liver homogenate in C_7-operated rats; Δ-----Δ, glucose content in liver homogenate in sham operated rats. Abscissa, time in min after operation; ordinate, glucose content in mg%. Each experimental group consisted of four animals. Each point represents mean value ± s.e.m.

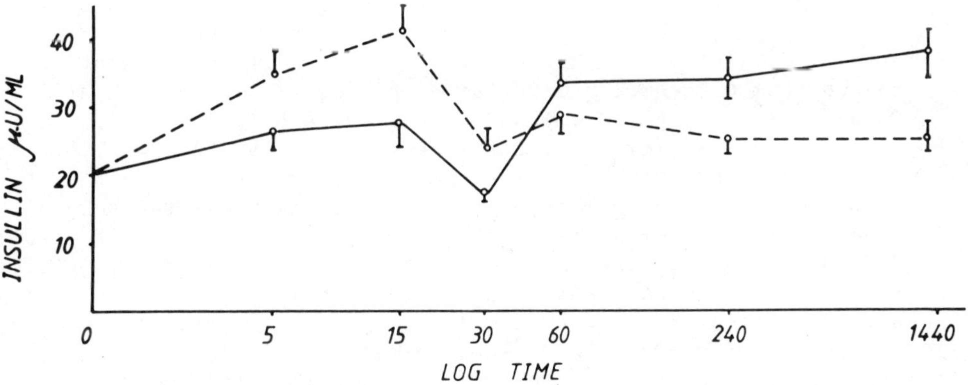

Fig. 7. Insulin concentration in plasma of C_7-sectioned (——) and sham (----) operated rats. Abscissa - log time, ordinate - insulin concentration in μU/ml. Each experimental group consisted of five animals. Each point represents mean value ± s.e.m.

value returning to normal at the 1st h after the sham operation. At the later terms insulinemia in sham-operated rats was normal. Therefore, sham operation elicits a biphasic change in insulinemia - an increase followed by a not very deep fall. In C_7-level sectioned rats the rise seen in sham operated animals at the 5th and 15th min was lacking. The fall at the 30th min however was much more pronounced, as compared to the sham-operated animals, and was highly significant ($p < 0.001$). One h after the transection of the spinal cord insulin concentration was significantly elevated above normal values and remained there to the 24th h. In sham operated animals the biphasic response of insulin to surgical stress can be ascribed to the interplay of beta-stimulatory and alpha-inhibitory influences of catecholamines taking place on the background of elevated glucocorticoids. The fall in insulin secretion at the 30th min after C_7-level transection of the spinal cord could be explained by a short-lived activation of the sympathetic system (below the segment of the lesion, too), leading to inhibition of insulin secretion via the alpha-adrenergic mechanism. The moderately pronounced but significant rise of insulinemia from the first to 24th h after C_7-section can be ascribed to the unrestrained secretagogue influence of the vagal nerve in respect to insulin secretion.

Now exists ample of evidence for the interaction between the effect of glucocorticoids and cyclic adenosine 3',5'-monophosphate (cAMP). Cyclic AMP, like glucocorticoids, is an inducer of TAT, although it is thought to act through a different mechanism and is not an obligatory mediator of glucocorticoid effects. The same holds for glucagon, which is considered to act through a cAMP-mediated mechanism. Now is generally accepted that glucocorticoids act at the level of transcription, whereas cAMP and glucagon act at post-transcriptional level.

We studied the effect of high level spinal cord section on the cAMP system. As shown in Fig. 8 cAMP level in rat liver was markedly altered by C_7-section of the spinal cord. Thus, its concentration decreased from 0.88 nmol/g liver at zero time to 0.36 nmol/g at 1 h (two-fold decrease, $p < 0.01$) and to 0.20 at 4 h (four-fold decrease, $p < 0.01$). The cAMP level had returned to normal at the 24 h. At the same periods after sham operation, no alteration in the hepatic cAMP could be detected. When glucagon (0.1 mg/rat) was injected subcutaneously in control animals 15 min before sacrifice, it induced a 10-fold increase in the cAMP level. When glucagon was administered at the 4th and 24th hour after spinal cord section, cAMP levels increased dramatically to 12 nmol/g liver (60-fold increase) and 19 nmol/g liver (24-fold increase), respectively. Thus, section of the spinal cord appeared to be followed by a four-fold decrease in the basal level of cAMP and by hyperreactivity of the cAMP system to exogenous glucagon. Among many possibilities which may explain the decrease in basal level of cAMP, the two most likely are an increase in phosphodiesterase activity, or a decrease in activity

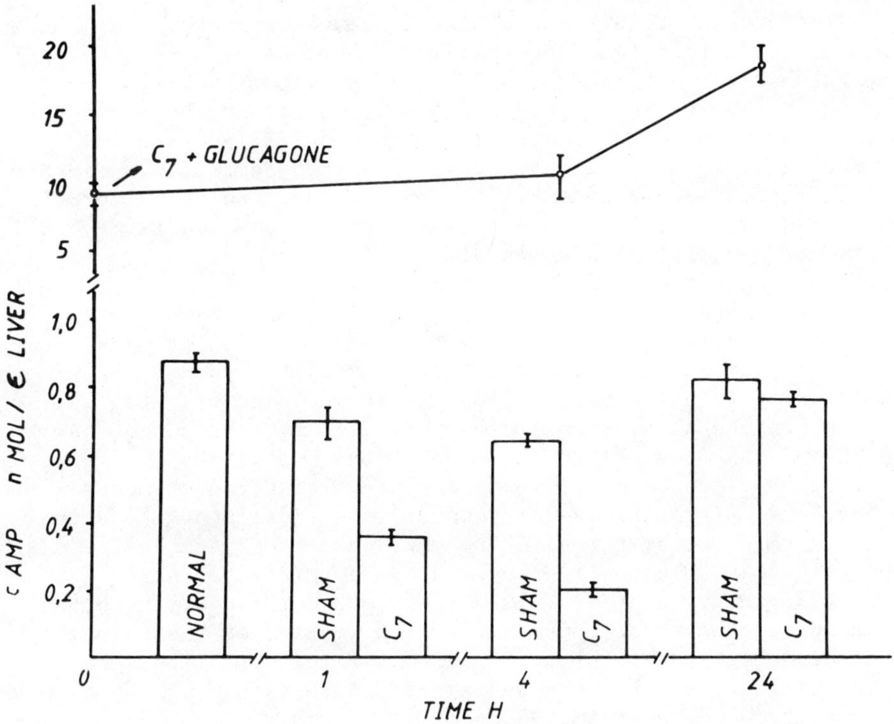

Fig. 8. Hepatic cAMP concentration after high level section of the spinal cord or sham operation. Ordinate, cAMP content in nmoles/g liver ± s.e.m.

of adenylate cyclase. No change in phosphodiesterase activity was detected either at 4th or at 24th h after spinal cord section or sham operation (Vaptzarova and Hanoune, 1977)

We therefore explored the possibility that the fall in hepatic cAMP concentration was due to a decreased basal activity of adenylate cyclase. The basal level of adenylate cyclase activity as well as its responsiveness to glucagon, epinephrine and fluoride were determined in a particulate fraction of liver at the 4th and 24th h after either C_7-level section of spinal cord or sham operation. The results obtained showed that neither the transection of the spinal cord nor the sham operation changed the basal activity of adenylate cyclase, or its sensitivity towards its activators i.e. glucagon, epinephrine and fluoride.

We assayed the quantity of acid-soluble nucleotides after spinal cord section at C_7-level. The concentration of ATP was not altered either in the early or in the late hours after high level spinal cord section (Vaptzarova et al., 1975b).

The present results show that C_7-level transection of the spinal cord causes a four-fold decrease in content of cAMP in the liver at the 4th h after the operation. It occurs concomitantly with the unresponsiveness of TAT to glucocorticoids. Whether these two phenomena are interdependent remains to be prouven. This dramatic decrease in the basal level of hepatic cAMP is unprecedented. Our experimental data excluded the possibility that an enhanced activity of nucleotide-specific phosphodiesterase or decreased activity of adenylate cyclase was responsible for the decrease in hepatic cAMP level at the 4th h after C_7-section of the spinal cord. We therefore favour the hypothesis that extrahepatic factors are primarily responsible for the changes in hepatic concentration of cAMP. Thus, during the first few hours after section of the spinal cord in rats, symptoms of spinal shock develop, which include an abated activity of the peripheral sympathetic nerves. It can be presumed that the decreased cAMP content in liver below the basal level, after C_7-chordotomy, is due to the lowered content of catecholamines in the sympathetic nerve terminals. However, the section of the spinal cord also affects the sympathetic innervation of the pancreas. Glucagon secretion was shown to increase by adrenergic stimulation (Bloom et al., 1973; Marliss et al., 1972). One could therefore hypothetize that during the first hours after high section of the spinal cord, the adrenergic input to the Langerhans islets is diminished. Indeed, in preliminary experiments we have found that the content of glucagon in plasma decreased from 530 pg/ml in controls to 200 pg/ml 4 h after section of the spinal cord, and was back to 440 pg/ml, i.e. a nearly normal level at 24 h.

What is the connection, if any, between the decreased liver cAMP concentration and unresponsiveness of liver TAT towards glucocorticoids? Cyclic AMP and its dibutyryl derivative is a TAT activity inducer at posttranscriptional level. Wicks et al. (1968) have shown that the inducing effect of cAMP and glucocorticoids on TAT activity are additive and, therefore, independent. There exist experimental data that phosphorylation of definite ribosomal proteins can influence their function and the process of association and dissociation of their subunits. It could be that lowered liver cAMP content causes ribosomal malfunction and, hence, the unresponsiveness of TAT to glucocorticoids. This effect however should be more general.

Although the relationship between cAMP and glucocorticoid receptors are not yet fully elucidated we studied the glucocorticoid receptors (GCR) after C_7-level spinal cord section. The chordotomy at C_7-level did not influence the quantity of GCRs, the formation and activation of hormone-receptor complex and its binding to the chromatin. However, the experiments in vitro eliminate many of the regulatory influences, taking part in vivo.

^{3}H-dexamethasone (^{3}H-DM), (specific activity 20 Ci/mmol) in a dose of 44 μCi/rat was injected i.p. in C_7-level chordotomized and

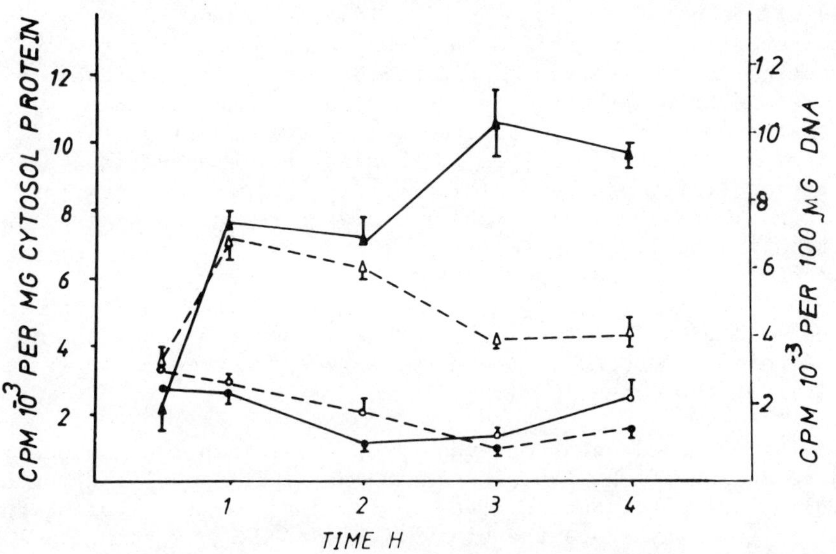

Fig. 9. Labelling of liver cytosol and nuclei in vivo in different terms after ^{3}H-DM administration and C_7-chordotomy. o- - -o binding of ^{3}H-DM by cytosol from control animals; •——• binding of ^{3}H-DM by cytosol of C_7-chordotomized rats; Δ- - -Δ binding of ^{3}H-DM by liver nuclei from control animals; ▲——▲ binding of ^{3}H-DM by liver nuclei from C_7-chordotomized rats.

control rats. The animals were killed by decapitation 30 min, 1, 2, 3 and 4 h after the operation. The labelled steroid was administered immediately after the operation. In Fig. 9 one can see that there does not exist any difference between the chordotomized and control animals in the radioactivity of cytosol (after treatment with charcoal) and, therefore, no difference in the quantity of GCRs in the cytoplasm.

The radioactivity of the thoroughly washed nuclei isolated after in vivo administration of the ^{3}H-DM and which is considered to be due to the radioactivity of hormone-receptor complexes bound to the chromatin, showed marked difference between C_7-operated and control animals. In control animals the highest radioactivity of the nuclei was observed at the first hour after the administration of the labelled DM. At later terms (2, 3 and 4 h after the injection) the radioactivity fell considerably. This time course of radioactivity is due to the normal turnover of hormone-receptor complexes and is in good agreement with the data of Bottoms and Gortsch (1967). One hour after C_7-level spinal cord section the radioactivity of the isolated nuclei was almost the same as in control animals. This finding demonstrates that the high level spinal cord section does not prevent the penetration of ^{3}H-DM into the hepatocytes and the formation and activation of the hormone-receptor complexes. Since the second hour after the transection of the spinal cord at C_7-level and later on we observed a retention of the labelled steroid in the nuclei. At the third and fourth hour after the operation the increase of radioactivity of the nuclei exceeds the two-fold mark ($p < 0.001$). We do not know the exact mechanism of the retention of the labelled steroid in the liver nuclei after the decentralization of the liver. Timoczko et al. (1982) showed that hormone-receptor complexes leave the nuclei after interaction with the synthesized under the influence of hormone mRNA. In other words mRNA synthesized under the influence of steroid hormone helps the hormone-receptor complex to leave the nucleus of the target cell.

The observed unresponsiveness of the TAT to the glucocorticoids and retention of the labelled DM in the hepatic nuclei after high level spinal cord section give us ground to surmise that C_7-chordotomy in some way stops the biosynthesis of TAT mRNA.

Spinal cord section brings about early (4h after surgery) and late (24h after surgery) changes in rat liver glucocorticoid-inducible enzymes TAT and TO. The observed unresponsiveness of TAT and TO to the glucocorticoids and retention of the labelled DM in the hepatic nuclei after high level spinal cord section are the early effects of C_7-chordotomy. Late effects (24h after surgery) consist in a nine-fold increase in TAT and two-fold increase in TO activity in animals with intact adrenals and a three-fold increase for both enzymes in adrenalectomized rats (Fig. 1, 2). In order to investigate the molecular events under the induction of TAT at 24 h after high level spinal cord section we carried out experiments planned to determine whether this induction is connected with activation of preformed TAT molecules or with new protein synthesis. Cycloheximide (1.6 mg/kg) was administered in non-adrenalectomized rats, immediately and at 1.5, 3, 6 and 20 h after C_7-level spinal cord section. All the animals were killed at 24th h after the operation and TAT activity was determined. In Fig. 10 can be seen that cycloheximide inhibits the induction of TAT activity to the same extent (about 80%) regardless of the time of injection. These results can be interpreted as a proof that the induction of TAT activity at 24 h after C_7-level spinal cord section is due to new biosynthesis of protein. In order to elucidate whether this induction of TAT requires new mRNA biosynthesis we administered actinomycin D (1 mg/kg) in different terms (immediately, 1.5, 3, 6 and 20 h after the operation).All animals were killed 24 h after the surgery. As shown in Fig. 10 the effect of actinomycin D (AMD) was clearly time-dependent: when injected immediately after the operation AMD caused a complete block of TAT induction; when given 1.5 h later the inhibition was 78% ($p < 0.001$), when administered 3 h after the operation - about 50% ($p < 0.001$), and applied later on - about 40% (p 0.01).

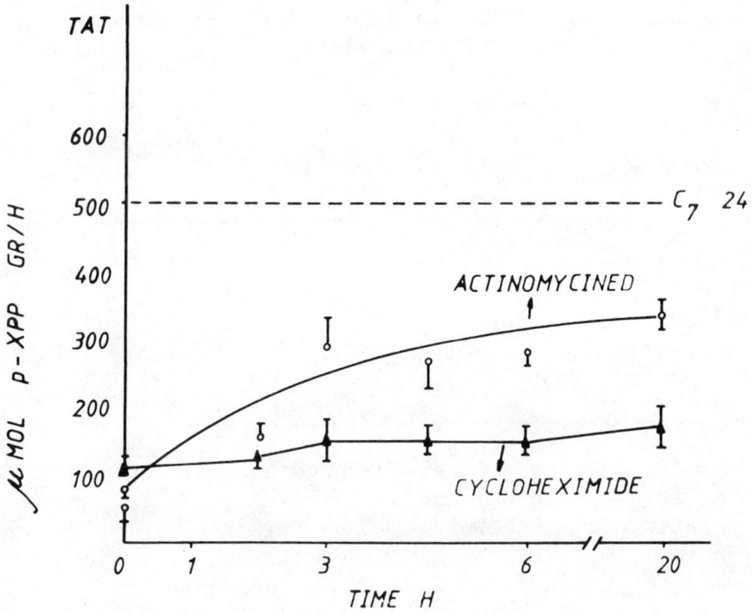

Fig. 10. Effect of actimomycin D and cycloheximide on TAT activity depending on the time of administration of the inhibitors. TAT activity is determined at the 24th h after C_7-level spinal cord section. Abscissa, time of administration of the inhibitors after surgery, ordinate, enzyme activity. Dashed line, - - - , TAT activity 24 h after C_7-level spinal cord section in absence of inhibitors. Each experimental group consisted of 5-11 animals. Each value is the mean ± s.e.m.

The results obtained with AMD can be interpreted if one assumes the existence of two mRNAs for liver TAT with different lifetime: short (about 1.5-3.0 h) and long (about 16 h or more).

Similar results were obtained with D-galactosamine and ethionine (Vaptzarova et al., 1975a; Vaptzarova et al., 1977). The late induction of TAT at the 24th h after high level spinal cord section can be interpreted as a result of an early disturbance (in the first 4 h after the operation) in TAT mRNA synthesis and/or in its release and transport from the nucleus to the cytoplasm. As a result of this disturbance one can suppose an amassing of untranslated TAT-m-RNA and its translation in later terms (e.g., at 24th h).

It was interesting to investigate the DNA synthesis in regenerating liver after high level section of the spinal cord, too. Group of 3-4 male rats were subjected to partial hepatectomy and/or C_7-

Table 1. DNA Synthesis in Regenerating Rat Liver after Spinal Cord C_7 Transection

Animals	DNA Synthesis (dpm $\pm$ s.e.)
Control	268 $\pm$ 45
Sham-operated	235 $\pm$ 38
Spinal cord section	142 $\pm$ 16
Hepatectomy	26175 $\pm$ 2410
Hepatectomy + spinal cord section	188 $\pm$ 15

Group of 3 male rats were subjected between 8.0 and 10.0 h to partial hepatectomy and/or spinal cord C_7-transection. 22 h later and 2 h before killing thymidine-2-^{14}C (1.5 μCi per animal) was injected i.p. and the incorporation of the label into the thymine of liver DNA was observed.

level spinal cord section. 22 h after the operation and 2 h before sacrifice the animals were injected with ^{14}C-thymidine and the incorporation of the label in DNA was estimated (see Table 1). DNA synthesis in regenerating rat liver (in rat with intact spinal cord) increases 12 h after the partial hepatectomy and reaches maximum at 24 h. Spinal cord transection at C_7-level in partially hepatectomized animals resulted in the depression of thymidine incorporation into hepatic DNA. This effect was best pronounced when transection was carried out immediately after partial hepatectomy. Even in animals at 16 h after hepatectomy, high level spinal cord section depressed the already enhanced DNA synthesis (Vaptzarova et al., 1973b).

In following experiments (Cihak and Vaptzarova, 1973c) we have found that the administration of reserpine to partially hepatectomized rats decreased the rate of thymidine uptake into liver DNA in a way similar to that observed after C_7-level spinal cord section. Reserpine causes depletion of noradrenaline from sympathetic terminals resulting in the decrease of sympathetic activity. It seems possible that transection of the spinal cord above the segments which innervate the liver and consequent interruption of descending neural activity to the relevant preganglionic sympathetic neurones results in the depletion of catecholamine content followed by depression of DNA synthesis.

GENERAL DISCUSSION

The high level transection of the spinal cord leads to a multitude of effects, the main among them being the following:

- a unresponsiveness of TO and TAT system to glucocorticoids in the early 4-5 h after the operation;
- an early (at the 4th h after the operation) drop in cAMP content of the liver and two-fold decrease in glucagonemia;
- retention in the liver nuclei of the labelled dexamethasone, administered in vivo (at the 4th h after the high level spinal cord section);
- a late (24 h after transection) manyfold induction of TO and TAT which is partially independent of the adrenals;
- depressed DNA biosynthesis in regenerating rat liver.

A possible common denominator of the effects of high level spinal cord section on the liver is the abrupt interruption of the sympathetic impulsation from the brain towards the preganglionic sympathetic neurons and consequent fall in sympathetic tonus in the peripheral organs, liver included.

The high level spinal cord section affects the sympathetic innervation of the pancreas, too. Adrenergic stimulation was shown to increase glucagon secretion. In our experiments (Vaptzarova and Hanoune, 1976) it was shown that the plasma level of pancreatic glucagon was decreased more than two-fold at the 4th h after C_7-chordotomy. After this operation the decreased levels of two activating agents, plasma glucagon and catecholamines from sympathetic terminals may result in a decrease of liver cAMP below its basal level. The "basal" level of hepatic cAMP (approximately 1 nmol/g liver) is maintained at its normal value probably by a permanent sympathetic tonus as well as by circulating glucagon, the level of the latter being influenced by the sympathetic impulsation, too.

The unresponsiveness of TAT and TO to the glucocorticoids is of obvious interest. We do not know the exact cause of this intriguing phenomenon, but it is tempting to link the unresponsiveness to the early decrease in liver cAMP content.

A relationship between some effects of glucocorticoids and cAMP system was suspected but was never firmly established (Munck and Leung, 1977). It is possible that there exists a relationship between the cAMP system (cAMP-dependent protein kinases) and the functional capacity of the glucocorticoid-receptors, especially the termination of their action in the nuclei.

CONCLUSION

The high level (C_7) transection of the spinal cord causes an early and transient unresponsiveness of TO and TAT towards glucocorticoids and a simultaneous block of the exit of the labelled glucocorticoids outside the nuclei. Depressed biosynthesis of DNA in regenerating liver is also seen after C_7-level spinal cord transaction.

REFERENCE

Baxter, J. D. and Tomkins, G. M., 1971, Specific cytoplasmic glucocorticoid receptors in hepatoma tissue culture cells, Proc. Natl.Acad.Sci., 68:932.

Berry, L. J., Goodrum, K. J., Resnik, I. G., and Ford, Ch. W., 1980, Endotoxin, liver enzyme and liver diseases, in: "The reticuloendothelial system and the pathogenesis of liver diseases", H. Liehr and M. Grun, eds., Elsevier/Northholland Biomedical Press, Amsterdam.

Bloom, R. S., Edwards, A. V., and Vaughan, N. J. A., 1973, The role of the sympathetic innervation in the control of plasma glucagon concentration in the calf, J.Physiol., 233:257.

Bottoms, G., and Coetsch, D. D., 1967, Subcellular distribution of the (^{3}H) corticosterone fraction in brain, thymus, heart and liver of the rat, Proc.Soc.Exptl.Biol.and Med., 124:662.

Burton, K., 1956, A study of the conditions and mechanisms of the diphenylamine reaction for the colorimetric estimation of deoxyribonucleic acid, Biochem.J., 62:315.

Čihak, A., and Vaptzarova K., 1973c, Decreased synthesis of DNA in regenerating rat liver after administration of reserpine, Br.J.Pharmacol., 49:253

Dabeva, M. D., Todorov, B. N., and Hadjiolov, A. A., 1976, Intranuclear distribution of ribosomal RNAs from rat liver, Biokhimia, 41:458.

Hanoune, J., Chambaut, A. M., and Josipowicz, A., 1971, The glucose effect of cortisone action upon rat liver metabolism, BBA, 244:338.

Hanoune, J., Lacombe, M. L., and Pecker, F., 1975, The epinephrine sensitive adenylate cyclase of rat liver plasma membranes, J.Biol.Chem., 250:4569.

Harding, H. R., and Rosen R., 1963, Effects of hypophysectomy and growth hormone (GH) on the endogenous levels and induction of two adaptive enzymes, Federat.Proceed., 22:409.

Kenney, F. T., 1967, Regulation of tyrosine-alpha-ketoglutarate transaminase in rat liver. V. Repression in growth hormone-treated rats, J.Biol.Chem., 242:4367.

Knox, W. E., Piras, M. M., and Tokuyama, K., 1966, Tryptophan pyrrolase of liver. I. Activation and assay in soluble extracts of rat liver, J.Biol.Chem., 241:297.

Liberti, J. P., Longman, E. S., Navon, R. S., 1970, Effects of hydrocortisone and growth hormone on tyrosine aminotransferase and tryptophan oxygenase levels in hypophysectomized rats, Endocrinology, 86: 1448.

Marliss, E. B., Girardier, L., Seydaux, J., Kanazawa, Y., Wollheim, C., Orci, L., Porte, D. Jr., 1972, Glucagon release by pancreatic nerve stimulation: further evidence for direct control of endocrine pancreatic secretion, Eur.J.Clin.Invest., 214:295.

Munck, A., and Leung, K., 1977, Glucocorticoid receptors and mechanism of action, in: "Receptors and mechanism of action of steroid hormones", G. R. Pasqualini, ed., Marcel Decker, New York.

Rosen, F., Harding, H. R., Milholland, R. J., and Nichol, C. A., 1963, Glucocorticoids and transaminase activity. IV. Comparison of the adaptive increase of alanine and tyrosine-alpha-ketoglutarate transaminase, J.Biol.Chem., 238:3725.

Sato, B., Kishimoto, S., and Matsumoto, K., 1983, Regulation of steroid receptor function, in: "Hormone receptors and receptor diseases", H. Imura and H. Kuziya, eds., Excerpta Medica, Amsterdam (1983).

Scatchard, G., 1949, The attraction of proteins for small molecules and ions, Ann.N.Y.Acad.Sci., 68:932.

Shapiro, S., 1968, Interaction between growth hormone and hydrocortisone on the regulation of liver tyrosine transaminase activity, Endocrinology, 83:475.

Silber, R. H., Busch, R. D., and Oslapas, R., 1958, Practical procedure for estimation of corticosterone and hydrocortisone, Clin.Chem., 4: 278.

Strashimirov, D., 1967, A method for transauricular hypophysectomy in rats, Exp.Med.i Morfol., 6:109.

Thomson, W. J., and Appleman, M. M., 1971, Characterization of cyclic nucleotide phosphodiesterase of rat tissues, J.Biol.Chem., 246:3145.

Tymoczko, J. L., Shapiro, J., Simenstad, D. J., and Nish, A. D., 1982, The effect of polyribonucleotides on the binding of dexamethasone-receptor complex to DNA, J.Steroid.Biochem., 16:595.

Vaptzarova, K. I., Davidov, M. S., Markov, D. V., Popov, P. G., and Galabov, G. P., 1969, The effect of spinal cord section on rat liver tryptophan pyrrolase activity, Life Sciences, 8:905.

Vaptzarova, K. I., Popov, P. G., and Galabov, G. P., 1973[a], Tyrosine-alpha-ketoglutarate aminotransferase activity in rat liver after spinal cord section, J.Neurochemistry, 31:291.

Vaptzarova, K. I., Popov, P. G., Vesely, J., and Čihak, A., 1973[b], Depressed synthesis of DNA in regenrating rat liver after spinal cord (C_7) transection, Experientia, 29:1505.

Vaptzarova, K. I., Popov, P. G., Dimova, R. N., Stoykova, A. S., Rosentall, L. H., and Chelibonova-Lorer, H., 1975[a], Alteration of tyrosine aminotransferase activity and ultrastructure of rat liver after high level spinal cord section and D-galactosamine administration, Compt.rend. Acad.bulg.Sci., 28:991.

Vaptzarova, K. I., Popov, P. G., Dimova, R. N., Rosentall, L. H., Stoykova, A. S., and Chelibinova-Lorer, H., 1975[b]. Effect of D-galactosamine and high level spinal cord section of nucleotide pool of rat liver, Compt.rend.Acad.bulg.Sci., 28:1117.

Vaptzarova, K. I., and Hanoune, J., 1976, Effect of high level section of the spinal cord on the cyclic AMP system in rat liver, BBA, 444:712.

Vaptzarova, K. I., Bachvarova, E. D., and Popov, P. G., 1980[a], High level section of the spinal cord causes unresponsiveness of rat liver tyrosine oxygenase to hydrocortisone induction, Compt.rend.Acad.bulg.Sci., 33:997.

Vaptzarova, K. I., Tarcolev, N., and Popov, P. G., 1980[b], Effect of high level spinal cord section on the insulinemia and glucosemia in rats, Compt.rend.Acad.Sci., 33:1001.

Wicks, W. P., 1968, Tyrosine-alpha-ketoglutarate transaminase induction by epinephrine and adenosine 3',5'-monophosphate, Science, 160:997.

REACTION OF NEUROENDOCRINE CELLS TO STRESS

Vladimir R. Pantić

Serbian Academy of Sciences and Arts
Belgrade, Yugoslavia

1. INTRODUCTION

The inhibitory effect of blood corticosteroid levels on ACTH release, caused by stress and the negative feedback exerted by corticosteroids on the hypothalamus, as pointed by Smelik, 1963, is the subject of recent advanced researches and serious discussions. Makara et al., 1970, examined ACTH release induced by traumatic stress in rats with unilateral spinal cord lesion. At that time Stark et al., 1970, paid attention to the afferent pathways of stressful stimuli. The major effect of cortisol on hypothalamic neurons, when applied directly to the cell membrane by microelectrophoresis, is inhibition of spontaneous activity (Kelly et al., 1982).

From the evolutionary and ontogenic point of view it might be acceptable that stressful stimuli are transfered by neuronal pathways through which they reach the specific brain neurons in which LPH, ACTH, MSH and opioid peptides are synthesised and released. It is often mentioned that these brain neurons are localised in the locus coerulens, amygdala, septum, preoptic area and some hypothalamic nuclei, and are innervated by norepinephine (NE) neurons(Barden and Dupont, 1982; Palkovits,1982).

Acustic, photo-sensory and somatosensory stimuli reach the hypothalamic nuclei, and other brain neurons, mainly through afferent neural pathway in which the median forebrain bundles and amygdala are involved (Feldman et al., 1972).

However, it is necessary to point out that peptidergic and aminergic fibers terminate in neurohypophysis and pars intermedia, that pars nervosa (PN) of pituitary modulates ACTH release in rats (Baertschi et al.,1980), that the content of nervous terminals might be transfered tc pars anterior (PA) by short portal blood vessels or by systemic circulation, etc.

The rapid extragenomic effect of the cortisol and synthesis of cortisol specific receptor protein occur, very likely, in neurons on the preformed specific mRNA (Kanazir et al.,1979). A modulation of the plasma membrane receptors for peptide hormone and catecholamine by glucocorticoids is suggested by Wolfe et al., 1976. Genomic effect of steroid -receptor complex has selective influence on the expression of serie of genes (Yu et al.,1977). In brain neurons, which are common target cells for both steroid and peptide hormones, steroids may modulate these cell responsiveness to peptide hormones and in brain common target cells subunit of steroid receptor might be involved in the regulation of calcium homeostasis (Kanazir, 1982). Antagonistic effect of corticosteroids on neuropeptides in the brain neurons is mentioned by

Edwards and Rousseau, 1982. Cortisol rapidly revearses the darkening effect of MSH by causing a centripetal movement of melanosomes in the dermal melanocytes and this effect is not dependent on new RNA and protein synthesis.

2. THE AIM OF PRESENTATION

The subject of this presentation is not to discuss questions as what is stress. The main aim is to present a point of view of the complexity of neuroendocrine cell reactions to stressful stimuli and agencies as are hormones. The attention will be paid on the hormones interdependence and complexed mechanisms influencing the pattern of differentiation and specificities of various cell type reactions.

For that purpose the results obtained up to now and based on the following investigations: treatment with steroid and peptide hormones during various stages of ontogenesis, after adrenalectomy, thyroidectomy, hypophysectomy and subsequent administration of corresponding hormones, irradiation with X-rays, or after organ transplantation will be briefly considered.

For better understanding of the differentiation of specific pituitary cells, their balanced interrelation, specificities and nature of responses to hormones and their properties during tumorogenesis, pituitary cells were divided into 3 groups (Pantić, 1975):

- The family of the first groups of hormones originating from known heptapeptide and evolved to prohormones, consisting of peptides. These peptides are involved in reactions to stress and synthetised mainly in specific brain neurons, pituitary - PI cells and ACTH cells of PA.

- To the second group of hormones belong prolactin (PRL) and growth hormone (GH) evolved from PRL-like molecules. These peptides are synthesised in the corresponding and specific pituitary (PRL and GH) cells.

- The third group of hormones are synthesised in glucoprotein producing (GTH and TSH) cells. In GTH cells both FSH and LH are synthesised. These cells are very sensitive and dependent on the activities of the first group of hormones, esspecially on ACTH and endorphines, but on PRL, as a hormone of the second group, as well.

3. BRAIN NEURONS AND PITUITARY CELLS AS A COMMON TARGET CELL FOR STEROIDS AND PEPTIDE HORMONES

Specific brain neurons and pituitary cells are common target cells for steroids, protein hormones, peptides, neurotransmitters and neuromodulators.

Both brain neurons and pituitary cells react specifically to feedback stimuli originated from different steroids and the effects are dependent on the serum concentration, the magnitude of the administred hormones, the number and the nature of receptors, etc. (Pantić, 1980, 1981).

The main peptides, closely related to stress, originate from hepapeptide. This peptide possesses ACTH and MSH activity (Li, 1972). Through the evolution from this peptide, as a precursor, prohormone molecule containing lipotropins (β and γ), MSH_s, CLIP, enkephalins and endorphins arised. These peptides might be stored in specific granules, or released from the cytoplasm into the capillaries influencing the activities of target cells, so that MSH influences melanocytes, ACTH steroidogenesis from adrenal cortex, etc.

In order to approach the mechanism of stressogenic effects various methods were used such as, the removal of the medial hypothalamus (Stark and Makara, 1981) implantation of pituitary grafts under kidney capsule (Pavić et al., 1977), administration of various doses of gonadal steroids into fishes, chicken, rats or piglets, or corticosteroids into rats during neonatal, juvenile or adult stages of development (Pantić,1974,1982,1984).

Characteristics and specificities of brain neurons and pituitary cell reactions after irradiation of head or total body and the effect of adrenocortical hormones were described (Hristić and Pantić, 1974).

3.1. Brain neurons

It is now known that stress causes elevation of vasopressin (VP) and corticotropin releasing hormone (CRH) influencing the release of ACTH and opiates. Both CRP and VP are synthesised in NSO and NPV.

However, besides Hpt, the extrahypothalamic neurons in the brain are involved in synthesis and release of the family of hormones which belong to the first group (Fig.1, 2, 3).

Our up to now obtained results showed, that NPV and NSO are very sensitive to corticosteroids and a close

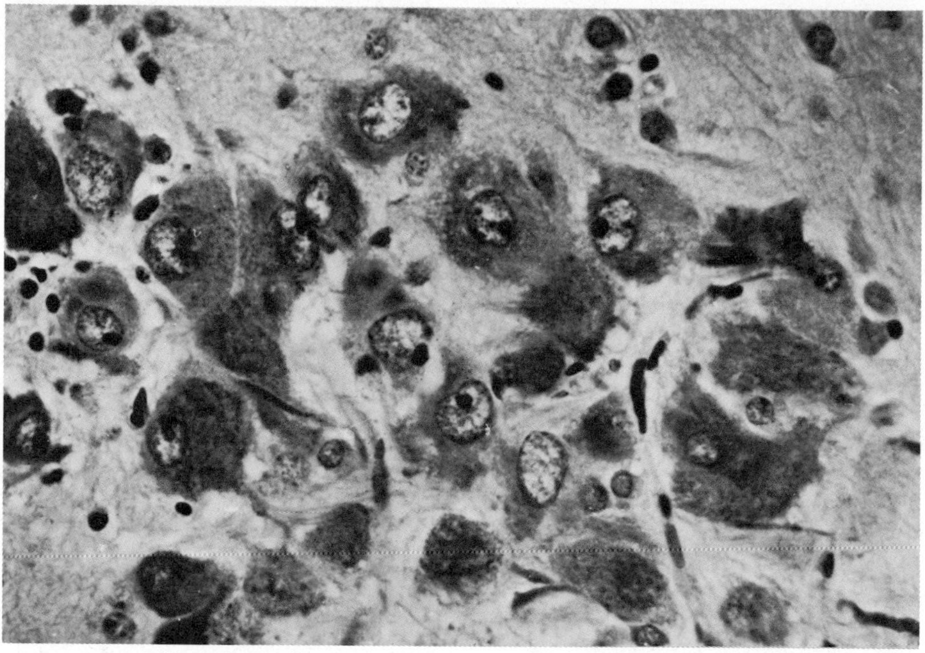

Fig.1. Neurosecretory cells of NPO in Serranus Scriba.

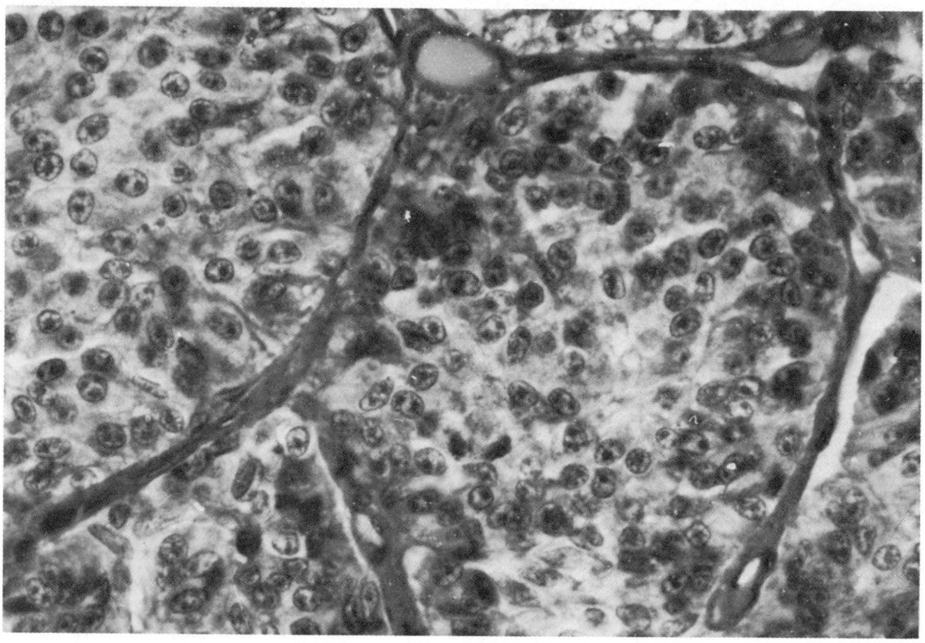

Fig.2. PI cells in the deer pituitary.

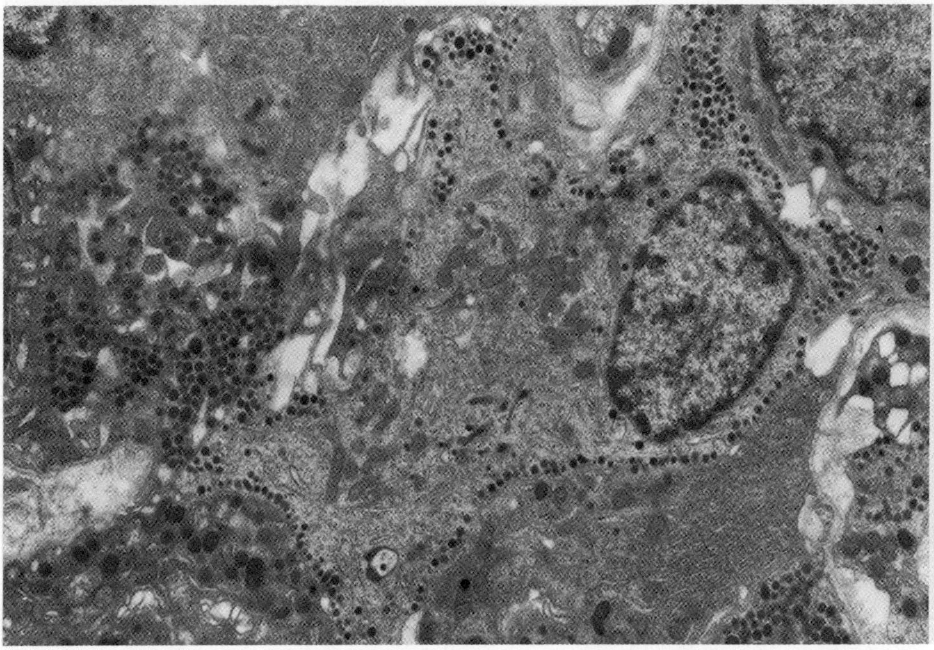

Fig.3. ACTH cell in PA of rat after transplantation.

relationship exists between neurosecretory cell structure and plasma concentration of corticosteroids.

Adrenalectomy (Adx) causes significant hypertrophy of NPV, NSO and NVM cells and an increased number of adrenalectomy cells, which are clearly expressed 15 days after the operation. On the other hand, if intact or Adx animals were treated with Hy or ACTH, neurosecretory substances in NSO, NPV, Me and pars nervosa (PN) are stored. The supresive effect of hydrocortisone (Hy), as an increase of the number and size of specific granules, is expressed in the ACTH cells, as well (Zgurić and Pantić, 1970).

Neurosecretory cells of these nuclei react after thyroidectomy and after the transplantation of X-ray irradiated thyroid into the anterior eye chamber. NPV,

NVM and ME showed that these nuclei are involved in synthesis of TRH and in regulation of TSH and thyroid follicular cell activities (Stošić et al., 1965; Pantić,1974). The changes in the neurosecretory cells, as a very sensitive cells to irradiation, are less pronounced after the treatment with corticosteroids (see Pantić, 1982). The role of this tripeptid in regulation of PRL and growth hormone producing cells (GH) releasing the corresponding hormones point to the interdependences of these hormones during evolution and during ontogenesis as well.

The role of peptide hormones originated from the ancestral heptapeptide is in focuss of recent discussions. This ancestral hormone might play a role in the evolution of LRH and other peptides as well. However, peptides, as LRH are established, not only in the brain neurons, but in testis (Sharpe and Frase, 1980), in ovary (Ying and Guillemin, 1979) and even in pancreas (Seppälä et al., 1979). It is of interest to mention that the affinity constants and specificity of the testicular GRH receptors are identical to GRH receptors in the pituitary cells (Jégou et al., 1984). Extra pituitary actions were examined and its inhibitory effects on the ovary and testis were observed (Sharpe, 1980, 1982).

3.2. PI cells

It has been shown that pars intermedia (PI) cells are closely dependent on nervous stimuli, neurotransmitters and neuromodulators, transported by peptidergic and aminergic fibers. The inervation is very rich, many unmyelinated axons terminate mostly at the periphery of lobes and have a synaptic like contact with PI cells (de Bold et al., 1980).

PI cells are sensitive to sufficiency or defficieny of gonadal steroids, as well (Pantić and Šimić,1977).The main product of these cells are ACTH, β-LPH, β-endorphin and corticotropin-like intermediate lobe peptides (CLIP). These cells react to stress activating proteases which split the prohormone molecules.

PI constitutes 70% of the total pituitary volume in squamata (Saint Gerons, 1961). This lobe is very developed in wild animals as for example deers and roe bucks (Pantić, 1974).

Stimulation of these cell activities and even hyperplasia are often mentioned. As a stellate cell their distribution is species specific, but often are localized between PRL and GH producing cells.

3.3. ACTH cells

The changes in ACTH of PA are highly specific in reaction to the defficiency or sufficiency of glucocorticoids and the responce is closely dependent on CRH.

The N-terminal portion of the ACTH molecule, which is responsible for corticosteroidogenesis, has remained relatively unaltered through the evolution, while the C-terminal has been the most liable to change (Lowry and Scott, 1975),

ACTH extracted from both PA and PI is biologically active, but ACTH stellate cells from PA paricipate, to a large extent, in the control of adrenal cortex (Stark and Makara, 1982). These cells produce β-LPH, β-endorphin and β-MSH as well (Fig.3). In the adult adrenalectomised (Adx) rats the number of ACTH cells increases, and from 15 days onwards adrenalectomy cells are more numerous. In these cells of Adx rat, 15-20 days after head irradiation with 1200 R, regression of GER and Golgi complex are observed and large granules are present. If such animals were treated with corticosteroids, a smaller number of ACTH cells degenerated (Pantić and Hristić,1975).

ACTH cells in neonatal rats are stimulated in response to maternal adrenalectomy (Nickerson et al., 1978). Corticosteroids from fetuses cross the placental barrier and enter the maternal circulation. At birth, the adrenal gland is hypertrophic and plasma level of this steroid is increased (Milković et al., 1973; Hristić et al., 1978).

ACTH cells contain nonspecific receptors and are capable of ACTH release in response to many peptides (Dallman and Ytes, 1969; Koch et al., 1979, 1980).Finding that the release of these peptides are less stimulated by VP than by medial basal hypothalamic (MBH) extract (Lutz-Bucher et al., 1977) undertook further researches, and recently new peptide with CRF activity was discovere The role of vasopressin and CRF in regulation of ACTH cell activities is the subject of recently opened discussion.

4. THE EFFECTS OF OPIATE PEPTIDES ON PRL CELLS AND GONADOTROPIC ACTIVITIES

The peptides from the first group of hormones produced

by brain neurons and pituitary cells have a role in differentiation and activities of two other groups of pituitary cells. In this article the effect of β-endorphin, met-enkephalin on PRL cells and gonadotropic activity will be considered.

4.1. The relationship between opiates and PRL cells

Both opiates and PRL are involved in reaction to stress but the effects of the opiate peptides in regulation of PRL release and synthesis is the subject of discussions from the point of view as:

-Opioid molecules, as β-endorphin, met-enkephalin and several analogues of met-enkephalin, may stimulate PRL and GH release from the corresponding second group of pituitary cells (Fig.4, 5)(Bruni et al.,1977; Krulich, 1979).

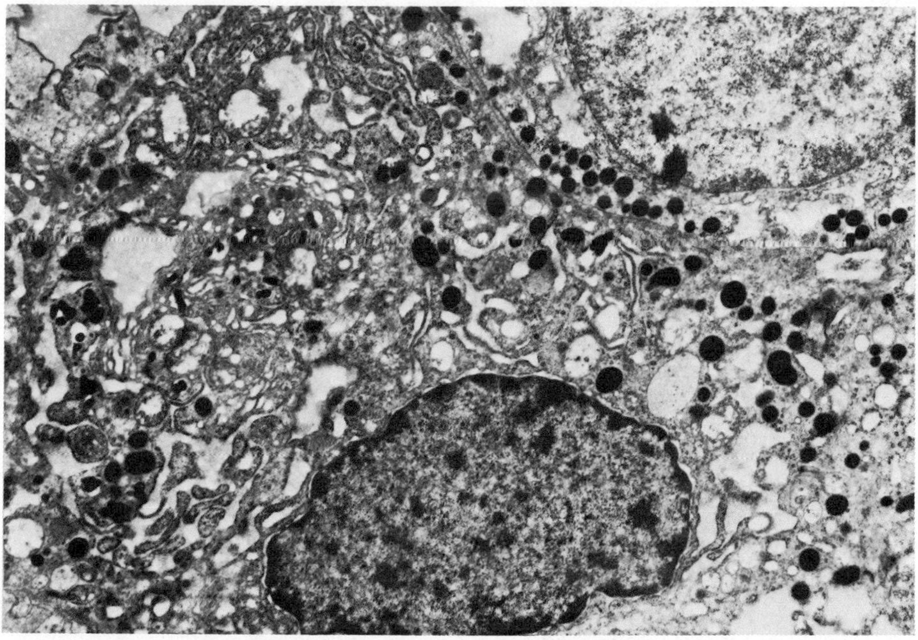

Fig.4. PRL cell with irregular specific granules.

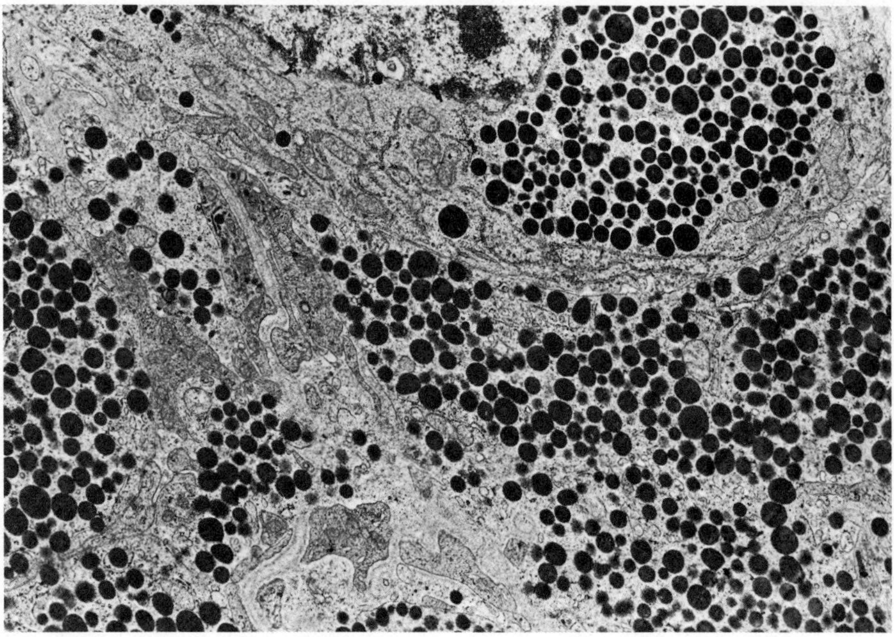

Fig.5. Growth hormone producing cells filled with specific granules.

- Analgetic activites of β-endorphin is more or less a unique property (Loh et al., 2975) and is mediated primarily by the so called μ receptors (Lord et al.,1977).

- PRL release can be modified by glucocorticoids (Sowers, 1977). On the other hand, opiates and opoide peptides supress the turnover and the release of dopamine (DA) into the portal vessels and this effect may in fact be involved with PRL release from the pituitary PRL cells (Shaar and Clemens, 1980).

- The release of PRL is regulated by TRH and Oe and is mainly inhibited by DA.

- In the regulation of PRL release TRH receptor complex activating cAMP, and Ca signalling system is involved (Gautvik et al., 1984).

- Met-enkephalin as a N-terminal fragment of β-endorphin appears to bind to the two types of brain receptors and is twenty times more active than normorphine.The role of met-enkephalin in ovulation in Lymnaca Stagnales was mentioned (see Roubos,1984).

- Morphine exerts testosterone like effects in the hypotalamus of the castrated male rats (Cicero et al., 1980).

4.2. The role of opiates in regulation of gonadotropin activities

Summarizing data related to catecholaminergic transmission, as an important mediator for interactions between steroid feedback and opiates action on LH release, Kalra, 1982, pointed that opoid peptides exert primarly anan inhibitory influence on LH release that can be modified by gonadal steroids milieu (Fig.6). The action of

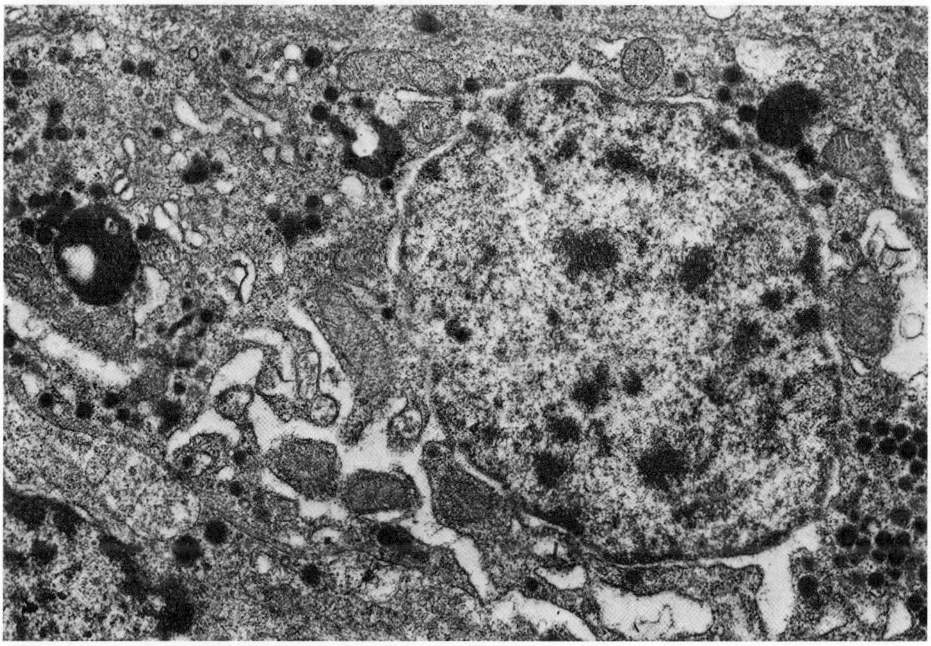

Fig.6. Gonadotropic cells of the rat pituitary after transplantation.

ment with glucocorticoids restore the synthesis of GH opiates can be attributed to functional links between opioid peptides and noradrenergic neurons occuring in close vicinity of the LRH neurons in the preoptic-tuberal pathway. He also revealed that privotal role of opioids in the chain of events, triggered by progesterone, is to stimulate hypersecretion of LRH in ovariectomized estrogen primed rats.

Opioid peptides may act at the level of LRH neurons to modulate DA action inhibiting DA induced release of these peptides from TIDA terminals in ME (Rotsztejn et al., 1978).

Opiate receptors have been demonstrated in regions innervated by monoaminergic neurons and on aminergic projections, which means that these two systems may interact to regulate several behavioral and neuroendocrine functions (Watson et al., 1980; Wamsley et al., 1980). The role of brain peptides as a neurotransmitter was mentioned by Snyder, 1980.

A close functional relationship exists between opioid peptides, norepinephrine (NE) and LRH containing neurons (Barry, 1979). Kalra, 1976, suggested that NE projections in the diencephalon may mediate the effects of opiates and their antagonists on LH release. It has been demonstrated that opioid peptides are modulators of LH secretion during sexual maturation as well (Blank et al.,1979).

The effects of these peptides are stimulatory for PRL secretion, but are inhibitory for gonadotropins, and in some species and under some experimental conditions, for TSH secretion and thyroid cell activities (Fig.7).

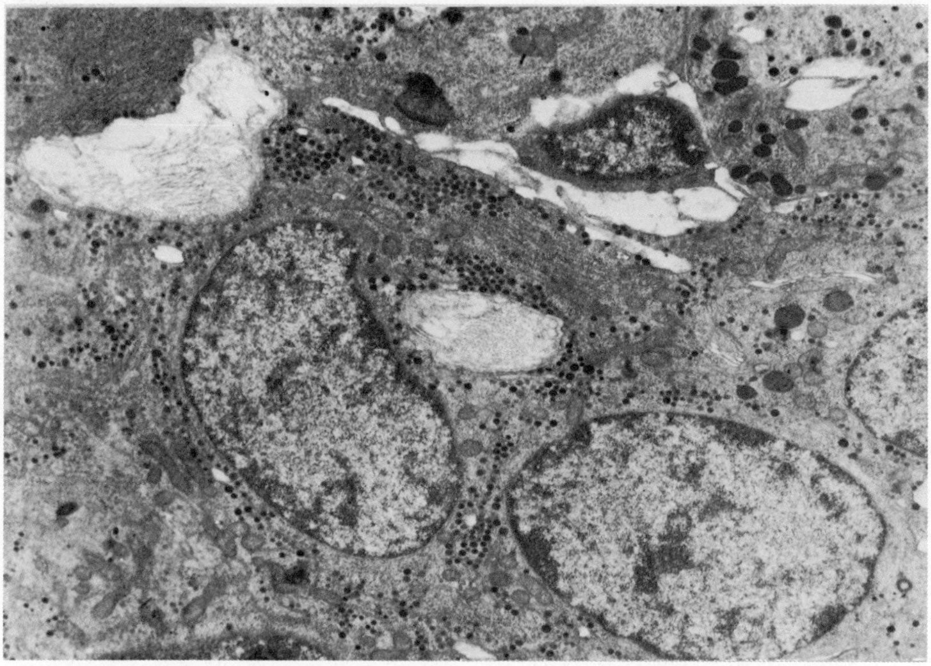

Fig.7. Thyrotropic cells of rats pituitary with increased intercellular spaces.

The effects of opiates, their antagonists and possibly of the endogenous opioid peptides on LH release might be mediated by the central norepinephrine neurons (Kalra, 1972; Kalra et al., 1972). The mode of opiates action inhibiting LH release is supported by the evidence that morphine can inhibit NE release from presynaptic nerve terminals (Stark et al., 1977). The basal plasma PRL levels and brain β-endorphin are significantly higher in old than in young rats (Barden and Dupont,1982).

5. THE EFFECTS OF ACTH AND PRL ON COMMON TARGET CELLS

A decrease of GH synthesis in the adrenalectomised rat is observed by Martial et al., 1977, 1982 and treat-

due to the increase of GH - mRNA synthesis (Yu et al., 1977).

Opiate molecules, as β-endorphine, play a very important role in stimulation of the release and the synthesis of PRL.

A common target cell for ACTH and PRL, as the hormones involved in stressogenic reaction, are adrenal cortex and mammary gland (Fig.6). Both opiates and PRL are inhibitors for the activities of glucoprotein producing cells esspecially gonadotrophs. These facts undoubtely show that the activities of GTH cells are dependent on the hormones of the two previous groups. Some results obtained examining adrenocortical cells as a target cell will be briefly mentioned.

The width of the adrenal cortex is diminished in all of the animals treated with a single injection of corticosteroids during early neonatal or with repeated doses administred during juvenile or perypubertal period of development. However, a decrease in the width of the adrenal cortex was observed in sexually mature female and male rats treated with large doses of Oe on day 3. or 6., and amounted from 18 to 24% in female rats (Pantić and Kilibarda, 1978; Kilibarda and Pantić, 1979). Such long term effect of Oe we considered from the point of feedback effect of this steroid on the maturation of brain target neurons affecting the differentiation and activities of ACTH and PRL producing cells, but other pituitary cells as well.

A significant decrease of zona reticularis is a result of the effect of Oe and PRL. Lesser width of adrenal cortex in the animals treated with Oe during juvenile and pubertal period, than in corresponding control, we considered from the point of view of lower responsiveness of adrenocortical cells to these steroids during juvenile than during neonatal period of life, even if they were treated with repeated doses of Oe. These data undoubtely suggested that sensitivity of hypothalamo-pituitary-adrenal axis is more pronounced in neonatal than in older examined period of development. For better understanding it is necessary to add that receptors for Oe and ACTH are present in cells of all cortical zones, while PRL receptors are in z.fasciculata and reticularis (Nolin , 1981). The reaction of adrenocortical cells in the Oe treated animals seems to be a result of the direct effect of gonadal steroid on these cells, but the effect is expressed via corresponding brain neurons and pituitary cells as well.

6. GONADES AS COMMON TARGET ORGANS FOR PRL, LRH, GTH AND STEROIDS

As parameters for character and degree of LRH and GTH cell reactions to hormones, both male and female gonads were examined and the obtained results were published in previous monographies and papers. Both steroidogenesis and gametogenesis are affected. The effect was dependent on the dose of steroids and stage of animal development, being most pronounced if they were administred during embriogenesis and neonatal period (Pantić, 1982).

It seems that both pituitary GTH and granulosa cell have the same pattern of LRH and PRL receptor complex and internalization by endocytosis. The nature of LRH receptors in the ovary was the subject of recent publication (Hazum, 1984).

Kalra and Kalra, 1982, pointed to the mode of involvement of gonadal steroids, adrenergic neurons and endogenic opioid peptides (EOP) system in the control of LRH secretion. These steroids modulate monoamine and neurons producing peptides and the responsiveness of LRH neurons as well. LH secretion is modified by NE action on LRH release (Ojeda et al., 1982). LRH neurons are localised in preoptic area (POA), nucleus arcuatus (NA) and ME. Brain neurons, as a major producer of EOP, are identified in the hypothalamus and POA.

Gonadal steroid can direct the accumulation of LRH as the most sensitive neurons. The action is dependent of their direct effect on LRH neurons as the clock responsible for LH secretion (Kalra and Kalra, 1982). Large doses of gonadal steroids administred into rats during neonatal, juvenile, peripubertal, adult and old period of life, affected directly LRH neurons, pituitary GTH cells, ovaries or testicles as well (Pantić, 1982, 1984). The reaction in rats and piglets differs and depends on the degree of differentiation of cells in brain neuron-pituitary-gonadal axis.

Accepting that high affinity and specific receptors of LRH exist in GTH cells, ovarian granulosa cells (Naor et al., 1980) and in testes as well, the extra-pituitary effect is clearly expressed on both steroidogenesis and gametogenesis in male and female gonads of rats treated with gonadal steroids. In addition, an increased blood concentration of PRL affect GTH cells and both gonads and finally, direct effect of gonadal steroids is expressed on steroidogenic cells and germ epithelium as well.

7. REACTION OF TARGET CELLS AT SUBCELLULAR LEVEL

Analizing the reaction of neuroendocrine cells in various stressogenic situtations, the cell reactions at subcellular and molecular level have to be considered. As it was mentioned the adrenal cortical cell reactions to corticosteroids and gonadal steroids are expressed and are dependent on the responses of brain neuron producing CRF, vasopressin, ACTH, prolactin and other hormones as well.

7.1. Hormone receptor complex

One of the contemporary problem of molecular biology is the role of hormone receptors with a specific capacity for receiving and transmission of information from extracellular enviroments affecting various cell activities as are: differentiation, growth, retrodifferentiation, determination of the cell cycle specificities, including reaction of noncyclic cells to division cycle or to return of cyclic cell to quiescences. Hormones, neurotransmitters and neuromodulators binded to receptors as a hormone-receptor complex include catalytic unit to its active, cAMP producing state, and other known intracellular events characteristical for responce to steroid or peptide hormones. The effects might be short or long term controlling cell activities during ontogenesis, being more pronounced during the early development, then in adult or old stages of life. The harmony of organisms of the animals, including man, with the environment may be altered in a different way so that brain neurons, endocrine and even other cell types may loose the ability to react at the appropriate time as they are adapted during development and adult stages. Usually hormones, neurotransmitters or neuromodulators affect plasma membrane complexities. For this process Mg ions are necessary and process dependent upon the integrity of its microenvironments for proper regulation (Kalra and Kalra, 1984).

7.2. Plasma membrane, cytoskeleton and cell organelle reaction

As a result of the repeated stressful stimuli, or influence of various agencies, the intracellular biochemical events occur and induce rearrangement of plasma membrane components, alteration circadian rhytmus of cell activities. As a result of gradual or even sudden loss of cell activities, error in programmed aging, senescence and different types of cell degenerations occur.

Plasma membrane activities is recycling during endocytosis or exocytosis and this is dependent on biophysical events as are presence of receptors, state of ionic channels, etc. For example, catecholamines have a role to contract cerebral arteries by depolarisation of the plasma membrane (see Harder and Waters, 1984). As it is known in the control of both endocytosis and exocytosis Ca ions have a very important role. These ions are stored in various cell organelles as are vesicles, cavities of ER, mitochondria, lysosomes, etc. More attention needs to be paid to the role of the cytoskeleton in the responses of target cells to hormones (Hall, 1984). Besides their important involvement in both endocytosis and exocytosis, the other intracellular events, as synthesis of new proteins which occur after the release, need to be in focus of molecular endocrinologists.

Steroids rapidly alter chromatin structure by activating genome and biosynthesis of proteins (Johnson et al.,1979). The mechanism of steroid feedback has been thought to involve DNA dependent RNA transcription in the hypothalamus and pituitary (McEwen and Luine, 1978).

Jutisz et al., 1984, pointed that the synthesis of gonadotropin subunits is controled by estradiol, GRH stimulated directly or indirectly by the biosynthesis of polypeptid chain of FSH and LH, but does not stimulate their glucosylation. However, for this effect the structural integrity of GTH cells is necessary (Khar et al., 1978). Justisz et al., 1984, concluded that the synthesis of gonadotropin subunits is under the dual control of GRH and Oe, which have opposite effects and they postulated that these hormones regulate the expression of the GTH subunits at the transcriptional level. However, it is necessary to point out that, besides direct action of GRH and Oe, the inhibitory effect of Oe on GTH cells via PRL cells, is of great importance (Pantić, 1984). The reaction of cell organelles in young chicken liver hepatocytes was observed after the treatment with a single large dose of Hy. Granular endoplasmic reticulum was less developed, Golgi zones occupied small areas and inclusion in the mitochondrial matrix were often observed (Pantić and Kosanović, unpublished) (Fig.8).

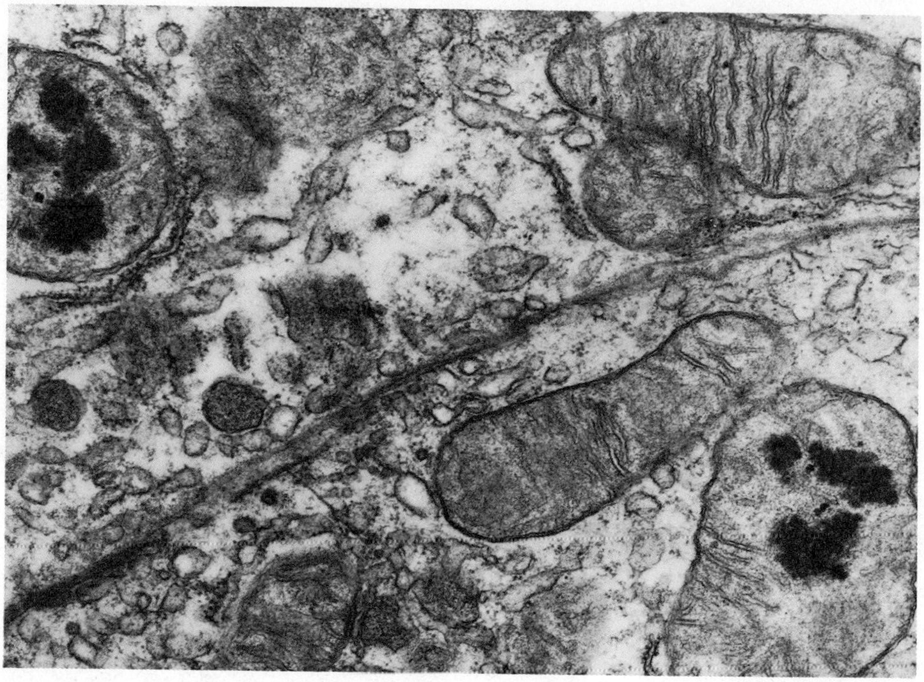

Fig.8. Cytoplasmic organelles in liver of young chicken treated with a large dose of Hy.

7.3. Neurotransmitters as modulators of steroid receptors

Peptide hormones and neurotransmitters, under some conditions, might stimulate the action of steroids or modulate the state of steroid receptors.

As it is known the receptors for peptidic and protein hormones are located at the external site of plasma membranes and for steroids in cytosoles. For example, adenylate cyclase appears to be located at multiple sites within plasma membrane of brain neurons and in the cell organelles as are endoplasmatic reticulum, nuclear membranes, lysosomes, Golgi zones, axones, synapses (Poeggel et al., 1984). Pietras and Szego, 1979,suggested the presence of uterine plasma membrane receptros for steroids, as well.

Changes in biochemical composition and physical state of membrane lipids may alter the properties of ionic channels on modified efficiency of receptors to peptides, neurotransmitters and other agencies (Dufy et al., 1982).

Harder and Waters, 1984, mentioned that, if the ion channels are blocked or inactivated, than many vasoactive agents are capable by bypassing the membrane to exert directly contractile elements.

Intracellular reaction to steroids in brain neurons, owing to the presence of blood brain barrier, is dependent on the dose of gonadal or cortical steroids. Cytoplasmic organelles respond on a specific and characteristical way. Proliferation of GER in PRL cells is clearly evident after treatment with both female and male gonadal steroids administered during all stages of ontogenesis being most expressed for a long period of time after a large, but single dose during neonatal development (Pantić, 1981, 1982). This may be interpreted as an evidence of PRL cell activation induced by the direct effect of Oe on these cell differentiations.

8. SUMMARY

Neuroendocrine cell reaction to stressfull stimuli and on constantly increasing number of agencies, arising from internal and external environmental factors, the role of these cells in the adaptation to an increased amount of endogenous or exogenous hormones, were considered and might be summarised as follows:

The family of the first group of stress responding hormones, evolved from heptapeptid to prohormones consisting of LPH_S, MSH_S, ACTH, CLIP, endorphins and encephalins, are synthesised and released from special brain neurons, PI cells and ACTH cells of PA.

The pituitary cells are specialized through the phylogenetic evolution to react on species specific ways on various stressful stimuli and agencies. The specificity of these cells depends on brain and pituitary differentiating cells, but they influence subsequently on the appearence of peptide producing cells from the second group and from the third group of pituitary cells producing glucoprotein hormones. Besides, these cells are common target cells for steroid and peptide hormones, brain neurons and PI cells, receive the signals from neurotransmitters and neuromodulators, as well.

Peptide hormones produced by the first group of cells affect the activities of the second and third group of pituitary cells. More data is necessary to elucidate the complexity of their influence and interrelationship. Recently it is often mentioned that met-enkephalin and β-endorphine stimulate prolactin cells to release and to synthesize PRL.

PRL cells as cells reacting to stressors are at the same time the common target cells for gonadal steroid and peptide hormones. These hormones influence the production of an increased amount of PRL, which inhibit the differentiation and the activity of GTH and to some extent TSH producing cells, and the reaction is dose dependent.

As hormones involved in reaction to stressors and in adaptation, ACTH and PRL, affect common target organs, such as adrenal cortex and mammary gland, PRL and GTH have receptors in testicular and ovarian target cells. These peripherial target organs are very convinient as parameters for better understanding of direct and indirect effects of peptide and steroid hormones.

The knowledge of complexed reactivity of neuroendocrine cells to various stressors, in the adaptation and the feedback influences of peripheral target organs on these specific cells, is rapidly increasing and more data is necessary to define their reaction at the molecular level.

In order to prevent unconvinient and not seldom fatal effects of some stressors, more attention needs to be paid to the nature and properties of plasma membrane organisation from the point of view of the presence of receptors for hormones, ion channels, cytosis, the role of cytoskeleton in internalisation, hormone release and synthesis, during specific cell differentiation, cell cycles and retrodifferentiation.

<u>In conclusion</u>, the intention of this article is to pay the attention to the species specific reactions of neuroendocrine cells on various stressors and to the complexity of the mechanisms involved in the adaptation. The rapidly increased number of stressors affect the gene expression of target cells and molecular organisation of their cell organelles and are dependent on the genetic determination. The reactions differ owing to the variability in sensitivity on the more and more uncontrolled

ecological conditions. The character and nature of response is potentiated by many medical drugs, as are the amount of internal or external steroids, peptide and other hormones. Sufficiency or defficiency of hormones lead to the debalance of neuroendocrine cells, expressed in many different abnormal processes and even in cancerogenesis.

Acknowledgment: Thanks to Meri Vasić for helping write the manuscript.

9. REFERENCES

Baertschi,A.J., Vallet,P., Baumann,J.B. and Girard,J., 1980. Neuronal lobe pituitary domuldates corticotropin releas in the rat, Endocrinology 106: 878.

Barden,N. and Dupont,A., 1982. Distribution and changes in peptides in the brain, in:"Hormonally Active Brain Peptide, Structure and Function",K.W.McKerns and V.Pantić, eds,Plenum Press, New York, p.307.

Barry,J., 1979. Immuno-histochemistry of luteinizing hormone-releasing hormone producing neurons of the vertebrates, Inter.Rev.Cytol. 60: 179.

Blank,M.S., Paneri,A.E, and Friesen,H.G., 1979. Opioid peptides modulate luteinizing hormone secretion during sexual maturation,Science 203: 1129.

Bruni,J.F., Van Vught,D., Marschall,S. and Meites,J., 1977. Effect of naloxone, morphine and methionine enkephalin on serum prolactin,luteinizing hormone, follicle stimulating hormone, thyroid stimulating hormone and growth hormone, Life Sci. 21: 461.

Cicero,T.J., Meyer,E.R., Gabriel,S.M., Bell,R.D. and Wilcox,C.E., 1980. Morphine exerts testosterone-like effects in the hypothalamus of the castrated male rats, Brain Res. 202: 151.

Dallman,M.F. and Yates,F.E., 1969, Dynamic asymmetries in the corticosteroid feedback path and distribution - metebolism - binding elements of the adrenocortical system, Ann.N.Y.Acad.Sci. 156: 696.

de Bold,A.J., de Bold,M.L. and Kraicer,J., 1980, Structural relationship between parenchymal and stromal elements in the pars intermedia of the rat adenohypophysis as demonstrated by extracellular space markers, Cell Tissue Res., 207 (3): 347.

Dufy,B., Dufy-Barbe,L., Arnauld,E. and Vincent,L.D., 1982, Steroids and Membrane-Associated Events in Neurons and Pituitary Cells, in:"Hormonally Active Brain Peptide Structure and Function", K.W.McKerns, and V.Pantić, eds, Plenum Press, New York, p .235.

Edwards,P.M. and Rousseau,G.G., 1982, Steroid Antagonism of Melanosome Movements Induced by Neuropeptides, in:"Hormonally Active Brain Peptide Structure and Function", K.W.McKerns and V.Pantić., eds. Plenum Press, New York, p .349.

Feldman,S., Conforti,N. and Chowers,I., 1972, Neural pathways mediating adrenocortical responses to photic and acoustic stimuli, Neuroendocrinology 10: 316.

Gautvik,K.M., Hang,E., Sand,O., Iversen,J., Johansen,P.W., Sletholt,K. and Gordeladze,J., 1984, Regulation of prolactin secretion by thyroliberin (TRH) in cultured rat pituitary tumor cells, in:"Regulation of Target Cell Responsiveness", K.W.McKerns, A.Aakvaag and V.Hansson, eds, Plenum Press, New York, p .23.

Hall,P.F., 1984, The role of the cytoskeleton in the responses of target cells to hormones, in:"Regulation of Target Cell Responsiveness"K.W.McKerns and A.Aakvaag and V.Hansson,eds,Plenum Press, New York p. 205.

Harder,D.R. and Waters,A., 1984. Electrical activation of arterial muscle, Inter.Rev.Cytol. 89: 138.

Hang,E., Gautvik,K.M., Sand,O., Iversen,J.G. and Kriz,M., 1982. Interaction between thyrotropin-releasing hormone and prolactin-producing cells, in:"Hormonally Active Brain Peptide, Structure and Function", K.W.McKerns and V.Pantić, eds,Plenum Press, New York, p.537.

Hazmun,A., 1984. Nature of the GnRH receptors in the ovary, in:"Regulation of Target Cell Responsiveness" K.W,McKerns, A.Aakvaag and V.Hansson,eds, Plenum Press, New York, p.23.

Hristić,M. and Pantić,V., 1974. Hypothalamus nuclei of rats after head irradiation and adrenocortical hormone treatment, Inter.J.Radiol.Biol. 26 (2): 147.

Hristić,M., Pantić,V. and Nickerson,P.A., 1978. Influence of maternal adrenalectomy on pituitary ACTH cells of fetal and neonatal rats, Acta Veterinaria (Belgrade) 18 (6): 231.

Jëgou,B., Le Gac,F., Hang,E., Torjesen,P.A. and Hansson, V., 1984. GnRH receptors and GnRH-like activity in the rat testis, in:"Regulation of Target Cell Responsiveness"K.W.McKerns, A.Aakvaag and V.Hansson,eds, Plenum Press, New York, p. 47.

Jutisz,M., Counis,R. and Corbani,M., 1984. Biosynthesis of pituitary gonadotropins and its regulation by gonadoliberin (GnRH) and estradiol, in:"Regulation of Target Cell Responsiveness"K.W.McKerns, A.Aakvaag and V.Hansson,eds, Plenum Press,New York, p. 385.

Kalra,P.S., Kalra,S.P., Krulich,L., Fawcett,C.P. and McCann,S.M., 1972. Involvement of norepinephrine in transmission of the stimulatory influence of progesterone on gonadotropin release, Endocrinology 90:1168

Kalra,S.P., 1976, Tissue levels of luteinizing hormone releasing hormone in the preoptic area and hypothalamus and serum concentration of gonadotropins following anterior hypothalamic deafferentiation and estrogen treatment of female rat, Endocrinology 99: 101.

Karla,P.S. and Kalra,S.P., 1982, Discriminative effects of testosterone on hypothalamic luteinizing hormone releasing hormone levels and LH secretion in castrated male rats : analysis of dose and duration characteristics, Endocrinology 111: 24.

Kalra,S.P., 1982, Mode of Opioid and Catecholamine Involvement in Regulating LH Secretion, in: "Hormonally Active Brain Peptides, Structure and Function", K.W.McKerns and V.Pantić, eds, Plenum Press, New York, p . 141.

Kalra,S.P. and Kalra,P.S., 1984, Hypothalamic microenvironment controlling LH RH secretion, in; "Regulation of Target Cell Responsiveness" K.W.McKerns, A. A.Aakvaag and V.Hansson,eds, Plenum Press, New York, p .127.

Kanazir,D.T., Ribarac-Stepić,N., Trajković,D., Blečić,G., Radojčić,M., Metlaš,R., Stefanović,D., Katan,M., Perišić,O., Popić,S. and Marković-Djordjević,R., 1979, Structure and regulatory functions of cortisol receptor. I. Extragenomic effect dependent on the cortisol receptor activation, J.Steroid Biochem. 11: 389.

Kanazir,D.T., 1982, The role of steroid receptors in the regulation and integration of steroid and peptide hormone actions in common target cells : Facts and speculations, in: "Hormonally Active Brain Peptides, Structure and Function", K.W.McKerns and V.Pantić, eds, Plenum Press, New York, p . 181,

Kelly,M.J., 1982, Electrical effects of steroids in neurons, in: "Hormonally Active Brain Peptides, Structure and Function", K.W.McKerns and V.Pantić, eds, Plenum Press, New York, p .253.

Khar,A., Debeljuk, L. and Jutisz,M., 1978, Biosynthesis of gonadotropins by rat pituitary cells in culture and pituitary homogenates : Effect of gonadotropin-releasing hormone, Mol.Cell Endocrinology 12: 53.

Kilibarda,M. and Pantić,V., 1979, The adrenal cortex of male rats treated with female gonadal steroids, Stereol.Yugosl.2: 65.

Koch,B., Lutz-Bucher,B., Briand,B. and Mialhe,C., 1979, Relationship between ACTH secretion and corticoid binding to specific receptors in perifused adenohypophysis, Neuroendocrinology 28: 169.

Koch,B., Lutz-Bucher,B. and Mialhe,C., 1980, Interaction of glucocorticoids, CRF and vasopressin in the regulation of ACTH secretion, in: "Synthesis and Release of Adenohypophyseal Hormones", M.Jutisz and K.W. McKerns, eds, Plenum Press, New York, p .561.

Krulisch,L., 1979, Central neurotransmitters and the secretion of prolactin, GH, LH and TSH, Ann.Rev. Physiol. 41: 603.

Li,H.C., 1972, Hormones of the adenohypophysis, Proc. Am.Philos.Soc.116: 365.

Loh,H.H., Tseng,L.F., Wie,E. and Li,C.H., 1976, Endorphin is a potent analgesic agent, Proc.Natl.Acad.Sci.USA 73: 2895.

Lord,J.A.H., Waterfield,A., Hughes,J. and Kosterlitz,H.W., 1977, Endogenous opioid peptides : Multiple agonists and receptors, Nature (London) 267: 495.

Lowry,P.J. and Scott,A.P., 1975, The evolution of vertebrate corticotrophin and melanocyte stimulating hormone, Gen.Comp.Endocrinol. 26: 16.

Lutz-Bucher,B., Koch,B. and Mailhe,C., 1977, Comparative *in vitro* activity of vasopressin and hypothalamic median eminence extract, Neuroendocrinology 23: 181.

Makara,G.B., Stark,E. and Mihaly,K., 1970, Corticotrophin release induced by traumatic stress in rats with unilateral spinal cord lesion, Acta Physiol.Acad.Sci. Hung. 38: 199.

Martial,J.A., Baxter,D.J., Goodman,M.H. and Seeburg,H.P., 1977, Regulation of growth hormone messenger RNA by thyroid and glucocorticoid hormones, Proc.Natl. Acad.Sci.USA 74: 1816.

Martial,J.A., Truong,A.T., Laverriere,J.N. and Morin,A., 1982, Structure and regulation of the prolactin gene, Program of the Europlan INSERM Symposium on "Multihormonal Regulation in Neuroendocrine Cells", Colmar (France) September 1-4, 53 (Abstr.32).

McEwen,B.S. and Luine,V.N., 1978, Specificity, mechanisms and functional significance of steroid-receptor interaction in the brain and pituitary, in: "Biologie Cellulaire des Processus Neurosécrétores Hypothalamique, J.D.Vincent and C.Kordon,eds, CNRS, Paris, p .239.

Milković,K., Paunović,J., Knïewald,Z., Milković,S.,1973, Maintenance of the plasma corticosterone concentration of adrenalectomized rat by the fetal adrenal gland, Endocrinology 93: 115.

Naor,Z., Clayton,R.N. and Catt,K.J., 1980, Characterization of gonadotropin releasing hormone receptors in cultured pituitary cells, Endocrinology 107: 1144.

Nickerson,P.A., Hristić,M. and Pantić,V., 1978, Influence of maternal adrenalectomy on the ultrastructure of the adrenal gland in neonatal rats, Cell Tissue Res. 189: 277.

Nolin,J., 1981, Profiles of target cells prolactin and adrenocorticotropin during lactation diestrus, in: "Reproductive Processes and Contraception", K.W. McKerns, ed, Plenum Press, New York, p.195.

Ojeda,S.R., Negro-Vilar,A. and McCann,S.M., 1982, Evidence for involvement of alpha-adrenerg-c receptors in norepinephrine - induced prostaglandin E_2 and luteinizing hormone-releasing hormone release and the median eminence, Endocrinology 110: 409.

Palkovits,M., 1982, Recent data on neuropeptide mapping in the central nervous system, in: "Hormonally Active Brain Peptides, Structure and Function", K.W. McKerns and V.Pantić, eds, Plenum Press, New York, p.279.

Pantić,V., 1974. Gonadal steroids and hypothalamo-pituitary-gonadal axis, Inter.Symp. on Sexual Endocrinol. of Perinatal Period, INSERM, Paris, 32: 97.

Pantić,V., 1975. The specificity of pituitary cells and regulation of their activities, Int.Rev.Cytology 40: 153.

Pantić,V.R. and Šimić,M., 1977, Sensitivity of pituitary pars intermedia to castration or gonadal steroids, Bull.Acad.Serbe Sci.Arts, T, LX (16): 67.

Pantić,V.R. and Kilibarda,M., 1978, Adrenal cortex of rats treated with oestradiol neonatally and during sexual maturity, Acta Veterinaria 28: 1.

Pantić,V.R., 1980, Adenohypophyseal cell specificities and gonadal steroids, in: "Synthesis and Release of Adenohypophyseač Hormones",M.Jutisz and K.W.McKerns, eds, Plenum Press, New York, p.335.

Pantić,V.R., 1981. Sensitivity of pituitary gonadotropic cells and gonads to hormones, in:"Reproductive Processes and Contraception", K.W.McKerns, ed. Plenum Press, New York, p .47.

Pantić,V.R., 1982. Genesis and properties of pituitary ACTH, MSH, prolactin and GH producing cells, in: "Hormonally Active Brain Peptides, Structure and Function", K.W.McKerns and V.Pantić, eds. Plenum Press, New York, p .504.

Pantić,V., 1984. Prolactin target cells in rats treated with gonadal steroids, in."Regulation of Target Cell Responsiveness" K.W.McKerns, A.Aakvaag and V.Hansson, eds. Plenum Press, New York, p . 283.

Pavić,D., Živković,N., Pantić,V. and Martinović,P.,1977. Glukoprotein synthesizing cells in the anterior pituitaries transplanted into hypophysectomized male rats, Arhiv bioloških nauka, 27, 1-2: 1.

Peck,E.J. and Kelner,K.L., 1984. Differential sensitivity of estrogen targets: Receptors and responses, in: "Regulation of Target Cell Responsiveness", K.W.McKerns, A.Aakvaag and V.Hansson,. eds. Plenum Press, New York, pg. 256.

Pietras,R.J. and Szego,C.M., 1979. Estrogen receptors in uterine plasma membrane, J.Steroid Biochem. 11:1471.

Poeggel,G., Luppa,H., Bernstein,H.E.G. and Weiss,J.,1984. Histochemistry of adenylate cyclase, Inter.Rev.Cytol. 89: 35.

Rotsztejn,W., Drouva,S., Pattou,E. and Kordon,C.,1978. Met-enkephalin inhibits in vitro dopamine-induced LHRH release from medio-basal hypothalamus of male rats, Nature (London) 274:281.

Roubos,E.W.,1984. Cytobiology of the ovulation-neurohormone producing neuroendocrine caudo-dorsal cells of Lymnaea stagnalis, Inter.Rev.Cytol., vol.89:295.

Saint Gerons,H., 1961. Particularites anatomiques et histologiques de l´hypophyse chez les Squamata, Arch. Biol. 72:211.

Seppälä,M., Wahlström,T. and Leppäluoto,J., 1979. Luteinizing hormone releasing factor (LFR)-like immunoreactivity in rat pancreatic islet cells, Life Sci. 25: 1489.

Shaar,C.J. and Clemens,J.A., 1980, The effect of opiate agonists on growth hormone and prolactin release in rats, Fed.Proc. 38: 2539.

Sharpe,R.M. and Fraser,H.M., 1980. Leydig cell receptors for luteinizing hormone releasing hormone and its agonists and their modulation by administration or deprivation of the releasing hormone, Biochem. Biophys.Res.Commun., 95: 256.

Sharpe,R.M., 1980. Extra-pituitary actions of LHRH and its agonists, Nature (London) 286: 12.

Sharpe,R.M., 1982. Cellular aspects of the inhibitory actions of LH-RH on the ovary and testes, J.Reprod. Fertility, 64: 517.

Smelik,P.G., 1963. Relation between blood level of corticoids and their inhibiting effect on the hypophyseal stress response, Proc.Soc.Exp.Biol.Med. 113: 616.

Snyder,S.H., 1980. Brain peptides as neurotransmitters, Science 209: 976.

Sowers,J.R., Carlson,H.E., Brautbar,N. and Hershman,J.M., 1977. Effect of dexamethason on prolactin and TSH responses to TRH and metoclopamide in man, J.Clin. Endocrinol.Metab. 44: 237.

Stark,E., Makara,G.B., Palkovits,M. and Mihály,K., 1970. Afferent pathways of stressful stimuli: Their dependence on strength and the time elapsed after the onset of stimulation, Acta Physiol.Acad.Sci.Hung.38:43.

Stark,E., Kárteszi,M., Rappay,G. and Makara,G.B., 1981. Effects of treatment with adrenocorticotrophin on the hypothalamo-pituitary-adrenal system,J.Endocrinol. 88: 131.

Stark,E., Makara,G.B., Marton,J. and Palković,M., 1973/74. ACTH release in rats after removal of the medial hypothalamus, Neuroendocrinology 13; 224.

Stark,K., Taube,H.D. and Borowski,E., 1977. Presynaptic receptor system in catecholaminergic transmission, Biochem.Phyrmacol. 26: 259.

Stark,E., and Makara,G.B., 1982. Stress, corticoliberin (CRF) and glucocorticoids in the regulation of ACTH release, in:"Hormonally Active Brain Peptide, Structure and Function", K.W.McKerns and V.Pantić,eds. Plenum Press, New York, p .157.

Stošić,N., Pantić,V., Pavlović-Hournac,M. and Radivojević, D., 1965.Investigation of hypothalamus and hypophysis of thyroidectomized rats after the transplantation of irradiated grafts thyroid gland, Iugoslav. Physiol.Pharmacol.Acta 1 (2): 194.

Jing,S.Y. et Guillemin,R.,1979. Gonadostatine et gonadocrinine, polypeptides d'origine ovarienne á activities hypophysiotropes, C.R.Hebd.Acad.Ser.D.(Paris) 289: 943.

Yu,L.Y., Tushinski,J.R. and Bancroft,F.C., 1977. Glucocorticoid induction of growth hormones synthesis in a strain of rat pituitary cells, J.Biol.Chem.252: 3870.

Wamsley,J., Young,W.S. and Kuhar,M.J., 1980. Immunohistochemical localization of enkephalin in rat forebrain, Brain Res. 190: 153.

Watson,S., Richards,G.W., Ciarvanello,R.D. and Barchas, J.D., 1980. Interaction of opiate peptides and noradrenalin system: Light microscopic studies, Peptides 1: 30.

Wolfe,B.B., Harden,K.T. and Molinoff,B.R., 1976.Adrenergic receptors in rat liver: Effect of Adrenalectomy, Proc.Natl.Acad.Sci.USA 73: 1343.

Žgurić,M. and Pantić,V., 1970. Hypothalamus and Hypophysis in rats following adrenalectomy and head irradiation with X-rays, Iugoslav.Physiol.Pharmacol. Acta 6, 3: 471.

CALCIUM-ACTIVATED PHOSPHOLIPID-DEPENDENT PROTEIN KINASE: A NOVEL SIGNAL TRANSDUCTION MECHANISM IN THE PITUITARY

Zvi Naor and Jacob Hermon

Department of Hormone Research
The Weizmann Institute of Science
Rehovot, 76100, Israel

INTRODUCTION

The hypothalamic peptide hormones exert their stimulatory effect upon the pituitary by elevation of intracellular cyclic AMP (cAMP) and/or calcium levels (for review see Naor, 1982; Gershengorn, 1982). cAMP was implicated as the second messenger for corticotropin-releasing factor (CRF) and growth hormone releasing hormone (GHRH) (Giguere et al., 1982; Brazeau et al., 1982). On the other hand, recent studies have suggested that increased phosphoinositide turnover and elevated Ca^{2+} levels are involved in the mechanism of action of gonadotropin releasing hormone (GnRH), thyrotropin releasing hormone (TRH) and GHRH (Naor, 1982; Snyder and Bleasdale, 1982; Gershengorn, 1982; Sutton and Martin, 1982; Rebecchi et al., 1983; Canonico et al., 1983; Kiesel and Catt, 1984; Raymond et al., 1984; Naor et al., 1984).

A new species of calcium-activated, phospholipid-dependent protein kinase (protein kinase C,) was recently discovered and characterized in the brain (Takai et al., 1979). Protein kinase C is activated by association with membrane phospholipids in particular phosphatidylserine (PS) in the presence of elevated Ca^{2+}. The presence of small amounts of unsaturated diacylglycerol (DG) increases the apparent affinity for PS and decreases the Ca^{2+} concentration needed for maximal enzyme activity (Kishimoto et al., 1980). A preliminary report on pituitary protein kinase C has recently appeared (Turgeon et al., 1984). Since GnRH, TRH and GHRH (and possibly other hypophysiotropic hormones) induce rapid phosphatidylinositol (PI) turnover during which DG is generated, it is tempting to suggest that protein kinase C plays a key role in transmembrane control of cellular activation in the pituitary.

The release of the stress hormone ACTH is regulated by complex interaction of CRF, vasopressin and catecholamines at the pituitary level (Axelrod and Reisine, 1984). Cyclic AMP and Ca^{2+} play a major role in mediating the release process. The recent recognition that protein kinase C might represent one branch of the Ca^{2+} messenger system (Zawalich et al., 1983) makes the enzyme an ideal candidate for signal transduction mechanisms involved in stress.

CHARACTERIZATION OF THE SOLUBLE ENZYME

The time course for enzyme activation using a crude cytosolic preparation is shown in Fig. 1. Reaction velocity is linear for the first 3 minutes, the time that was chosen for all experiments. Enzyme velocity is linear with protein concentrations as shown in Fig. 2. The range of 10-20 µg protein of crude cytosol preparation was used routinely.

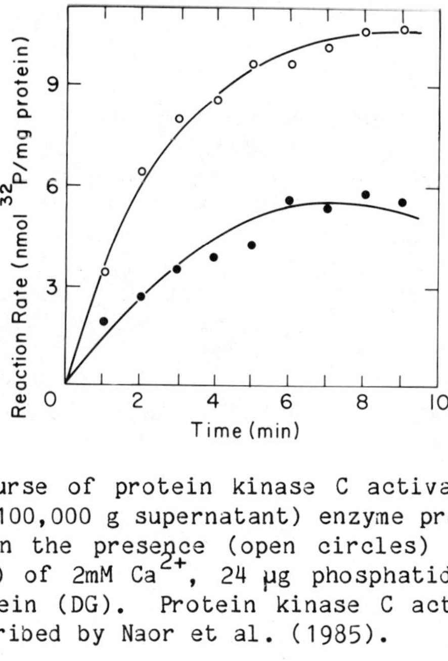

Fig. 1. Time-course of protein kinase C activation. Crude cytosolic (100,000 g supernatant) enzyme preparation was incubated in the presence (open circles) or absence (closed circles) of 2mM Ca^{2+}, 24 µg phosphatidylserine (PS); 0.8 µg diolein (DG). Protein kinase C activity was measured as described by Naor et al. (1985).

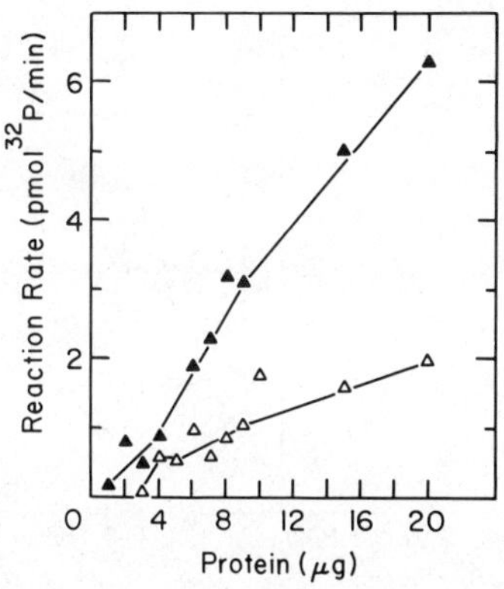

Fig. 2. Protein kinase C activation as a function of protein concentration. Enzyme assay was carried out for 3 min at 30° C in the presence (closed triangles) or absence (open triangles) of 2 mM Ca^{2+}, 24 μg phosphatidylserine and 0.8 μg diolein.

Protein kinase C is activated by phosphatidylserine (PS) and an unsaturated diacylglycerol such as diolein (DG), as shown in Fig. 3. The enzyme is absolutely dependent on the simultaneous presence of Ca^{2+} and PS, whereas Ca^{2+} and diolein alone are not sufficient for enzyme activation. Phosphatidylserine alone increased enzyme activity in the presence of calcium (Ka = 30 μg/ml). However, the presence of small amounts of DG (1.6 μg/ml) significantly reduced the Ka for PS from 30 to 15 μg/ml and also slightly increased maximal enzyme activity. Only in the presence of both Ca^{2+} and PS, a dose-response curve for DG activation of protein kinase C could be demonstrated (Ka = 0.8 μg/ml). The role of PS seems unique since other phospholipids tested in this reaction, phosphatidylethanolamine, phosphatidylinositol or phosphatidylcholine, could only partially support enzyme activity.

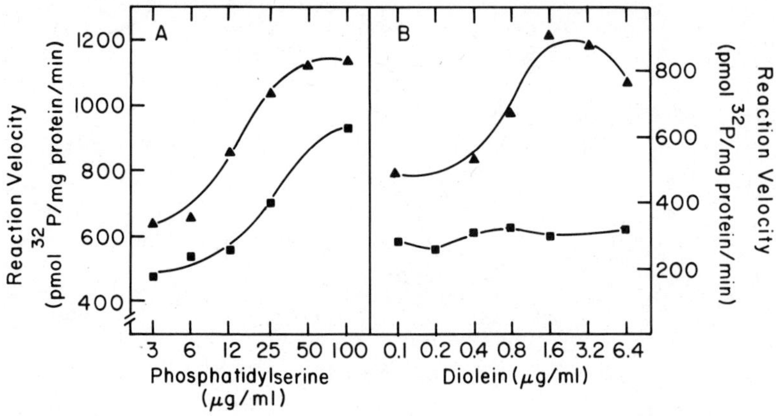

Fig. 3. Effect of phosphatidylserine (PS) and diolein (DG) on protein kinase C activity. Activity was determined in the presence of various concentrations of PS (A) in the presence of Ca^{2+} (10 uM, squares) or in the presence of Ca^{2+} (10 μM) and diolein (1.6 μg/ml, triangles), or (B) at various concentrations of diolein and Ca^{2+} alone (1 mM, squares) or Ca^{2+} (1 mM) and PS (12 μg/ml, triangles).

The reaction rates of protein kinase C in the presence of DG or PS alone or in the presence of both DG and PS were tested at various Ca^{2+} concentrations (Fig. 4). DG slightly increased enzyme activity, whereas PS produced a remarkable increase in enzyme activity. The presence of DG in addition to PS reduced the K_a for Ca^{2+} from 32 μM to 10 μM with little or no effect on maximal reaction velocity at saturating Ca^{2+} concentration.

A comparison of protein kinase C and other kinase activities present in crude pituitary cytosol is shown in Fig. 5. Only the simultaneous presence of calcium and PS markedly increase protein kinase C activity, as demonstrated previously, and the addition of DG increased maximal velocity at micromolar calcium concentration.

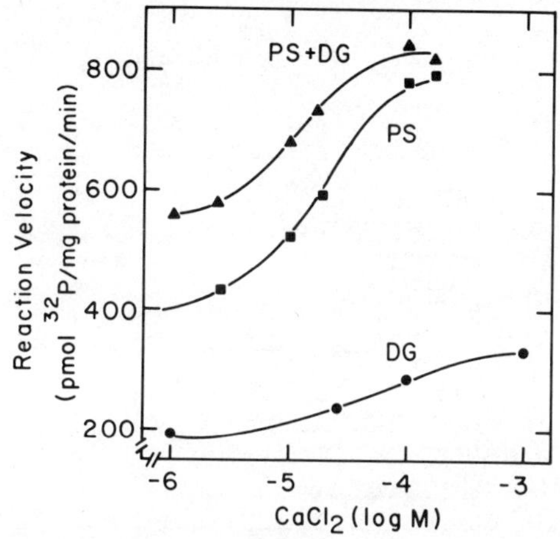

Fig. 4. Effect of diolein (DG) on the affinity of protein kinase C for calcium. Various concentrations of calcium were added with diolein (DG) alone (6.4 µg/ml), or with PS alone (8 µg/ml), or with DG and PS together. The Ca^{2+} concentrations indicated represent the added $CaCl_2$, not necessarily the actual free Ca^{2+} present in the assay.

cAMP-dependent protein kinase when fully activated reaches about 80% of maximal protein kinase C activity and cGMP- and calmodulin-dependent kinase activities represent 30 and 55% of protein kinase C activity respectively, when histone H1 + H2B is used as phosphate acceptor.

Partial purification of pituitary protein kinase C on DEAE cellulose chromatography yielded a major peak of activity eluted at 0.17 M NaCl (Fig. 6). Most of the cyclic-AMP dependent protein kinase (protein kinase A) eluted immediately after protein kinase C, coinciding with a peak of a Ca^{2+}-independent protein kinase which is not activated by PS or DG. The major peak of protein kinase C was 3.5 fold greater than the peak of protein kinase A when assayed with histone (H1 + H2B) as the phosphate acceptor.

PROTEIN KINASE C AND SIGNAL TRANSDUCTION IN THE PITUITARY

Neurotransmitters, peptide hormones, growth factors and other regulatory agents achieve certain of their biological effects by

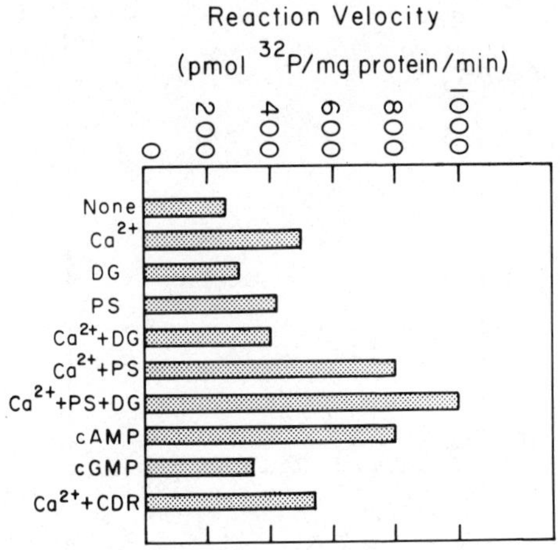

Fig. 5. Comparative activities of the various kinases present in crude pituitary cytosol preparation and contribution of Ca^{2+}, diolein and phosphatidylserine to protein kinase activity. None (EGTA 0.5 mM); Ca^{2+} (10 µM); DG (diolein, 3.2 µg/ml + EGTA 0.5 mM); PS (phosphatidylserine 50 µg/ml + EGTA 0.5 mM); Ca^{2+} + DG (10 µM, 3.2 µg/ml); Ca^{2+} + PS (10 µM, 50 µg/ml); Ca^{2+} + PS + DG (10 µM, 50 µg/ml, 3.2 µg/ml); cAMP (0.5 µM); cGMP (0.5 µM); Ca^{2+} + CDR (2 mM + calmodulin 0.8 µg/ml).

altering the phosphorylation of specific proteins (Greengard, 1978). Following the binding of the regulatory agent to its specific membrane receptor a 'second messenger' is generated and is responsible for protein phosphorylation (Greengard, 1978). cAMP, cGMP and calcium are considered classical second messengers and are capable of activating a respective protein kinase. A new protein kinase (protein kinase C) was recently discovered and characterized in rat brain (Takai et al., 1979; Kishimoto et al., 1980; Nishizuka, 1984). The enzyme is cAMP-independent but activated by calcium and phosphotidylserine. However, the presence of unsaturated diacylglycerol reduces the calcium concentration needed for maximal enzyme stimulation.

Some hypothalamic hormones do not act by activation of the cAMP-dependent protein kinase cascade (Gershengorn, 1982; Naor, 1982), but stimulate Ca^{2+} uptake and phosphatidylinositol turnover during which diacylglycerol is generated (e.g. GnRH and TRH) (Snyder and Bleasdale, 1982; Gershengorn, 1982; Sutton and Martin, 1982; Re-

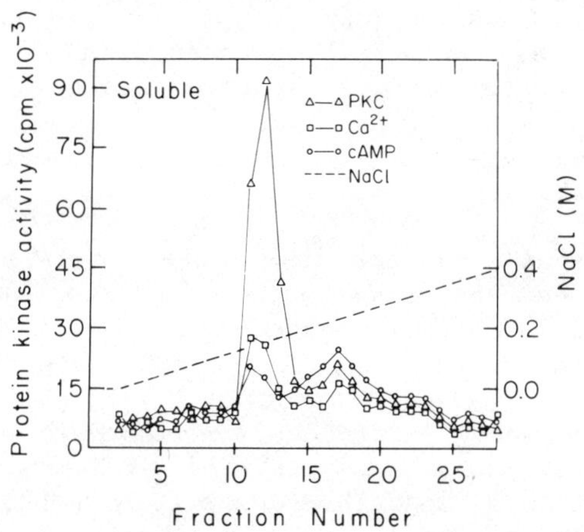

Fig. 6. DEAE-cellulose (DE-52) chromatography of pituitary protein kinase C. The 100,000 x g supernatant was prepared from thirty three anterior pituitaries. The column was first washed with 15 ml of column Buffer and protein kinases were eluted with a 30 ml linear gradient of NaCl (0-0.4 M). Fractions of 1 ml were collected and 50 µl samples were assayed for cAMP-dependent protein kinase A (0.5 µM cAMP), for Ca^{2+}-dependent protein kinase (1 mM Ca^{2+}), and for protein kinase C (Ca^{2+} 1 mM, PS 50 µg/ml, and DG 3.2 µg/ml).

becchi et al., 1983; Raymond et al., 1984; Kiesel and Catt, 1984; Naor et al., 1984). The case of GHRH seems more complex, since both cAMP and PI turnover were implicated in its action (Brazeau et al., 1982; Canonico et al., 1983). Protein kinase C present in rat pituitary preparation, is therefore an ideal mediator for transmembrane signal transduction for the hypothalamic peptide hormones that act via a Ca^{2+} generating system.

The activation of protein kinase C is most likely associated with enhanced phosphatidylinositol turnover and DG formation in the plasma membrane after hormonal challenge. Thus the liberated DG can bring about activation of the enzyme in the face of micromolar concentrations of calcium and a relatively high concentration of PS present in the cell membrane. However, since most of the pituitary enzyme is soluble, it is likely that the inactive enzyme is recruited to the membrane by the activated hormone-receptor complex (Naor et al., 1985). Such translocation by phorbol ester in parietal yolk sacs cells was recently proposed (Kraft and Anderson, 1983).

Protein kinase C was mostly studied in the brain (Nishizuka, 1984). However, its widespread occurrence in various tissues and phyla of the animal kingdom was reported (Kuo et al., 1980; 1984). Nevertheless, little is known about the pituitary enzyme where it might serve a key regulatory role in the mechanism of action of certain hypophysiotropic hormones.

The physiological substrates for protein kinase C are still not known but a few endogenous proteins were recently reported to be phosphorylated by the enzyme, among them a 40 K protein in human platelets (Kaibuchi et al., 1983), the cytoskeletal protein vinculin (Werth et al., 1983), 80 K protein in 3T3 cell line (Rozengurt et al., 1983) and smooth muscle heavy meromyosin (Nishikawa et al., 1982). It is also known that multiple phosphorylation of H1 histone occurs in late G1 through M phase (Langan and Hohmann, 1974), suggesting that endogenous H1 might be a natural substrate for the enzyme.

Protein kinase C was recently reported to be activated by phorbol ester (Castanga et al., 1982). and more recently it was found that the phorbol ester receptor and C-kinase from rat brain co-purify suggesting that the enzyme is the phorbol ester receptor (Niedel et al., 1983). The tumor promotor phorbol ester binds and activates pituitary cells and causes the release of various pituitary hormones (Naor and Catt, 1981; Smith and Vale, 1981; Jacken et al., 1981), lending support to our proposal that pituitary protein kinase C is a potential key biochemical event in pituitary function.

Pituitary protein kinase C is a distinct and unique Ca^{2+}-dependent protein kinase for several reasons. It is fully activated only in the simultaneous presence of Ca^{2+}, PS and DG. Neither Ca^{2+} alone, nor Ca^{2+} + calmodulin can account for the activity found when Ca^{2+}, PS and DG are present. Its substrate specificity differs from that of cAMP-dependent protein kinase. While protein kinase C preferentially phosphorylates H1 histone, cAMP-dependent protein kinase favors histone H2B as its substrate. The possibility that protein kinase C activity results from a dissociated free catalytic subunit of cAMP-dependent protein kinase which becomes cAMP-independent is ruled out since elevated Ca^{2+} and PS will inhibit such activity (Iwasa and Hosey, 1983). The possibility that the activity of protein kinase C observed in the pituitary resulted from a dissociated catalytic subunit of protein kinase C (protein kinase M) is ruled out since protein kinase M is fully active even in the absence of Ca^{2+}, PS and DG (Nishizuka, 1984).

SUMMARY

A new species of calcium-activated phospholipid-dependent protein kinase (protein kinase C) recently characterized in the brain is present in rat pituitary cytosol. This enzyme is more active than pituitary cyclic AMP-, cyclic GMP-, or Ca^{2+}-calmodulin dependent protein kinases with histone (H1+H2B) as phosphate acceptor. Activity of soluble protein kinase C present in the pituitary is absolutely dependent on the simultaneous presence of Ca^{2+} and phosphatidylserine (PS). Other phospholipids such as phosphatidylcholine, phosphatidylethanolamine or phosphatidylinositol could only partially substitute for PS in supporting enzyme activity. Unsaturated diacylglycerol such as diolein greatly increases the apparent affinity of the enzyme for Ca^{2+} and PS. Partial purification on DEAE-cellulose chromatography yielded a major peak of activity that was separated from most of the cyclic AMP dependent protein kinase. It is suggested that pituitary protein kinase C might play a key regulatory role in signal transduction in pituitary cells stimulated by hypothalamic hormones which operate via stimulation of phosphoinositide turnover during which diacylglycerol is liberated. Since ACTH release from the pituitary is mediated by both cAMP and Ca^{2+}, it is suggested that protein kinase C might play a role in the biochemical pathways involved in stress.

ACKNOWLEDGEMENTS

The technical assistance of Mrs. Yona Eli, Tamar Hannoch and Anat Azrad is greatly appreciated. We also thank Dr. Yoram Salomon for the interest taken in this study and Mrs. M. Kopelowitz for typing the manuscript. Supported by NIH grant HD-16279 and by the United States Israel Binational Science Foundation.

REFERENCES

Axelrod, J., and Reisine, T.D., 1984, Stress hormones: their interaction and regulation. Science, 224:452.

Bradford, M.M., 1976, A rapid and sensitive method for the quantitation of microgram quantities of protein utilizing the principle of protein-dye binding. Anal. Biochem., 72:248.

Brazeau, P., Ling, N., Esch, F., Bohlen, P., Mougin, C., and Guillemin, R., 1982, Somatocrinin (growth hormone releasing factor) in vitro bioactivity: Ca^{2+} involvement, cAMP mediated action and additivity of effect with PGE_2. Biochem. Biophys. Res. Commun., 109:588.

Canonico, P.L., Cronin, M.J., Thorner, M.O., Macleod, R.M., 1983, Human pancreatic GRF stimulates phosphatidylinositol labeling in cultured anterior pituitary cells. Am. J. Physiol., 245:E587.

Castanga, M., Takai, Y., Kaibuchi, K., Sano, K., Kikkawa, U., and Nishizuka, Y., 1982, Direct activation of calcium-activated phospholipid-dependent protein kinase by tumor promoting phorbol esters. J. Biol. Chem., 257:7847.

Gershengorn, M.C., 1982, Thyrotropin releasing hormone. Mol. Cell. Biochem., 45:163.

Giguere, V., Labrie, F., Cote, J., Coy, D.H., Sueiras-diaz, J., and Schally, A.V., 1982, Stimulation of cyclic AMP accumulation and corticotropin release by synthetic ovine corticotropin releasing factor in rat anterior pituitary cells: site of glucocorticoid action. Proc. Natl. Acad. Sci. USA., 79:3466.

Greengard, P., 1978, Phosphorylated proteins as physiological effectors. Science, 199:146.

Iwasa, Y., and Hosey, M.M., 1983, Acidic phospholipids stimulate the autophosphorylation of the catalytic subunit of cyclic AMP-dependent protein kinase. Biochem. Biophys. Res. Commun., 113:916.

Jacken, S., Tashjian, A.H. Jr., and Blumberg, P.M., 1981, Characterization of phorbol ester receptors and their down-modulation in GH_4C_1 rat pituitary cells. Cancer Res., 41:2175.

Kaibuchi, K., Takai, Y., Sawamura, M., Hoshijima, M., Fujikura, T., and Nishizuka, Y., 1983, Synergistic functions of protein phosphorylation and calcium mobilization in platelet activation. J. Biol. Chem., 258:6701.

Kiesel, L., and Catt, K.J., 1984, Phosphatidic acid and the calcium-dependent actions of gonadotropin-releasing hormone in pituitary gonadotrophs. Arch. Biochem. Biophys., 231:202.

Kishimoto, A., Takai, Y., Mori, T., Kikkawa, U., and Nishizuka, Y., 1980, Activation of calcium and phospholipid dependent protein kinase by diacylglycerol; its possible relation to phosphatidylinositol turnover. J. Biol. Chem., 255:2273.

Kraft, A.S., and Anderson, W.B., 1983, Phorbol ester increase the amount of Ca^{2+}, phospholipid-dependent protein kinase associated with plasma membrane. Nature, 301:621.

Kuo, J.F., Andersson, R.G.G., Wise, B.C., Mackerlova, L., Salomonsson, I., Brackett, N.L., Katoh, N., Shou, M., and Wrenn, A.W., 1980, Calcium dependent protein kinase: Widespread occurrence in various tissues and phyla of the animal kingdom and comparison of effects of phospholipid, calmodulin and trifluoperazinine. Proc. Natl. Acad. Sci. USA, 77:7039.

Kuo, J.F., Schatzmann, R.C., Turner, R.S., and Mazzei, G.J., 1984, Phospholipid-sensitive Ca^{2+}-dependent protein kinase: a major protein phosphorylation system. Mol. Cell. Endocrinol., 35:65.

Langan, T.A., and Hohmann, P., 1974, Phosphorylation of threonine and serine residue of leucine rich histone in growing cells. Fed. Proc., 33:1597

Naor, Z., 1982, Cyclic nucleotide production and hormonal control of anterior pituitary cells. in: "Multihormonal Regulation in Neuroendocrine Cells", A. Tixier-Vidal and P. Richard, eds., Inserm, 110:395.

Naor, Z. and Catt, K.J., 1981, Mechanism of action of gonadotropin releasing hormone: involvement of phospholipid turnover in luteinizing hormone release. J. Biol. Chem., 256:2226.

Naor, Z., Molcho, J., Zilberstein, M., and Zakut, H., 1984, Phospholipid turnover in gonadotropin releasing hormone target cells: Comparative studies. in: "Hormonal Control of the Hypothalamo-pituitary-gonadal Axis", K.W. McKerns, and Z. Naor, eds., Plenum Press, p. 493.

Naor, Z., Azrad, A., Zer, J., Hannoch, T., Zakut, H. and Hermone, J., 1985, Characterization of pituitary calcium-activated phospholipid dependent protein kinase: Redistribution by gonadotropin releasing hormone. Proc. Natl. Acad. Sci. USA, (in press).

Niedel, J.E., Kuhn, L.J., and Vanderbark, G.R., 1983, Phorbol diester receptor copurifies with protein kinase C. Proc. Natl. Acad. Sci. USA, 80:36.

Nishikawa, M., Hidaka, H., and Adelstein, R.S., 1983, Phosphorylation of smooth muscle heavy meromyosin by calcium activated phospholipid dependent protein kinase. J. Biol. Chem., 258:14069.

Nishizuka, Y., 1984, The role of protein kinase C in cell surface signal transduction and tumor promotion. Nature, 308:693.

Raymond, V., Leung, P.C.K., Veilleux, R., Lefevre, G., and Labrie, F., 1984, LHRH rapidly stimulates phosphatidylinositol metabolism in enriched gonadotrophs. Mol. Cell. Endocrinol., 36:157.

Rebecchi, M.J., Kolesnick, R.N., and Gershengorn, M.C., 1983, Thyrotropin releasing hormone stimulates rapid loss of phosphatidylinositol and its conversion to 1,2-diacylglycerol and phosphatidic acid in rat mammotropic pituitary cells. J. Biol. Chem., 258:227.

Rozengurt, E., Rodriguez-Pena, M., and Smith, K.A., 1983, Phorbol esters, phospholipase C and growth factors rapidly stimulate the phosphorylation of Mr 80,000 protein in intact quiescent 3T3 cells. Proc. Natl. Acad. Sci. USA, 80:7244.

Smith, M.A., and Vale, W.W., 1981, Desensitization to gonadotropin releasing hormone observed in superfused pituitary cells on cytodex beads. Endocrinology, 108:752.

Snyder, G.D., and Bleasdale, J.E., 1982, Effect of LHRH on incorporation of [^{32}P]-orthophosphate into phosphatidylinositol by dispersed anterior pituitary cells. Mol. Cell. Endocrinol., 28:55.

Sutton, C.A., and Martin, T.F.J., 1982, Thyrotropin releasing hormone (TRH) selectively and rapidly stimulates phosphatidylinositol turnover in GH pituitary cells: A possible second step of TRH action. Endocrinology, 110:1273.

Takai, Y., Kishimoto, A., Iwasa, Y., Kawahara, Y., Mori, T., and Nishizuka, Y., 1979, Calcium-dependent activation of a multifunctional protein kinase by membrane phospholipids. J. Biol. Chem., 254:3692.

Turgeon, J.L., Ashcroft, S.J.H., Waring, D.W., Milewski, M.A., and Walsh, D.A., 1984, Characteristics of adenohypophyseal Ca^{2+}-phospholipid dependent protein kinase. Mol. Cell. Endocrinol., 34:107.

Werth, D.K., Niedel, J.E., and Pastan, I., 1983, Vinculin, a cytoskeletal substrate of protein kinase C. _J. Biol. Chem._, 258:11423.

Zawalich, W., Brown, C., and Rasmussen, H., 1983, Insulin secretion: Combined effects of phorbol ester and A23187. _Biochem. Biophys. Res. Commun._, 117:448.

INDEX